BASIC PRINCIPLES OF ĀYURVEDA

ṬOḌARĀNANDA-ĀYURVEDA SAUKHYAṀ SERIES

Edited by

Vaidya Bhagwan Dash

Vaidya Lalitesh Kashyap

No. 1 Materia Medica of Āyurveda, Rs. 500
No. 2 Basic Principles of Āyurveda, Rs. 500
No. 3 Diagnosis and Treatment of Diseases in Āyurveda Vol. I Rs. 500
No. 4 Diagnosis and Treatment of Diseases in Āyurveda Vol. II Rs. 500
No. 5 Diagnosis and Treatment of Diseases in Āyurveda Vol. III, Rs. 500
No. 6 Diagnosis and Treatment of Diseases in Āyurveda Vol. IV, Rs. 500
No. 7 Diagnosis and Treatment of Diseases in Āyurveda Vol. V, Rs. 500
No. 8 Five Specialised Therapies of Āyurveda (*Pañca Karma*), Rs. 500
No. 9 Iatro-Chemistry of Āyurveda (*Rasa Sāstra*), Rs. 500

Also

Alchemy and Metallic Medicines in Āyurveda by **Vaidya Bhagwan Dash,** Rs. 160
A Hand Book of Āyurveda by **Vaidya Bhagwan Dash** and **Acharya Manfred M. Junius,** Rs. 90

PAÑCAKARMA THERAPY OF AYURVEDA SERIES

BY

Vaidya Bhagwan Dash

No. 1 Massage Therapy in Ayurveda, Rs. 200
No. 2 आयुर्वेद के मूलभूत सिद्धान्त (प्रेस में)

Ṭoḍarānanda-Āyurveda Saukhyaṁ Series, No. 2

BASIC PRINCIPLES OF ĀYURVEDA

BASED ON

ĀYURVEDA SAUKHYAṀ OF ṬOḌARĀNANDA

by

VAIDYA BHAGWAN DASH

D.A.M.S., H.P.A., M.A., Ph. D.
Deputy Adviser (Ayurveda)
Ministry of Health &
Family Welfare
New Delhi

VAIDYA LALITESH KASHYAP

B.I.M.S., Ph. D.
Senior Physician (Ayurveda)
Central Govt. Health Scheme
Directorate General of Health Services,
New Delhi

CONCEPT PUBLISHING COMPANY, NEW DELHI-110059

ISBN 81-7022-024-6 (Set)
ISBN 81-7022-257-5 (No. 2)

First Published 1980
Reprinted 1989, 1994, 2003

Published and Printed by
Ashok Kumar Mittal
Concept Publishing Company
A/15-16, Commercial Block, Mohan Garden
NEW DELHI-110059 (India)

Phones : 25351460, 25351794
Fax : 091-11-25357103
Email : publishing@conceptpub.com

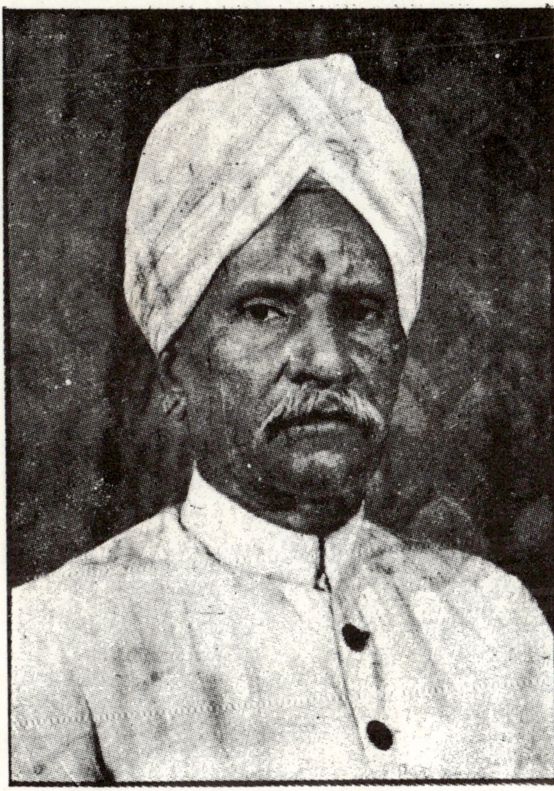

Dedicated to the memory
of

Late PANDIT RAM PRASAD SHARMA
Ex-Rajavaidya of Patiala
in
Grateful acknowledgement of his erudite scholarship and unwearied services for the revival and development of Ayurveda

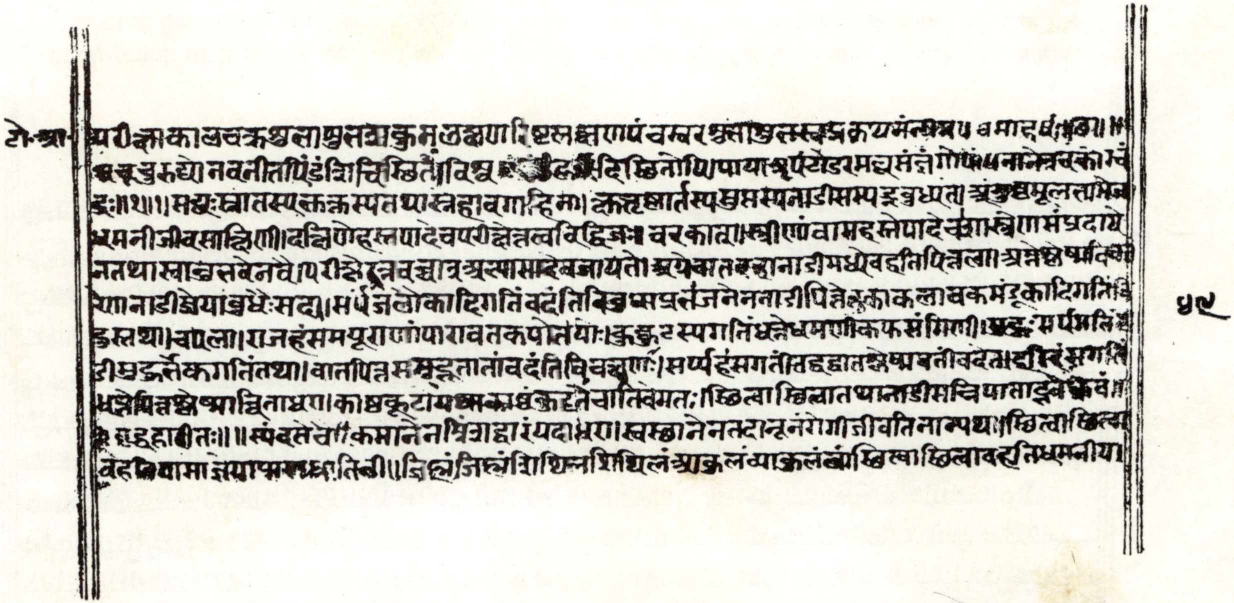

Photograph of the page no. 49 from *ms.* no. 1 in which a reference from *Caraka* (*saṁhitā*) is quoted describing *Nāḍi parikṣā* (pulse examination). In the extant editions of *Caraka saṁhitā* this reference is not available. (Ref. pp. 489-491 of this volume).

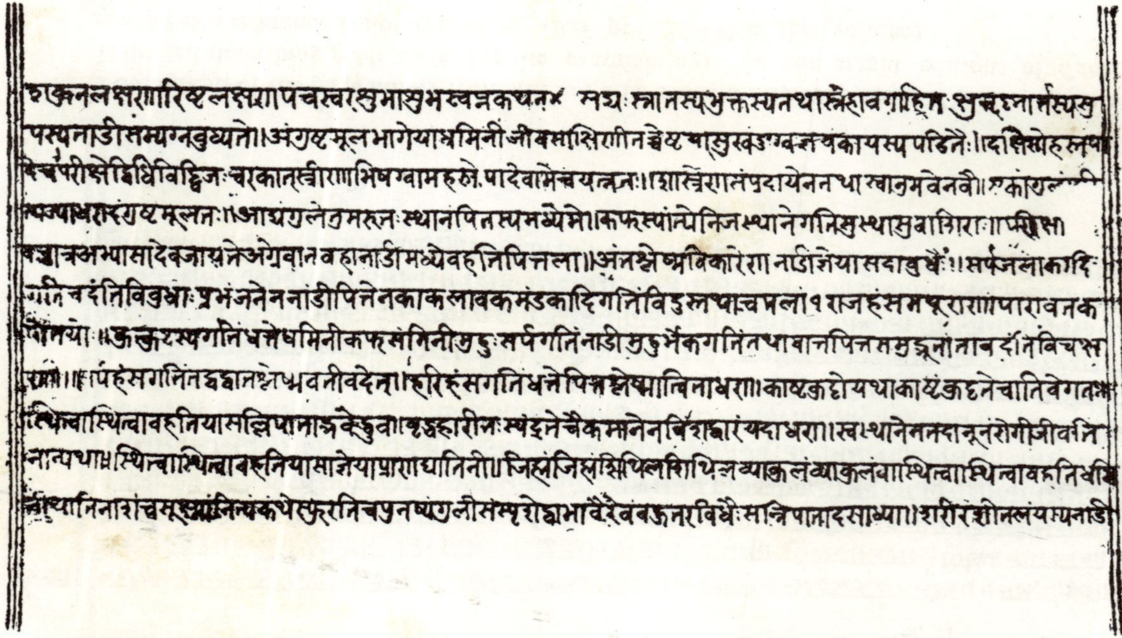

Photograph of the page no. 48 from *ms.* no VI in which a reference from *Caraka* (*saṁhitā*) is quoted describing *Nāḍi parikṣā* (pulse examination). In the extant editions of *Caraka saṁhitā* this reference is not available. (Ref. pp. 489-491 of thi svolume)

भूमिका
(FOREWORD)

श्रीः

अथेदमभिदृश्यते यत् प्रागन्यत्र शिक्षित एव स्थापत्यकलाज्ञाता विशिष्ट-नगरादिनिर्माणाय नियुज्यते। स च स्थपतिः पूर्वोपार्जितानुभवजन्यस्मृतिद्वारा नगरादिनिर्माणाय प्रयतते। तथैव एतद् विश्वस्रष्टा ब्रह्मापि प्रागन्यत्र पूर्वकल्पे प्राप्तं विश्वनिर्माणज्ञानं समुपादाय एतद् विश्वं निर्ममे। एतद् विश्वं दिवारात्रि-चक्रवत् सर्गं प्रलयं च चक्रगत्या प्राप्नोति क्रमशः इति दृष्ट्वा केचित् स्वभाव-वादिनः खलु स्वभावादेव जगदिदं प्रचलतीति मन्यन्ते। यत्रेदमुक्तम् स्वभाव-वादितर्कोदाहरणम् यत्—

"किमीहः किं कायः स खलु किमुपायस्त्रिभुवनम्।

किमाधारो धाता सृजति किमुपादान इति च॥"

किन्तु वस्तुस्वभावं ज्ञात्वा यथा अद्यतनीनाः वैज्ञानिकाः उत्तरोत्तरं नवीनवस्तु-निर्माणाय प्रयतन्ते सफलाश्च भवन्ति तथैव प्राक् सर्गे शिक्षितं विज्ञानमाश्रित्य ब्रह्माऽपि जगत्स्रष्टा वस्तुज्ञानपूर्वकं जगदिदं निर्ममे। एवं च जगतोऽस्य निर्माणप्रसङ्गे **"वेदेभ्य एव सर्वं जगदिदं निर्ममे"** इत्याह स्वयम्भुः मनुः। तथैव च आयुर्वेदावतरणप्रसङ्गेऽपि जगतोऽस्य निर्माणात् प्रागेव **"शतसहस्त्रश्लोकमायु-र्वेदं रचितवान् ब्रह्मा"** इत्युक्तम्। युक्तं चैतत् गुरुपरम्परा प्राप्तत्वाद् आयुर्वेद-स्येति।

प्रायो लक्षश्लोकात्मकपठं सुविस्तृतमायुर्वेदमुत्तरोत्तरम् जिज्ञासूनां सामर्थ्या-नुसारं तथा प्रयोजनानुसारं च अष्टधा कृत्वा विभागं आयुर्वेदस्येति अष्टाङ्गः आयुर्वेदः प्रसिद्धः।

तत्र यथा सामान्यतः संक्षेपत् प्रथमत अष्टांगमायुर्वेदं पठित्वा पश्चात् तत्तद् विशिष्टांगेषु प्रयतन्ते मनीषिणः इति कृत्वा सामान्यत आयुर्वेदजिज्ञासूनां कृते अष्टांगसंग्रहग्रन्थम् ततश्च ततोऽपि सारमादाय पुनरपि अष्टाङ्गहृदयग्रन्थम्

निर्ममे वाग्भटः। इत्थम् विविधविस्तृतानेकग्रन्थेभ्यः सारवचनान्यादाय प्रायः प्रयोजनपरम्परां पूरयितुम् यवनसम्राज अकव्वरस्य प्रमुखसहायेन श्रीमता टोडरमल्लेन तदानीन्तनविद्वद्वैद्यद्वारा ग्रन्थोऽयम् **"टोडरानन्दः"** प्रकटीकृतः। तस्य सुविस्तृतस्य "टोडरानन्द"ग्रन्थस्य आत्मसौख्यप्रकरणस्य द्वितीयो विभागः पाठकसमक्षं प्रापितो हस्तलिखितानाम् षट्संख्यकानां प्रयत्नोपलब्धप्रतीकपुस्तकानामादर्शमादाय सुवाच्यमुद्राक्षरैः प्रकाशनस्य सर्वप्रथमोऽयं प्रयास इति परमः प्रसन्नतावसरोऽयमस्माकम्। यत्र तत्र विकीर्णानामायुर्वेदग्रन्थानां सूक्तिमुक्तावलीरूपस्यास्य "टोडरानन्द"ग्रन्थस्य सूत्रस्थानरूपोऽयं भाग एवायम् अस्मत् समक्षम् प्रमोदपारावारप्लावनाय प्रकाशितोऽस्ति।

पुस्तकस्यास्य पर्यवेक्षणेन प्रतीताः **पाठकप्रमोदप्रकटनपटवः पद्यपल्लवाः** कतिपये प्रस्तूयन्ते। तद् यथा—

पुस्तकस्यास्य ६६ पृष्ठत आरभ्य ७८ पृष्ठपर्यन्तम्—वैद्यव्यवहारायुर्वेदो वस्तुतो वैद्येन सफलतासाधनाय प्रागेव पठनीयो भवतीति कृत्वा सम्यङ् मननीयो भवति। तत्रापि विशेषतः—

"पञ्च वा सप्त वा वैद्यो यो न वेत्तीह संहिताः।

राज्ञा दुर्भिषजस्तस्य छेत्तव्यो दक्षिणः करः॥"

इत्येवं ७२पृष्ठे वचनस्य कालेऽस्मिन्नप्यस्ति विचारणीयता। अयं भावः—यथा कस्यचिद् सद्वैद्यस्य भृत्यो निरक्षरोऽपि सन् सद्वैद्यद्वारा तेषु तेषु विविधचिकित्साकर्मसु सहायकत्वेन नियुक्तः कियता कालेन प्रयोजनवशात् स्वग्रामं गतस्तत्र कमपि रुग्णं प्राप्य तस्य चिकित्सां करोति, किन्तु कस्यामवस्थायां रोगस्य किं किं करणीयमिति शास्त्रज्ञानशून्यो विनाप्रयोजनम् किमपि कर्म कृत्वा व्याधितं मारयत्येवेति शास्त्रज्ञानरहितः केवलं कर्मज्ञानमात्रेण व्यवहरन् चिकित्सको राजदण्डभयभाग् भवतीति सूचितमनेन पद्येन। अतएव सुश्रुतेऽपि प्रोक्तम् **"वधं चार्हति राजतः"** इति। अत्र पंच वा सप्तसंहिताग्रन्थज्ञानन्तु विविधावश्यकज्ञानदायकसंहिताग्रन्थसंख्यासंकेत एव। यत्रेदमुक्तम्—**एकं शास्त्रमधीयानो न विद्याच्छास्त्रनिश्चयमिति**। शास्त्रं संहितामित्यर्थः। न तु संख्यानियमः।

तथा ८०तमे पृष्ठे—दोषशोधनमहत्वं दोषशोधनत्यागे हानिं च कथयन् ग्रन्थकारः—

"अविशुद्धशरीराणां देहिनां च "भवान्तरे"।
सर्वथा हि प्रसर्पन्ति तस्माच्छोधनमाचरेत्"

तथा "न केवलं भवान्तरे किन्तु अशोधनादन्वयेऽपि प्रचरन्ति न चान्यथा" अर्थात् दोषाणां शोधनं यदि यथाकालं न क्रियते तर्हि ते रोगारम्भका दोषा रुग्णस्य अन्वयेऽपि कुलेऽपि प्रचरन्ति इति। सम्भावितोऽपि विशेषोऽयम् अन्यत्रासंकेतित इति।

तथा असाध्यरोगप्रसङ्गे ८२ पृष्ठे "च्युतधनस्य" इति कथयता ग्रन्थकृता असाध्यरोगकारणविशेषः सूचितः प्रेक्षकाणां समवधानीयो भवत्येव। तथा सति संचितधनक्षयात् के के रोगाः प्रसरन्तीति।

अपि च ११०तमे पृष्ठे व्यानवायुवर्णनप्रसङ्गे प्राणापानसमानोदानवायु-वर्णनवत् प्राकृतानां व्यानवायुकार्याणां वर्णनं चरकादिसंहिता संकेतितं विहाय केवलं दुष्टव्यानवायुकार्याणामेव वर्णनम् :—

"व्यानो विनाशयेदङ्गं व्यानो रोगप्रकोपकः।
प्रीतिं नाशयते वायुस्तेनैव व्यान उच्यते॥"

इति ग्रन्थसंकलयितुः कौशलं कलयति किमु ? उपलब्धसंहितासु तु—

"व्यानो हृदिस्थितः सर्वदेहचारी महाजवः।"
गत्यपक्षेपणोत्क्षेपनिमेषोन्मेषणादिकाः।
प्रायः सर्वाः क्रियास्तस्मिन् प्रतिबद्धाः शरीरिणाम्॥"

इत्यादिना प्राकृतव्यानवायुकार्यमहत्वम् सूचितम्।

अथ च १११तमे पृष्ठे पञ्चवायुरूपनिरूपणम् प्रकटयता ग्रन्थकर्त्रा योग तन्त्रसाधकसूचितोऽयं श्लोकः संकलितः—

"द्रुततारनिभं रक्तं इन्द्रगोपसमप्रभम्।
क्षीराभं स्फटिकाभं च पञ्चानां रूपलक्षणम्॥"

इत्थं प्राणापानसमानोदानव्यानानां यथाक्रमं प्राणस्य द्रुतरजतनिभम्, अपानस्य रक्तम्, समानस्य इन्द्रगोपसमम्, उदानवायोः क्षीराभम् तथा व्यानवायोः स्फटिकाभम् रूपम् संकेतितम्। अत्रार्थे यद्यपि न्यायशास्त्रे **"रूपरहितस्पर्शवान् वायुः"** तथा चरकेऽपि **"अमूर्तत्वम् वायोः"** इत्युक्तम् तथापि समाधिदृष्ट्या योगिनः स्वशरीरे संचरतः पञ्चधा स्थानकार्यभेदेन भिन्नस्य वायोः प्राणादिस्थानेषु मनः-संयमसमाधिद्वारा प्राणादिरूपभेदविवेकः सूचितः। यतोऽपांचभौतिके शुद्धे वायौ न रूपम् किन्तु शारीरे पाञ्चभौतिके वायौ सूक्ष्मरूपदर्शनं संभाव्यते। अतएव नीरूपोऽप्याकाशः पांचभौतिकतया **"नीलं नभ"** इति प्रत्यक्षीक्रियते।

१३६पृष्ठे ग्रन्थकर्त्रा वातादिदोषाणां परस्परसंसर्गजन्यरोगाणां चिकित्सायाम् द्विदोषसंसर्गशोधनाय यथायथं तत्तत् पंचकर्मणां प्रयोगसंकेतः प्रकटीकृतो जेज्जटवचनमुद्धरता, तथाहि—

"कफपित्तप्रकोपे वमननस्यविरेचनानि पित्तवातप्रकोपेतु रेचनं बस्तिकर्म च कफवातप्रकोपे हि वमननस्यबस्तयः। सन्निपातेऽमूनि सर्वाणि यथायोग्यं प्रयोजयेत्" इति।

जेज्जटवचनमिदं ग्रन्थेऽस्मिन्नेव समुपलब्धम् पञ्चकर्मचिकित्सायामत्युपयुक्तं चेति वैशिष्ट्यम्।

तथा अस्मिन्नेव १३६पृष्ठे निराममलरुजावर्णनम् विशेषतोऽस्ति समवधानीयम्, तद् यथा—

भुक्ते जीर्यति जीर्णेऽन्ने, इत्यनेन, भुक्तभोजनस्य तत्कालं निरामवातरुजा न जायते, जीर्यति भोजने निरामवातरुजा स्वल्पा भवति, तथा जीर्णेऽन्ने निरामवातरुक्प्रचुरता संभाव्यते प्रायः। तथैव निरामपित्तरुजा जीर्णे भोजने प्रायो न प्रकटी भवति, भुक्ते भोजने स्वल्पाभवति, जीर्यति भोजने च वर्धते। एवं निरामकफपीडा जीर्णे भोजने प्रायो न प्रकटी भवति, जीर्यति भोजने स्वल्पा, भुक्तमात्रे च समधिका संभाव्यते। किन्तु सामदोषजन्या पीडा तु एतद् वैपरीत्येन भवति इति सामनिरामवातादिदोषज्ञानाय उपशयप्रकारः प्रकटितः परीक्षकाणां कृते रोगमूलदोषज्ञानाय।

तथा १३९पृष्ठे श्लोकोऽयं विशेषत समवधानीयोऽस्ति :—

"आलस्य-तन्द्रा-हृदयाविशुद्धि-दोषाप्रवृत्याकुलमूत्रताभिः ।

गुरूदरत्वारुचिसुप्तताभिरामान्वितं व्याधिमुदाहरन्ति"

दोषाप्रवृतिः पुरीषाप्रवृतिः आकुलमूत्रता आविलमूत्रता ॥

१४७ पृष्ठे—

"पित्तासृक् सहितो वायुः पाददाहं करोति वै ।

कुर्यादसृक्पित्तहरां क्रियां तत्र सुखप्रदाम् ।।"

श्लोकोऽयं विशेषतः समवधानीयोऽस्ति । २१० पृष्ठे प्रक्षीणदोषवर्धकं द्रव्यं संशमनमिति यदत्रिवचनमुद्धरता ग्रन्थकर्त्रा संकेतितम् तद् विचारणीयमस्ति । यतः **"शोधनं शमनं चेति समासादौषधं द्विधा"** इति सर्वसम्मतवचनानुसारं शोधनं विनैव दोषप्रकोपनिवारकं द्रव्यं संशमनमिति व्यावहारिकम् यथा छर्दिरोगे कफशोधनं विनैव गुडूचीस्वरसप्रयोगः । तस्माद् संशमनशब्दार्थमतभेद एवायम् प्रतीयते ।

तथा २२२पृष्ठे वीर्यमहत्त्वसूचकाः ८१-८२-८३श्लोकाः सन्ति विशेषतः समवधानीयाः वीर्यकार्योदाहरणसूचकाश्च । तथा—

"मृदुरूक्षगुरुस्निग्धतीक्ष्णोष्णलघुशीतलम् ।

बलमष्टविधं त्वेतद् द्रव्याणां वीर्यमुच्यते" ।।

इति च ।

किन्तु चरके तु **"वीर्यन्तु क्रियते येन या क्रिया"** इत्युक्तम् ।

२२६पृष्ठे विपाकविवेचनप्रकरणे विशेषतः सोदाहरणं विवेचनं विशेषतः समवधानीयमस्त्येव । विदग्धकफलवणतोदाहरणप्रभृतिविचारस्तु विदग्धपाकस्य वास्तविकविपाकाभावात् समुपेक्षणीय एव ।

अपि च ग्रन्थकर्त्रा कृतः दोषपाचनद्रव्यस्य तथा दीपनद्रव्यस्य च परस्परं भेदवर्णनस्य विचारः सम्यग् सोदाहरणं वर्णितः २०६पृष्ठतः २१०पृष्ठपर्यन्तम् विशेषतः समवधानीयोऽस्ति ।

२२६पृष्ठे **"तस्करः स्नायुज मूलं"** इति पाठः प्राप्तः विचारदृष्ट्या "तस्करस्नायुः" इत्येकमेव द्रव्यम् तथाहि धन्वन्तरिनिघण्टौ—

"काकनासा ध्वांक्षनासा काकतुण्डफला च सा ।

सुरङ्गी तस्करस्नायुः" इति काकनासापर्यायाः ।।

तथा राजनिघण्टावपि—

"काकनासा ध्वांक्षनासा काकतुण्डा च वायसी ।

सुरङ्गी तस्करस्नायुः" ॥

इति काकनासापर्याय एव तस्करस्नायुः इति समवधानीयमस्ति ॥

२७९पृष्ठे स्वस्थवृत्तप्रकरणे पुष्पधारणप्रसङ्गे कानि पुष्पाणि कियत् कालं सुरक्षितसुगन्धानि सन्ति इति सूचयता ग्रन्थकर्त्रा पुष्पविज्ञाने स्वानुभवः प्रकटितः ।

अपि च **नाडीपरीक्षा**वर्णनप्रसङ्गे चरकवचनानाम् उल्लेखः प्राप्यते ग्रन्थेऽस्मिन् । किन्तूपलब्धचरकग्रन्थे नाडीपरीक्षावचनानामुल्लेखो न प्राप्यते । ग्रन्थेऽस्मिन् महर्षि**कणादकृत नाडीविज्ञान**ग्रन्थप्राप्ताः श्लोकास्तु सन्ति । परं तद् वचनानां कणादनाम्ना सम्मुल्लेखः कथमिति न कृतः ?

मूत्रपरीक्षाप्रकरणे च कस्माद् ग्रन्थात् संगृहीतानि तानि वचनानीति विशेषतो नोपलभ्यते । केवलं ४९९पृष्ठे **"गोपुरात्"** इत्युक्तम् । **गोपुरग्रन्थो** नाधुना प्राप्यते । अंशतः योगरत्नाकरादिग्रन्थेषु कथितमपि विशेषतो विचारयोग्य मूत्रपरीक्षाप्रकरणम् रोगसाध्यासाध्यतायामुपयोगि भवत्येव ।

पुरीषपरीक्षाप्रकरणमपि विशेषतः प्रचारयोग्यमस्ति । समुपलब्धेषु ग्रन्थान्तरेषु पुरीषपरीक्षावर्णनम् सविस्तरं नोपलभ्यते । तस्माद् ग्रन्थेऽस्मिन् समुल्लिखिता पुरीषपरीक्षा विकृतिविज्ञानाय विशिष्टमुदाहरणं प्रकटीकरोति ।

ग्रन्थेऽस्मिन् प्रोक्ता **नेत्रपरीक्षा**ऽपि विकृतिविज्ञानोपयुक्ताऽस्ति न तु नेत्ररोग-परीक्षायाम् । तथैव **जिह्वापरीक्षा दन्तपरीक्षा त्वचापरीक्षा नखपरीक्षा**ऽपि विविध-रोगविकृतिसूचनायोपयुक्ता विशेषतः पठनपाठनप्रयुक्ता चिकित्साकर्मणि सहायभूता प्रचारयोग्यास्त्येवेति नात्र सन्देहः । **मंत्रयंत्रादिद्वारा रुग्णस्यायुःपरीक्षायाः** प्रकारोऽपि वर्तमानकाले लुप्तप्रायः पुनरपि सावधानतया परीक्षणीयो व्यवहार-दृष्ट्या प्रचारणीयो भवत्येव ।

तदित्थं सामान्यतः टोडरानन्दग्रन्थस्यायं प्रकटितः द्वितीयोभागः पठनपाठन-द्वारा प्रचारयोग्यः एतावत् कालं जिज्ञासूनां कृते दुष्प्राप्योऽपि डा० भगवानदासेन

डा० ललितेशकाश्यपेन च प्रायो लेखकप्रमादप्रचुराशुद्धपाठयुक्तानां खण्डित-पृष्ठपाठबहुलानां यथा कथंचित् समुपलब्धानां षट्संख्यकानां ग्रन्थप्रतीनाम् साहाय्येन महता परिश्रमेण साम्प्रतिकमुद्रायंत्रप्रक्रियाद्वारा प्रसिद्धिं प्रापितः अनुसन्धान-प्रियाणाम् जिज्ञासूनां मनोमोदावहः समुल्लसतीति स्तुत्यः प्रयासोऽयम् ।

निदेशकः
मूलचान्दखैरातिराम-चिकित्सालयः
लाजपतनगरः
नवदेहली

वैद्यो हरिदत्तः शास्त्री

दिनाङ्कः १४-७-१९८०

PREFACE

We are very happy to present before our esteemed readers and learned scholars this work on "Basic Principles of Āyurveda". This is the second volume in the series *Ṭodarānanda—Āyurveda Saukhyaṁ*, the first being "Materia Medica of Āyurveda" published early this year.

Āyurveda Saukhyaṁ contains 97 chapters whose details are given in the Introduction to the present work. The various aspects of āyurveda are unfortunately, scattered in different places in this encyclopedic work and even the topics of each chapter are sometimes haphazardly tossed together without any visibly systematic arrangement. One may hazard a guess that perhaps the work was not finally edited, and immediately after the compilation of the material, further work was discontinued.

The present volume is prepared on the basis of the first six chapters of *Āyurveda Saukhyaṁ*. These chapters primarily deal with the basic principles of ayurveda and allied topics.

In the 'Introduction' to the present work, the life of Rājā Ṭodara malla and his intimate relationship with this work have been explained. After this book was printed, we have come across a book on "Raja Todar Mal" written by Kumud ranjan Das, published in 1979 by Saraswat Library, Calcutta. This is, perhaps, the first book of its genre and scholars interested in the biographical details of this great statesman, administrator and scholar, may refer to this book.

The first chapter of the present work deals with various specialities of this system of medicine. The attributes of genuine drugs, physicians, nurses as well as patients are described in this chapter in detail. Medical ethics, classification of diseases and their complications and methods of examination of the patient are also described here.

The second chapter deals with various stages of the process of the manifestation of diseases which are called *kriyā kālas*. Various aspects of *doṣas, dhātus* and *malas* are described in detail. The classification of *deśa* or locality and the characteristics of different types of physical constitution are also given.

The third chapter is concerned with different therapeutic measures and the attributes of different categories of drugs. The basic theories of *Rasa, Guṇa, Vīrya, Vipāka* and *Prabhāva* are elucidated and the regimens that should be followed in different seasons and in the day time and epidemics along with their management are also described. The general conduct conducive to the well being of human beings is also explained here.

The fourth chapter deals with embryology, maternity and various anatomical as well as physiological topics. The process of metabolism and *marmas* or vital organs are described in detail in this chapter.

In the fifth chapter prognostic signs, messengers, dreams and omens which are conducive to the recovery of the disease are described in detail.

The sixth chapter describes various methods for the examination of patients. The examination of pulse, urine, stool, the eyes, the tongue, the teeth and nails are described in detail. In addition, the tantric methods for determining the prognosis of a disease and the future health and ill-health of patients are also elaborated in this chapter.

As is familiar to scholars, exact English equivalents of many Sanskrit terms are not available. Providing such explanations repeatedly as and when they appear in the text would have made the reading of this book quite cumbersome. In view of this, besides the index, a glossary of such terms is given at the end. Certain terms with controversial meanings and some other terms indicating the names of plants, animals etc., which are not clearly identified are also included in this glossary for the benefit of the readers.

Manuscripts which were utilised for the collation and edition of this work were full of calligraphic errors. Most of the original texts referred to in this work are not available now. Therefore, it was difficult to ascertain the correct reading in many places. Any correction without authentic textual support might mislead the reader. Keeping this in view, corrections of some such Sanskrit texts in this book have not been attempted. The English translation of these texts is based on the Hindi translation which was attempted on one of these MSS. Where the text was absolutely unintelligible, the English translation has been omitted and this has been indicated below the Sanskrit text within square brackets.

Acknowledgements

The late Pandit Shiv Sharma, ex-President of the Central Council of Indian Medicine, encouraged us to undertake this work and supplied us with two manuscripts from the collections of his illustrious father the late Vaidya Rama Prasad Sharma, who was the Raj Vaidya of Patiala. Panditji is no more with us. He has left for his heavenly abode. May his Soul rest in peace and continue to bless us in the pursuit of our mission for the development of Ayurveda.

Vaidya Hari Dutta Shastry, Director of the Mool Chand Khairaiti Ram Hospital in New Delhi, has guided us in the preparation of this work and has written its Foreword. We are greatly honoured to acknowledge our debt of gratitude to him.

For the preparation of this work, manuscripts available at the Abhilekhalaya, Kathmandu, Royal Asiatic Society Library and Government Sanskrit College Library both at Calcutta, were consulted. We are thankful to the curators of these Libraries for supplying us copies of these manuscripts.

Shri Subhash Gupta, Kumari Kanchan Gupta and Kumari Sharada Gupta have provided us considerable assistance in the preparation of this work and we are extremely thankful to them too.

CONTENTS

---

*Figures inside the square bracket indicate the verse/paragraph numbers of the respective chapters.

INDO-ROMANIC EQUIVALENTS OF DEVANAGARI

अ	a	क	ka	ढ	ḍha	र	ra
आ	ā	ख	kha	ण	ṇa	ल	la
इ	i	ग	ga	त	ta	व	va
ई	ī	घ	gha	थ	tha	श	śa
उ	u	ङ	ṅa	द	da	ष	ṣa
ऊ	ū	च	ca	ध	dha	स	sa
ऋ	ṛ	छ	cha	न	na	ह	ha
ए	e	ज	ja	प	pa		
ऐ	ai	झ	jha	फ	pha		
ओ	o	ञ	ña	ब	ba		
औ	au	ट	ṭa	भ	bha		
अं	ṁ	ठ	ṭha	म	ma		
अः	ḥ	ड	da	य	ya		

INTRODUCTION

According to the Indian tradition, the four primary objectives of human life are (i) *Dharma* or performance of such rites as are conducive to the well-being of the individual as well as his society, (ii) *Artha* or the collection of the means of livelihood (iii) *Kāma* or the satisfaction of the mundane desires and (iv) *Mokṣa* or the attainment of salvation. Good health is considered to be the *sine qua non* for the achievement of all these four fold objectives. The man has therefore, eternally endeavoured to keep himself healthy and free from miseries. These miseries are of the following three types :

(1) *Ādhyātmika duḥkha* or miseries that arise out of factors which operate from within the living organism. This is again of two types namely *śārīrika* or somatic and *mānasika* or psychic;

(2) *Ādhibhautika duḥkha* or miseries caused by factors which operate on the living organism from outside; and

(3) *Ādhidaivika duḥkha* or miseries effected by providential causes or acts of the gods, that is factors that are beyond human control.

Like all systems of Indian sciences, the science of medicine has taken origin from the gods. According to Indian mythology, Āyurveda was first perceived (not composed) by Brahmā, and he taught this science to Dakṣa-Prajāpati, who taught it to the Aśvini-Kumāras, and they taught it to Indra. About the further hierarchy of Āyurvedic propounders, different Āyurvedic texts vary. According to *Suśruta Saṁhitā*, Lord Dhanvantari learned it from Indra and according to *Caraka Saṁhitā*, Bharadvāja (also Ātreya) learnt it from Indra. According to *Brahma Vaivarta Purāṇa*, Bhāskara composed Āyurveda as the fifth Veda on the advice of Prajāpati.

While *Brahma Vaivarta Purāṇa* considers Āyurveda to be the fifth Veda, Caraka, Suśruta and Kāśyapa have described its allegiance to the Atharva Veda. On the other hand, *Caraṇa vyūha* and *Prasthāna bheda*, where the term Āyurveda was used perhaps for the first time, have described Āyurveda as an *Upaveda* of the *Ṛk Veda*.

The Vedas are the most ancient repository of human knowledge. All the subjects of science and arts have therefore their original source in the Vedas.

An analysis of the material in the Vedas reveals that all the four Vedas are replete with references to various aspects of medicine. The gods like Rudra, Agni, Varuṇa, Indra and Maruta were designated as the celestial physicians. The most famous physicians at that time were the Aśvins. In the Vedas many miraculous achievements in the field of medicine and surgery had been attributed to them. Revitalisation of individuals and saints, correction of sterility, giving longevity and cure of serious diseases like *Yakṣmā* (Tuberculosis) are attributed to them. Many surgical performances like transplantation of the head of a horse in a human trunk and its subsequent replacement by the human head, providing artificial limbs, connecting the head of Yajña to his trunk etc., are described in several places. In the Vedas, the fundamental principles of the science of medicine including the *tri-doṣa* concept, *sapta dhātu* concept, the concept of digestion and metabolism, anatomical descriptions and descriptions of several diseases are available. Different types of bacteria that are responsible for the causation of diseases are also described in detail. Some of these bacteria are stated to be invisible to the naked eye. The process of delivery, cauterization, toxins, correcting the seizures of evil spirits, rejuvenation therapies and aphrodisiacs are described in many places. Medicinal plants, their different parts and therapeutic effects are also described. About 28 diseases alongwith their medicines are also described. The method of preparation of medicines is available only in brief. In the *Ṛk Veda*, there is a description of 67 medicinal plants. In the *Yajur Veda*, 81 medicinal plants are described. Two hundred ninety medicinal plants are described in the *Atharva Veda* alone. In addition, description of about 130 medicinal plants is available in *Brāhmaṇa* literature. It is described in the *Ṛk Veda* that Viśpalā, wife of Khela king, lost her legs during a war. She was supplied with a pair of artificial legs, and they were fitted to the body through prosthetic surgery.

The most ancient Āyurvedic classics that are available today are *Caraka saṁhitā* and *Suśruta saṁhitā*. They were composed, according to scholars entitled to an opinion, during the 7th century B.C. It is during the mediaeval period, in about the 3rd century after Christ that Iatro-chemistry or *Rasa Śāstra* came in a big way to be incorporated into Āyurveda. Thereafter, India was subjected to number of foreign attacks and internal conflicts. There was very little time for people to think of science. They were engaged in fighting for the security of the country. Original thinking was completely at a stand still. Science by nature is progressive. It is more so in the case of a medical science. Any arrest of this progress in original thinking leads to dogmas, prejudices and accumulation of superstitious ideas. This is exactly what happened to Āyurveda during this period. During foreign invasions and internal frictions, many original Āyurvedic works, among others, were destroyed. Whatever remained had to be preserved and explained with the help of commentaries and notes. This was exactly the position in the 16th century A.D. when Ṭoḍara malla wanted to preserve the ancient knowledge from the then available mutilated Āyurvedic works and took initiative for the composition of the work '*Āyurveda saukhyaṁ*' by compiling material from different authentic sources.

Eight specialised branches of Āyurveda

In the post-vedic period eight specialised branches of Āyurveda were developed. Eminent scholars of these specialities composed works in their respective fields. It is said in the first chapter of *Āyurveda saukhyaṁ* :

सृष्ट्युत्पादनचित्तेन स्मृतः पूर्वं स्वयंभुवा ।

श्लोकानां शतसाहस्रं सहस्राध्यायसंयुतम् ।

ततोऽल्पादल्पमेघस्त्वं ज्ञात्वा नृणां सुनिश्चितम् ।

अष्टधा कारयामास भगवान् कालमर्दनः ॥

शल्यं शालाक्यमगदं कुमारभरणं तथा ।

कायभूतक्रियावाजीकरणं च रसायनम् ॥

Lord Brahmā, during the process of creation of the universe, brought out the science of medicine in one thousand chapters containing one lakh verses. Thereafter, realising the declining wisdom of human beings, he divided the scripture into eight parts. Several authentic texts were thereafter composed by experts and specialists in these fields. They are as follows :

I. *Kāyacikitsā* or Internal medicine

(a) Agniveśa Saṁhitā

(b) Hārīta Saṁhitā

(c) Bhela Saṁhitā

(d) Jatukarṇa Saṁhitā

(e) Kṣārapāṇi Saṁhitā

(f) Parāśara Saṁhitā

(g) Kharanāda Saṁhitā

(h) Viśvāmitra Saṁhitā

(i) Aṣṭāṅga hṛdaya

(j) Aṣṭāṅga saṁgraha

(k) Caraka Saṁhitā

(l) Dāruvāha Saṁhitā

(m) Bharadvāja Saṁhitā

(n) Aśvinī Kumāra Saṁhitā

II. *Śalya* or General surgery

(a) Dhanvantarī Saṁhitā

(b) Suśruta Saṁhitā

(c) Aupadhenava Tantra

(d) Aurabhra Tantra

(e) Pauṣkalāvata Tantra

(f) Vaitarāja Tantra

(g) Vṛddha Bhoja Tantra

(h) Kṛtavīrya Tantra
(i) Bhoja Tantra
(j) Karavīrya Tantra
(k) Gopura Rakṣita Tantra
(l) Bhāluki Tantra
(m) Kapila Tantra
(n) Gautama Tantra

III. *Śālakya* or the treatment of diseases of the Head and Neck

(a) Videha Tantra
(b) Nimi Tantra
(c) Kaṅkāyana Tantra
(d) Gārgya Tantra
(e) Gālava Tantra
(f) Sātyaki Tantra
(g) Bhadra Śaunaka Tantra
(h) Śaunaka Tantra
(i) Karāla Tantra
(j) Cakṣuṣya Tantra
(k) Kṛṣṇātreya Tantra
(l) Kātyāyana Tantra

IV. *Kaumāra Bhṛtya* or Paediatrics

(a) Vṛddha Kāśyapa Saṁhitā
(b) Kāśyapa Saṁhitā or Vṛddha Jīvaka Tantra
(c) Parvataka Tantra
(d) Bauddhaka Tantra
(e) Hiraṇākṣa Tantra
(f) Kumāra Tantra

V. *Agada Tantra* or Toxicology

(a) Vṛddha Kāśyapa Saṁhitā
(b) Kāśyapa Saṁhitā

(c) Sanaka Saṁhitā
(d) Lāṭyāyana Saṁhitā
(e) Ālamhāyana Saṁhitā
(f) Uśanaḥ Saṁhitā
(g) Bṛhaspati Saṁhitā
(h) Garuḍa Saṁhitā

VI. *Vājikaraṇa Tantra* or the Science of Aphrodisiacs

(a) Kucumāra Tantra

VII. *Rasāyana Tantra* or the Science of Rejuvenation

VIII. *Bhūta Vidyā* or Psychiatry including treatment of diseases caused by evil spirits

References to these specialised branches are available in important Āyurvedic classics like *Caraka Saṁhitā* and *Suśruta Saṁhitā*. In *Hārita Saṁhitā* these are described in a slightly different way. In respect of some of these specialised branches names of works are not available. Most of the works mentioned above are also not available. References to them are available in the commentaries.

Most of the extant works are available only in a mutilated form. Even *Caraka Saṁhitā* which was originally written by Agniveśa has undergone many changes inasmuch as it was redacted by Caraka and subsequently non-available portions were supplemented by Dṛḍhabala.

During the period when Ṭoḍarānanda was compiled, the scholars might have realised this problem of paucity of authentic Āyurvedic texts, specially the problem of the mutilated ones. There must have been an effort to reconstruct an Āyurvedic text by compiling from different authentic sources material on various topics of Āyurveda. Ṭoḍara malla who had a broader view must have encouraged scholars to make the work as comprehensive as possible with a view to proving its authenticity and dependability. This effort is clearly discernible from the first six chapters of *Āyurveda Saukhyaṁ* in Ṭoḍarānanda which are given in this work.

ṬOḌARA MALLA & HIS WORK

Life of Ṭoḍara malla

Ṭoḍara malla who hailed from Oudh, was a *Kṣatriya* by caste and he belonged to the clan *Ṭaṇḍaṇa.* About his place of birth, there are two different views. One section of scholars hold the view that he was born in Lahore. This is based on the information provided in *Ain-i-Akbari* of Abul Fazal. However, the vocal section of scholars hold the view that he was born at Lahar Pur in Oudh.

The surname *Ṭaṇḍaṇa* or *Ṭaṇḍana* or *Ṭannan* is used by people of two different castes viz., *Kṣatriyas* and *Kāyasthas* of Punjab as well as Uttara Pradesh. It is very clear from the invocations provided in the *Āyurveda saukhyaṁ* that Ṭoḍara malla belonged to *Kṣatriya* caste and *Ṭaṇḍaṇa* clan.

He is popularly known as Rājā Ṭoḍara malla because he belonged to the family of ex-rulers or Zamindars of Oudh. His ancestors were as follows :

Bāla
|
Attali
|
Dāmodara
|
Assū
|
Dvārakā dāsa
|
Dvija malla
|
Bhagavati dāsa
|
Ṭoḍara malla

Ṭoḍara malla's father Bhagavati dāsa died when the former was very young. The family was in pecuniary difficulty for which he undertook a clerical job in the finance department of the then govt. of Akbar to maintain the widow mother and other members of his family.

Ṭoḍara malla's date of birth is not known. However, it is clear from the *Ain-i-Akbari* that he joined service of Akbar in 1573. His devoted and sincere work coupled with intellect and wisdom soon drew the attention of Akbar. The state of Gujerat was then annexed to Akbar's kingdom, and to settle its affairs, Ṭoḍara malla was sent there. His achievements in that state made him very popular and he enjoyed the confidence of Akbar as an able Administrator.

In 1574, he was sent to Bihar and Bengal alongwith Munim Khān and successfully carried out the mission. In the battle of Dāud Khān-i-Kararānī when Khān Ālam had been killed and Munim Khān's horse had run away, he faced the war bravely and became victorious. In 1577 he was again sent to Gujerat, and in 1582 he was appointed as the Vazir or Dewan of the empire. In 1589 he tendered his resignation from Govt. service because of old age and sickness which Akbar accepted reluctantly. Ṭoḍara malla retired to the bank of the Ganges with a desire to die there. But Akbar called him again from Haradwar and told him that looking after duties was more virtuous than retiring. Ṭoḍara malla unwillingly acceded to the request of his master and joined his duties. His death took place on 10th Nov. 1589.

He rose from the position of a Clerk to the Dewan of the state because of his strict integrity, administrative ability and valour. Because of his strict adherance to his religious belief and independence in thinking, he had many enemies. He made his coreligionists to learn Persian and join Govt. services to which Hindus originally had a strong aversion. He succeeded in his mission inasmuch as before the end of 18th century the Hindus had almost become the Persian teachers of the Muhammedans. His advice to Hindus to learn Persian language had made many enemies for him among his coreligionists also. In 1587, a person who was *Kṣatriya* by caste made an unsuccessful attempt on the life of Ṭoḍara malla.

Religious belief

Ṭoḍara malla was a great devotee of Lord Kṛṣṇa. He spent all his earnings on charities, in building temples and in consecrating images of the gods. The invocations in the beginning of each *harṣa* (chapter) of *Āyurveda Saukhyaṁ* and his other works are replete with references to the adoration of Lord Kṛṣṇa. Images of Viṣṇu and Śāligrāma were held in great veneration by him and he was spending considerable time in offering *Pūjā* to them.

There is an anecdote about his devotion to Lord Kṛṣṇa and his *Pūjā*. Once he was to go for war in Punjab, and in hurry, he left his images at home. When this fact was discovered by him, the next day morning, he did not take any food and drink in spite of strong persuation by his master Akbar. His fast continued till his images were brought back to him.

Works of Ṭoḍara malla

The series of works composed under the patronage of Ṭoḍara malla are collectively called *Ṭoḍarānanda*. This word '*Ṭoḍarānanda*' means the work which delights Ṭoḍara(malla). The series contains the following works :

(1) *Sarga saukhyaṁ* or the work on the creation of the universe;

(2) *Avatāra saukhyaṁ* or the work dealing with the ten incarnations of Viṣṇu;

(3) *Kālagaṇanā saukhyaṁ* or the work on the calculation of the time;

(4) *Kālanirṇaya saukhyaṁ* or the work on the fixation of suitable time and date for the performance of various religious rites;

(5) *Deśa saukhyaṁ* or the work on the determination of suitable places for the construction of the houses, temples etc.;

(6) *Saṁskāra saukhyaṁ* or the work dealing with various rites (*saṁskāra*) for the twice-born (*dvijas*);

(7) *Ācāra saukhyaṁ* or the work dealing with daily conduct;

(8) *Śuddhi saukhyaṁ* or the work dealing with purity and impurity as a result of the birth or death of a person in the family;

(9) *Śrāddha saukhyaṁ* or the work dealing with the annual or periodical offerings to the dead *pitṛs*;

(10) *Varṣakṛtya saukhyaṁ* or the work dealing with the observances during the year;

(11) *Vrata saukhyaṁ* or the work dealing with various religious vows;

(12) *Pratiṣṭhā saukhyaṁ* or the work dealing with the rituals for the installation of the images and idols of the gods;

(13) *Devapūjā saukhyaṁ* or the work dealing with the rituals to be performed for the daily worship of deities;

(14) *Dāna saukhyaṁ* or the work dealing with charity;

(15) *Śānti karma saukhyaṁ* or the work dealing with the pacification of deities and performance of rituals to bring about prosperity;

(16) *Yātrā saukhyaṁ* or the work dealing with pilgrimage to holy places;

(17) *Vivāha saukhyaṁ* or the work dealing with the rituals to be performed in marriage;

(18) *Vyavahāra saukhyaṁ* or the work dealing with the legal procedures;

(19) *Rājanīti saukhyaṁ* or the work dealing with politics and state craft;

(20) *Prāyaścitta saukhyaṁ* or the work dealing with the rituals to be performed for the expiation of sinful deeds;

(21) *Karmavipāka saukhyaṁ* or the work dealing with the fruits of good and bad work to be experienced in the next life;

(22) *Āyurveda saukhyaṁ* or the work dealing with the science of medicine; and

(23) *Āgama saukhyaṁ* or the work dealing with the *mantra śāstra*.

All these works in the series of *Ṭoḍarānanda* are divided into several chapters called *harṣas*. Some of these works are not available even in manuscript form. Some of the available works are in a mutilated form. Of these, the *Sarga saukhyaṁ* and the *Avatāra saukhyaṁ*—the first two sections of this famous encyclopaedic series called *Ṭoḍarānanda* have been published. Others including the *Āyurveda saukhyaṁ* have not so far been brought out in modern print.

All these works of this series are based on the ancient works of India and it is estimated that they had in total 80,000 verses/paragraphs.

Authorship

From the colophons given at the end of each chapter of *Āyurveda saukhyaṁ* and also at the end of this book, it appears that the author of this work was Ṭoḍara malla. But in the invocations in the beginning of each chapter, prayer has been offered to Lord Kṛṣṇa for the long and prosperous life of Ṭoḍara malla himself. Obviously Ṭoḍara malla himself could not have written such type of invocations which is against the scholarship and the tradition of humility among the mediaeval and ancient authors. Therefore, it can safely be presumed that this work and similar other works under the series of *Ṭoḍarānanda* were composed by different scholars under the patronage and financial assistance from this statesman Ṭoḍara malla. In the past, it was the tradition in this country that rich people and kings used to patronize scholars, and the latters used to attribute the authorship of their original works to their financiers. The same might have been the case here also and out of Ṭoḍara malla's love for Hinduism and Indian tradition the real authors might have omitted their own names and given the authorship to Ṭoḍara malla. In the series *Ṭoḍarānanda* there is compilation covering various facets of Indian culture including *smṛti śāstras*, *purāṇas*, astronomy, astrology, mathematics, politics, philosophy, *mantra śāstra* and medicine. Ṭoḍara malla no doubt was an intellectual giant. But for him to study all these subjects in depth and to find time for their selection and compilation appears to be well nay impossible. He was extremely busy in wars and administrative matters for which he was moving from Gujerat to Bengal very often. For him, to carry the huge source material for study, selection and compilation was an impossible task.

During his frequent travels, he got to know the scholars of Varanasi. During this period there were four families of erudite scholars in Benaras. They were the *Bhaṭṭas* the *Dharmādhikāris*, the *Maunis* and the *Śeṣas*. The foremost among these scholars was Pandit Nārāyaṇa Bhaṭṭa who was venerated with the title of Jagadguru. It was this Nārāyaṇa Bhaṭṭa who induced Ṭoḍara malla to renovate the Viśvanātha temple. This Nārāyaṇa Bhaṭṭa was perhaps the chief editor of the series and they were all compiled in Varanasi itself. All the works in this series including *Āyurveda saukhyaṁ* were composed between 1572 A.D. and 1589 A.D.

The colophon at the end of *Āyurveda saukhyaṁ* is given below with a view to showing that it is the Akbar's Minister Rājā Ṭoḍara malla who patronised the compilation of this encyclopaedic work and also to show the high esteem in which he was venerated by the scholars of those days. Verses and the prose paragraphs in this colophon are replete with grammatical and syntactical errors and they are reproduced below without editing or correction.

पूर्णं सौख्यमिदं शिवं वितनुतां श्री टोडरेंद्रे सदा।
धन्यं वृत्तिकरं सुधर्म्माभिभवं प्राणिप्रियं शर्म्मदं।
आयुर्वेदसमुद्रजं सुरतरो रूपं द्वितीयं परम्।
भूमावंकुरितं प्रयोगसुदलं नैरुज्य भूयः फलं ॥१॥

यो वेदार्थसमूहमौक्तिकगणैः श्रीटोडरानंदकः।
पूर्णो वारिधिरेष सर्व्वजगतां वर्व्वत्ति धर्म्मार्थदः।
अंतर्वाणिविभूषणैरुपरितो गीर्व्वाणतुल्यैः शिवै-
रालोड्यार्थतरंगवान् विरचितः शास्त्राणि राजाज्ञया ॥२॥

विश्वेषां परमार्थदोऽखिलजनां ज्ञानांधकारे रविः।
सद्धर्म्माब्जसुबोधने च शशिवत्तापत्रये राजते।
श्री गोविंदपदारविन्दे वसतामानंददोऽयं सतां-
मन्वर्थं भजते सुनामसकलं भूयान्मुदे सर्व्वदा ॥

इति श्रीमद्विविधविरुदावलीविराजमानदेरघुमांधातृभरतादिसमय-
प्रवृत्तपदवीप्रवर्त्तकांत्ययुगाभिःकृतश्रीमूर्त्तिमहद्दरिद्राविदुखःवद्धकाक्रांतः ब्राह्मणादि-
पक्षिगणाश्रयःकल्पपादपःसमस्तशरणपलतासंपौषणाद्दौर्द्दंडदुष्टप्रदमनःतिाविकटप्रो-
च्चदुर्गमनित्रक्षपणक्षमकोपकटाक्षः हस्तिहयहीरहेमादिदानविस्मारितहरिश्चंद्रादि-
चक्रवर्त्तिवर्गो दुदन्वदंतरावर्त्तिविश्वंभराधिनाथप्रतापलीढा विप्लुष्टदिगंतस्थपरिपंथि
सीमंतिनीहृद्गर्भ श्रीमदकवरसाहिपुरःसर भारोद्धरणक्षम प्रचंडदोर्दंडनिरंतरधर्म्मा-
नुरक्तांतःकरणः द्वितीययुधिष्ठिर श्रीमद्गोविंदपादारविंदार्प्पितसमस्तमनोवृत्यंवरीष-
प्रह्लादादिसदाग्रहाखिलक्षत्रवंशावतंसमूर्द्धन्यललामकरुणाकूपारगरिमा चलप्रवरागा-
धांतःकरणातिप्रसिद्धटंडणवंशपारावारोद्भूत भूचंद्रमा महाराजाधिराज श्रीटोडर-
मलविरचिते टोडरानंदे आयुर्वेदसौख्ये एकनवतितमोहर्षः (?) ॥ शुभमस्तु ॥
मांगल्यं भूयात् ॥ श्री श्री ॥ लिखितं कायस्थ माथुरमेवरि गोपाचलीठा हरिवंशुत-
त्पुत्रदयालदासलिखितम् ॥

॥ श्रीगोपीजनवल्लभाय नमः ॥

Manuscripts consulted for study

It was with great deal of difficulty, six manuscripts of this work could be located. Out of them only one *ms.* was partially complete. It was in wooden block litho. Two of these *mss.* were copied recently and they were written in ordinary paper and blue black ink. These *mss.* were serially numbered from I to VI for sake of convenience of reference. Details about these *mss.* are furnished below :

Ms. No. I

This was kindly given by Pandit. Shiv Sharma and it was originally collected by the verteran Āyurvedic physician of Patiala, Pandit Ram Prasad Sharma. It is written in clean and beautiful handwriting. It is a wooden block litho print on Nepali paper.

There are some marginal notes which were perhaps subsequently inserted. Each chapter in this *ms.* starts with an invocation to Lord Kṛṣṇa and ends with a colophon. At the end of *ms.* a detailed colophon eulogising Ṭoḍara malla is given. Most of these colophons are printed in red ink.

It starts with ॥ श्री गरोशाय नमः ॥ ॥ श्री सरस्वत्यै नमः ॥ and it ends with ॥ शुभमस्तु ॥ ॥ छ ॥ ॥ छ ॥ ॥ मांगल्यं भूयात् ॥ ॥ छ ॥ श्री श्री ॥ ॥ लिषितं कायस्थ माथुरमेवरि गोपाचलीठा हरिवंशु तत्पुत्रदयालदास लिखितं ॥ ॥ श्री गोपीजनवल्लभायनमः ॥

In the left hand top corner of each folio "टो० श्रा०" is written and folio numbers are given at the middle of the right side space of the recto of the folio. Each topic and the names of the author or the book referred to in the text are also written in red ink.

Marginal notes are in black ink written in the space above, below, right and left side of the *ms*. In some notes some signs are also given in the text which indicates that some body had attempted to correct the *ms*. after comparing it with some other available *mss*. or some other extant Āyurvedic texts.

In total it has 545 folios. The size of each folio is $11'' \times 4\frac{2}{3}''$. There are approximately 11 lines in each folio, each line containing about 17 words.

This is perhaps the best *ms*. for reference but there are many grammatical as well as syntactical errors in it.

The colophon at the end of this *ms*. indicates that this was copied by Śrī Dayāla Dāsa the son of Śrī Gopāla Cāliṭhā Harivaṁśu belonging to the clan of *Kāyastha Māthura*.

Ms. No. II

This *ms*. was also kindly supplied by Pandit Shiv Sharma and it originally belonged to his illustrious father Pandit Ram Prasad Sharma, the royal physician to the ex-ruler of Patiala. It is written in ordinary ruled paper of brown colour in blue black ink. The paper has become very fragile. *Śloka* as well as paragraph numbers are given with side headings, some of which are not available in the *ms*. No. I.

The size of the paper is $13'' \times 8\frac{1}{2}''$. There are approximately 29 lines in each page and each line has about six words. The line normally ends by the verse or the prose paragraph. The first chapter is however written in a running manner and each line has about 10 words. The last few chapters are written in black ink leaving sufficient space between two verses. In some places '............' signs are given indicating non—availability of the text. It begins with "॥ श्री गणेशाय नमः ॥ ॥ टोडरानन्दः ॥" It has an abrupt ending while dealing with the chapter on *śūla roga* (while describing *pariṇāma śūla*). The colophon of this chapter is also not given which indicates that the writer could not complete his mission.

In the *ms.*, invocation is provided only at the beginning of the first chapter. Unlike the first *ms.* invocation is not given at the beginning of each and every chapter. Colophons are also missing at the end of many chapters and in some chapters they are incomplete.

Some side headings to topics are given in red/blue black ink and in some places topics are underlined in red. These are made in different hand writings which indicates that several scholars have attempted to edit this work at different intervals of time. The *ms.* is incomplete and has fewer mistakes in comparison to the *ms.* no. I.

Ms. No. III

This *ms.* was available in the Library of the Sanskrit College, Calcutta. A photostat copy was obtained. It has 78 folios. However, at the end of the *ms.* the folio number is given as 80 which indicates that two folios which were available in this *ms.* when copied originally, were subsequently lost. The hand writing is illegible and there are many cuttings in the *ms.* The folio numbers are given in the left hand top corner as well as the right hand bottom corner in the recto of the folio. In the right hand side of the folio, above the folio number, the word 'राम' is inscribed.

There are many marginal notes in this *ms.* which are equally illegible.

It abruptly begins from the middle of 13th chapter without any invocation and ends in the middle of the chapter dealing with 'संग्रहणी'.

In the beginning of the complete chapters invocations are given and at the end of these chapters, colophon has also been provided. This is on the line followed in *ms*. I.

Apart from the illegibility of the hand writing there are several grammatical and syntactical mistakes in this *ms.*

Each page of this *Ms.* is 9″×4″ in size. There are about 12 lines in each page, each line having about 17 words.

Ms. No. IV

This is the photostat copy of a *ms.* available in the Library of the Royal Asiatic Society, Calcutta. It is written in clear and beautiful handwriting. There are 416 folios in total. In the left hand top corner of each folio the page number is given along with 'टो० द०'. The page number is also given in the right hand bottom corner below the word 'राम'. Each folio has about nine lines and each line has about 25 words. The text is written in running manner.

It begins with 'श्री गणेशाय नमः' and ends in '।। श्री रामचन्द्राय नमः ।।'. The beginning and the end indicates that the calligrapher considered it to be a complete *ms.* of *Ṭoḍarānanda.* Actually it starts from the eighth chapter and ends in the chapter dealing with 'निदानरोगपरीक्षाचिकित्साकथनम्' (that is the 89th chapter). Unlike *ms.* I, invocation has not been provided in the beginning of each chapter. However, colophons are given at the end of these chapters.

In some places in this *ms.* words are missing which are indicated by '———' marks. Unlike previous *mss.* there are no marginal notes. There are many grammatical mistakes in this *ms.*

Ms. No. V

This hand written script was obtained from Varanasi. It is

written in thick brown paper. The text is written in bold and thick letters and below the śloka its meaning in Hindi is given. This translation varies from place to place in so far as the ink and the hand writing are concerned. There are several marginal notes and corrections of the text as well as the translations. Translation is not available in all chapters. Even in some chapters some paragraphs are left untranslated. However, space has been provided below the concerned verse or prose paragraph for the subsequent insertion of the translation. Serial numbers of the *ślokas* are not given. All these indicate that several scholars had attempted to translate and edit this *ms.* which remained miserably incomplete.

It has ninety-one chapters. It begins with 'ॐ नमः' and ends with the colophon to the chapter 91. Below that some body has written in Hindi, "11th and 15th chapters are not available in this *ms.* and eighteenth chapter is in three sections. This is perhaps the omission by mistake." Page number of this *ms.* is given chapter wise.

The paper is very fragile. Each page is 10″ × 7″ in size. Each page has approximately 27 lines and each line has approximately 10 words.

There are some mistakes in the text of this work and many passages as well as words are missing. Each chapter has its invocation and colophons on the lines of the *ms.* No. I.

Ms. No. VI

This *ms.* was available in the *Abhilekhālaya* of Kathamandu and a calligraphic copy was obtained. It begins with 'श्री गणेशाय नमः' and ends in 'शुभम्'. It has 89 chapters from the very beginning. It has invocations in the beginning of each chapter and colophons at the end of each chapter.

The *ms.* is full of grammatical and syntactical mistakes. It is difficult to ascertain if these mistakes were present in the original *ms.* of the *Abhilekhālaya* or subsequently inserted by the calligrapher.

Chapters in the manuscripts

As has been mentioned before, some of these *mss.* are incomplete. Even the complete *mss.* had different numbers of chapters. In some cases, some chapters were also repeated because of calligraphic errors. The colophons of some chapters of these *mss.* have also different types of reading. The order of chapters has also been changed in some *mss.* Providing all these details, a statement in respect of all these six *mss.* is given below.

Mss. Consulted and Their Contents

A—Available

NA—Not available

Chapter No.	Contents	Ms. I	Ms. II	Ms. III	Ms. IV	Ms. V	Ms. VI
1.	आयुर्वेदप्रयोजन-अष्टचिकित्सालक्षण-वैद्यावैद्यप्रतिरूपिकवैद्यलक्षण-वैद्यदीक्षा-रोगलक्षणकथनम्	A	A	NA	NA	A	A
2.	दोषपञ्चात्मक-दोषस्थानकर्म-अविकृत-लक्षणविकृतदोषोपचयगतिहेतुप्रकोप-लक्षणोपशमनदोषावस्था-दोषवेदना-दोषधातुक्षयलक्षणभेषजपरीक्षा-देश-लक्षण-भूमिलक्षण-नानाप्रकृतिलक्षण-कथनम्	A	A	NA	NA	A	A

		I	II	III	IV	V	VI
3.	पञ्चात्मकद्रव्यलक्षण-पाचनादिपृथक् द्रव्योदाहरणरसवीर्यविपाकलक्षण-ऋतुचर्या-वयोबलसात्म्यपरीक्षाकथनम्	A	A	NA	NA	A	A
4.	शारीरकथनम्	A	A	NA	NA	A	A
5.	शुभाशुभदूतपरीक्षा-कालशुभाशुभ-शकुनलक्षण-अरिष्टलक्षण-पञ्चस्वर-शुभाशुभस्वप्नकथनम्	A	A	NA	NA	A	A
6.	नाडीपरीक्षा-मूत्रपरीक्षा-मलपरीक्षा-नेत्रपरीक्षा-जिह्वापरीक्षा-दीपदेवता-वरणवैकुण्ठद्वादशाक्षरीकालज्ञानविद्या-कथनम्	A	A	NA	NA	A	A
7.	परिभाषाकथनम् (परिमाणकथनम् Ms. II)	A	A	NA	NA	A	A
8.	द्रव्यगुण-वमन-विरेचनकथनम्	A	A	NA	A (incomplete)	A	A

		I	II	III	IV	V	VI
9.	रसशोधन-अष्टसंस्कार-गौरीयन्त्र-वज्र-मूषामृत्तिका-साधन-क्षुद्‌वोधकरण-सोमानलयंत्रनिगडद्रवजारण-दरदोत्थ-रसग्रहणोपायरसमारणभक्षण-रसदोष-मृतसूतज-दोषोपशमन-गंधकोत्पत्ति-जातिलक्षण-शोधन-अभ्रकोत्पत्ति-जाति-शोधन-मारण-सत्त्वपातन-सत्त्वमारणकथनम्	A	A	NA	A	A	NA
10.	लोहोपलोहशोधनमारण-गुणागुण-सन्निपातादौविशेषधातुमारण-जसदमारण-स्फुटितधातुमृदुकरणम्	A	A	NA	A	A	NA
11.	रसोपरस-महारस-मणि-रत्न-शोधन-मारण-सत्त्वपातन-सत्त्वमारण-द्रुतिकरण-गुणागुण-विषलक्षण-दिंव्यौषधादिलक्षणवह्निलक्षण-तैलापातनकथनम	A	A	NA	A	NA	NA

		I	II	III	IV	V	VI
12.	गणोद्देशकथनम्	A	A	NA	NA	A	NA
13.	रोगविज्ञानप्रकारः	A	A	A	NA	A	A
14.	सर्वरोगेषुलंघनादिषडुपक्रमकथनम्	A	A	A	NA	A	A
15.	समस्तरसक्रियासूत्रकथनम्	A	A	A	NA	NA	A
16.	ज्वरनिदानचिकित्साकथनम्	A	A	A	A (incomplete)	A	A
17.	अतिसारनिदानचिकित्साकथनम्	A	A	A	A	A	A
18.	संग्रहणीनिदानचिकित्साकथनम्	A	A	A	A (incomplete)	A	A
19.	अर्शोनिदानचिकित्साकथनम्	A	A	NA } both given in one chap.		A	A
20.	अग्निमान्द्याजीर्णविसूचिकानिदानचिकित्साकथनम्	A	A	NA }		A	A
21.	कृमिनिदानचिकित्साकथनम्	A	A	NA	A	NA	A
22.	पाण्डुरोगनिदानचिकित्साकथनम्	A	A	NA	NA	A	A
23.	रक्तपित्तनिदानचिकित्साकथनम्	A	A	NA	A	A	A

		I	II	III	IV	V	VI
24.	राजयक्ष्माक्षतक्षयनिदान चिकित्सा-कथनम्	A	A	NA	NA	A	A
25.	कासनिदानचिकित्साकथनम्	A	A	NA	A	A	A
26.	हिक्काश्वासनिदानचिकित्साकथनम्	A	A	NA	A	A	A
27.	स्वरभेदनिदानचिकित्साकथनम्	A	A	NA	A	A	A
28.	अरोचकनिदानचिकित्साकथनम्	A	A	NA	A (incomplete)	A	A
29.	छर्दिनिदानचिकित्साकथनम्	A	A	NA	A	A	A
30.	तृष्णानिदानचिकित्साकथनम्	A	A	NA	A	A	A
31.	मूर्छानिदानचिकित्साकथनम्	A	A	NA	A	A	A
32.	दाहनिदानचिकित्साकथनम्	A	A	NA	A	A	A
33.	मदात्ययनिदानचिकित्साकथनम् (पानात्यय in *ms.* II & IV)	A	A	NA	NA	A	A
34.	उन्मादनिदानचिकित्साकथनम्	A	A	NA	A	A	A
35.	अपस्मारनिदानचिकित्साकथनम्	A	A	NA	A	A	A

		I	II	III	IV	V	VI
36.	वातव्याधिनिदानचिकित्साकथनम्	A	A	NA	A	A	A
37.	वातरक्तनिदानचिकित्साकथनम्	A	A	NA	A	A	A
38.	उरुस्तम्भनिदानचिकित्साकथनम्	A	A	NA	A (Repeated)	A	A
39.	आमवातनिदानचिकित्साकथनम्	A	A	NA	A	A	A
40.	शूलनिदानचिकित्साकथनम्	A	A	NA	A	A	A
41.	परिणामशूलनिदानचिकित्साकथनम्	A	NA	NA	A	A	A
42.	उदावर्तनिदानचिकित्साकथनम्	A	NA	NA	A	A	A
43.	गुल्मनिदानचिकित्साकथनम्	A	NA	NA	A	A	A
44.	हृद्रोगनिदानचिकित्साकथनम्	A	NA	NA	A	NA	A
45.	मूत्रकृच्छ्रनिदानचिकित्साकथनम्	A	NA	NA	A	A	A
46.	मूत्रघातनिदानचिकित्साकथनम्	A	NA	NA	A	A	A
47.	अश्मरीनिदानचिकित्साकथनम्	A	NA	NA	A	A	A

		I	II	III	IV	V	VI
48.	प्रमेहमधुमेहपिडकानिदानचिकित्सा-कथनम्	A	NA	NA	A	A	A
49.	मेदोरोगनिदानचिकित्साकथनम्	A	NA	NA	A	A	A
50.	कृशरोगनिदानचिकित्साकथनम्	A	NA	NA	A	A	A
51.	उदरनिदानचिकित्साकथनम्	A	NA	NA	A	A	A
52.	शोथनिदानचिकित्साकथनम्	A	NA	NA	A	A	A
53.	आन्त्रवृद्धिकुरण्डकवर्ध्मनिदान-चिकित्साकथनम्	A	NA	NA	A	A	A
54.	गलगण्ड-गण्डमाला-अपची-ग्रन्थ्यर्बुद-निदानचिकित्साकथनम्	A	NA	NA	A	A	A
55.	श्लीपदनिदानचिकित्साकथनम्	A	NA	NA	A	A	A
56.	विद्रधिनिदानचिकित्साकथनम्	A	NA	NA	A	A	A

		I	II	III	IV	V	VI
57.	शोफव्रण-शारीरव्रण-सद्योव्रण-नासिका-संधानवहि्नदग्ध-भग्ननिदान-चिकित्साकथनम्	A	NA	NA	A	A	A
58.	नाडीव्रणनिदानचिकित्साकथनम्	A	NA	NA	A	A	NA
59.	भगन्दरनिदानचिकित्साकथनम्	A	NA	NA	A	A	NA
60.	उपदंशनिदानचिकित्साकथनम्	A	NA	NA	A	A	NA
61.	शूकदोषनिदानचिकित्साकथनम्	A	NA	NA	A	A	NA
62.	कुष्ठनिदानचिकित्साकथनम्	A	NA	NA	A	A	NA
63.	उदर्दकोठशीतपित्तनिदानचिकित्सा-कथनम्	A	NA	NA	A	A	NA
64.	अम्लपित्तनिदानचिकित्साकथनम्	A	NA	NA	A	A	NA
65.	विसर्पनिदानचिकित्साकथनम्	A	NA	NA	A	A	NA
66.	विस्फोटनिदानचिकित्साकथनम्	A	NA	NA	A	A	NA
67.	स्नायुनिदानचिकित्साकथनम्	A	NA	NA	A	A	NA

		I	II	III	IV	V	VI
68.	मसूरिकानिदानचिकित्साकथनम्	A	NA	NA	A	A	A
69.	क्षुद्ररोगनिदानचिकित्साकथनम्	A	NA	NA	A	A	A
70.	श्रोष्ठदन्तजिह्वागलमुखरोगनिदान-चिकित्साकथनम्	A	NA	NA	A	A	A
71.	कर्णरोगनिदानचिकित्साकथनम्	A	NA	NA	A	A	A
72.	नासारोगनिदानचिकित्साकथनम्	A	NA	NA	A	A	A
73.	नेत्ररोगनिदानचिकित्साकथनम्	A	NA	NA	A	A	A
74.	शिरोरोगनिदानचिकित्साकथनम्	A	NA	NA	A	A	A
75.	सोमरोगनिदानचिकित्साकथनम्	NA	NA	NA	NA	NA	A
76.	श्रसृग्दरनिदानचिकित्साकथनम् (प्रदर in *ms.* IV)	A	NA	NA	A	A	NA
77.	योनिव्यापद्योनिकन्दनिदानचिकित्सा-कथनम्	A	NA	NA	A	A	A
78.	मूढगर्भनिदानचिकित्साकथनम्	A	NA	NA	A	A	A

		I	II	III	IV	V	VI
79.	सूतिकारोगनिदानचिकित्साकथनम्	A	NA	NA	A	A	A
80.	स्तनरोगनिदानचिकित्साकथनम्	NA	NA	NA	A	NA	NA
81.	बालरोगनिदानचिकित्साकथनम्	A	NA	NA	A	A	A
82.	विषनिदानचिकित्साकथनम्	A	NA	NA	A	A	A
83.	रसायनाधिकारः	A	NA	NA	A	A } Both taken in one chapter	
84.	वाजीकरणाधिकारः	A	NA	NA	A	A }	
85.	स्नेहपानकथनम्	A	NA	NA	A	A	A
86.	वमन-विरेक-नस्य-धूमपान-गण्डूष-कवल-प्रतिसारणाधिकारः (Reference chapter—8)	NA	NA	NA	A	A (Without Vamana & Virecana)	A
87.	शोणितस्रावविधिः	A	NA	NA	A	A	A
88.	वस्तिविधि-निरूहण-अनुवासनयुक्त-रसवस्तिकथनम्	A	NA	NA	A	A	A

		I	II	III	IV	V	VI
89.	निदान-रोगपरीक्षा-चिकित्साकथनम्	A	NA	NA	A	A	A
90.	निघण्टौ अभयादिकः	NA	NA	NA	NA	A	A
91.	निघण्टौ शुण्ठ्यादिकः	A	NA	NA	NA	A	NA
92.	निघण्टौ कर्पूरादिवर्गः	A	NA	NA	NA	A	A
93.	निघण्टौ स्वर्णादिवर्गः	A	NA	NA	NA	A	A
94.	निघण्टौ वनस्पतिवर्गः	A	NA	NA	NA	A	A
95.	निघण्टौ फलवर्गः	A	NA	NA	NA	A	A
96.	निघण्टौ शाकवर्गः	A	NA	NA	NA	A	A
97.	अन्नपानवर्गः	A	NA	NA	NA	A	NA

Āyurveda saukhyaṁ in *Ṭoḍarānanda* is virtually a compilation from different authentic sources. Most of these source works are not readily available now. Some of these important works are given in the statement below :

Authors and works quoted in the First seven chapters of the Āyurveda saukhyaṁ in Ṭoḍarānanda :

Name of the Author/Work		*Reference in Āyurveda saukhyaṁ*
1. Agniveśa	...	1 : 50, 111, 130; 2 : 38, 63, 167; 3 : 6-9, 66, 130-131, 197, 226, 373, 380; 4 : 51, 95, 117, 142, 159, 188, 193, 205; 5 : 55, 101; 7 : 142, 198, 396, 413, 479;
2. Ātreya	...	1 : 73; 2 : 127, 205; 3 : 79, 116, 122, 152, 156, 157, 376; 4 : 177, 184, 186, 201; 5 : 7, 131; 7 : 136, 154, 167, 252, 390, 393;
3. Kāśyapa	...	7 : 169;
4. Kṛṣṇātreya	...	3 : 30, 179, 370; 4 : 10, 151, 185, 189; 7 : 53, 59, 65, 70, 78, 125, 174, 267, 401;
5. Kṣārapāṇi	...	7 : 147;
6. Kharanāda	...	1 : 60; 2 : 84, 203; 4 : 319; 7 : 187;

7. Garga		4 : 287;
8. Gopura	...	3 : 34; 4 : 129; 5 : 57; 6 : 42; 7 : 85, 214, 292;
9. Gorakṣa	...	7 : 49, 487, 488, 490;
10. Candra nandana	...	7 : 118;
11. Candrikā	...	7 : 305;
12. Caraka	...	1 : 153; 3 : 95, 150, 364, 365, 366; 4 : 44, 102, 254; 6 : 4; 7 : 141, 144, 171, 228, 245, 410;
13. Carpaṭi	...	6 : 32;
14. Cikitsā kalikā	...	2 : 52, 53, 54, 76;
15. Cikitsā sāra saṁgraha	...	4 : 56, 57, 58, 59;
16. Cintāmaṇi	...	7 : 52;
17. Jejjaṭa	...	2 : 85, 86; 7 : 417;
18. Dalhaṇa	...	2 : 148; 4 : 20; 7 : 262;
19. Narapati caryā	...	6 : 118, 119, 120, 121, 122;
20. Nala	...	7 : 202, 203, 204, 327;
21. Nāgārjuna	...	7 : 442, 526;
22. Padmā	...	1 : 51;
23. Puṣkalāvata	...	7 : 90;
24. Prayoga pārijāta	...	3 : 141;

25. Bhadra śaunaka ... 7 : 107, 295, 395;

26. Bhālluki ... 4 : 11, 12, 13, 14;

27. Bhela ... 7 : 95, 151, 152, 229;

28. Bhoja ... 4 : 147, 266, 267;
7 : 95;

29. Mārkaṇḍeya purāṇa ... 4 : 163;

30. Yoga pradīpa ... 4 : 128;

31. Yoga ratnāvalī ... 6 : 140;

32. Yoga śārīra ... 4 : 125;

33. Ratnākara ... 4 : 143, 229, 279;
7 : 452;

34. Rasa ratnākara ... 7 : 476;

35. Rasa sāra ... 7 : 502, 503, 504, 505, 506, 507. 508, 509, 510, 511, 512;

36. Rasa siddhānta ... 7 : 557;

37. Rasāṅkuśa ... 7 : 450;

38. Rasārṇava ... 6 : 125, 126, 127, 128, 129, 130, 131;
7 : 59, 75, 176, 438, 454;

39. Rudra kautuka ... 2 : 55;

40. Rāja caṇḍeśvara ... 5 : 38;

41. Rudra tantra ... 6 : 70;

42. Raudrāṁsa ... 7 : 495, 496;

43. Varāha mihira ... 7 : 145;

44. Vaśiṣṭha ... 4 : 27, 28, 88, 97, 180, 257, 312;
7 : 210, 232;

45. Vāgbhaṭa	...	1 : 10, 77; 2 : 36, 82, 110, 146, 204; 3 : 74, 75, 76, 77, 89, 94, 124, 125, 126, 127, 128, 148, 158; 7 : 214, 244;
46. Vācaspati	...	7 : 308;
47. Videha	...	1 : 26; 4 : 121;
48. Viveka mārtaṇḍa	...	2 : 8, 9, 10, 11;
49. Viśvā mitra	...	7 : 91;
50. Vīrabhadra	...	3 : 195;
51. Vṛddha bhoja	...	1 : 25; 7 : 340;
52. Vṛddha vāhaṭa (Vāgbhaṭa)	...	2 : 187; 4 : 74, 243, 343, 344, 7 : 114, 223;
53. Vṛddha śaunaka	...	7 : 303;
54. Vṛddha suśruta	...	7 : 196, 240, 266, 285, 311, 335, 393;
55. Vṛddhātreya	...	4 : 68, 167;
56. Vṛddha hārīta	...	6 : 13; 7 : 62, 63, 497, 498, 499;
57. Vaikhānasa	...	4 : 124;
58. Vaidyālaṅkāra	...	7 : 487;
59. Vaiśvānara	...	4 : 25, 26;
60. Śārṅgadhara	...	7 : 4, 5, 6, 7, 8, 9, 10, 11, 12,13, 14, 15, 16, 17, 18, 19, 20, 21, 22, 23, 24, 25, 26 27, 28, 29, 30, 31, 32, 33, 34, 35,36, 37, 38, 39, 40, 41;

61. Śivāgama	...	6 : 54;
62. Śaivāla	...	7 : 479;
63. Śiva mekhalā	...	7 : 397;
64. Śaunaka	...	7 : 344, 391;
65. Sarvāṅga sundara	...	4 : 231;
66. Siddha sāra	...	7 : 181;
67. Suśruta	...	1 : 18, 70, 71, 72, 148, 151; 2 : 46, 47, 48, 49, 50, 51, 59, 60, 61, 111, 114, 123, 133, 185, 186; 3 : 117, 118, 129, 188, 225, 385, 386, 387; 4 : 18, 19, 37, 38, 63, 73, 81, 98, 99, 119, 127, 131, 140, 141, 158, 161, 162, 164, 178, 196, 197, 198, 199, 200, 216, 236, 248, 249, 250, 251, 252, 253, 254, 255, 256, 349; 7 : 97, 113, 170, 194, 255, 263, 283;
68. Hariścandra	...	4 : 237;
69. Hārīta	...	7 : 185.

Method followed for preparation of critical edition

As has been mentioned before, six *ms*s. collected from different parts of the country and abroad were utilised for this critical study. It has already been stated that all these *ms*s. were full of grammatical and syntactical errors. In total there were 97 chapters (*harṣas*). *Ms*s. differ in giving numbers to some chapters both in the beginning and at the end of each chapter. Contents of these chapters and their availability in different *ms*s. are already given in the form of a statement. The later chapters mostly deal with drugs and diseases including their diagnosis and treatment. The most important portion of this work dealing with fundamental principles, and the lesser known but more important aspect of Āyurveda that is the *rogi parīkṣā* are elucidated in the first six chapters. Because of this and also with a view to avoiding the enormous size of the work (that would have accrued had all the chapters been taken together) it was felt necessary to confine to the first six chapters for the purpose of this book.

As has been mentioned before, under the patronage of Ṭodara malla, scholars prepared this work mainly by the compilation from different authentic sources which were then extant. During this process and during the subsequent process of copying, many calligraphic errors have crept into this work. Source books which were utilised by them and which are available now have also under gone many transformations, mutilations and corruptions. Some of the texts quoted in *Ṭodarānanda* are not available now, but similar texts are available in other extant works. Keeping all the above in view, an attempt has been made to present the most appropriate and the correct text of various topics in these six chapters. Variant readings available in other *mss*. on this work are given in the notes (*ṭippaṇi*) at the end of each chapter. However, such variant readings which were conspicuously errors-either calligraphic or otherwise—have not been taken note of.

There are many and orthographic peculiarities by which ख has been written as ष, ष as ख, न as ण, ण as न, ब as व, व as ब, प as य, य as प, त्त as त, त as त्त, ज as य, य as ज, र व as ख, ख as र व, श as स, स as श, म as भ and भ as म. In many places there is also a duplicationof म and य specially after 'r'. Attempts have been made to correct these calligraphic errors in the present critical edition. However, some proper nouns like वशिष्ठ and वसिष्ठ are intentionally left out without any correction.

In the same chapter, there were different readings in different *mss*. and attempt has been made to reconcile them. Therefore, the serial numbers of verses and paragraphs of the original *mss*. (which were obviously at variant) have not been taken into account. On the other hand, continuous number of these verses and paragraphs appropriate to their locations in the chapter has been given. The authors have taken the liberty of giving one number to a verse having only three lines or even one line, even though this procedure doesn't confirm to the established tradition of poetics. This has been done simply to indicate the end of the topic.

In some of the *mss.* side headings of different topics are given. In respect of some topics such headings are missing. These missing side-headings are provided by the authors. But such insertions by the authors are always indicated by the mark [.........].

At the end of these topics in some *mss.* foot notes are provided. They are kept as such in this critical study because of their significance and importance.

As will be seen from the texts, the names of the texts/authors from where these references have been compiled are originally provided in the left hand top corner as side-headings. Some of these are available in the extant texts and the exact references—the name of the text, the *sthāna* (section) number and the verse/paragraph number are located by the authors and given in the right hand side bottom of the topic. These insertions by the authors are also given with the mark [...] to facilitate their easy identification and the portions of these texts to which the reference is related, are given within the marks "..."

In *Ṭoḍarānanda,* extant works like *Caraka, Suśruta, Vāgbhaṭa* are profusely quoted. Even though these texts are available now, in some places the exact references are either not available or are available in a different form. Notes on these are provided at the end of each chapter under *ṭippaṇi* by providing a corresponding neumarical cross reference in the text.

In some places, even though a reference is quoted from one of the extant texts, such references are actually not available. But they are available in another extant text. These references are given along with the names of the text, *sthāna* (section) number & verse/paragraph number at the end of the topics in the right hand bottom and they are also kept within the mark [...] to facilitate their identification.

Inside the text, in the *mss.*, certain portions/words are missing. These are replenished either from the allied text or by the author, keeping in view the syntax and the topic of discussion. These are also indicated inside the text by the mark [...].

Portions of the text which are missing in any of the *mss.* but are available in other *mss.* or extant texts are given within quotation marks ('...'). The *ms.* where these texts are available, are indicated in the *ṭippaṇi* at the end of the chapter.

Compiler's own Comment

Ṭoḍarānanda is primarily composed by compiling material on different topics from various authentic sources. The original author has however given his own comments at several important places.

According to verse numbers 38 in the first *harṣa*, *Agada tantra* is explained as the specialised branch dealing with various types of *Basti* (medicated enema). According to Atri quoted in verse 37 of this *harṣa*, *Basti cikitsā* is treated as the ninth specialised branch of Āyurveda. But the author has explained his own view in this connection in paragraph numbers 39 and 40. According to him *Basti cikitsā* constitutes a part of *kāya cikitsā* and it is not correct either to interpret it as *Agada tantra* or to keep it as a separate specialised branch. He has therefore, concluded that there are only eight branches of Āyurveda which is traditionally accepted in *Caraka*, *Suśruta*, *and Vāgbhaṭa*. Similar comments of the author are available in other places also.

Important and Significant Topics

In this work several important and significant topics are discussed. Some of them are not available in extant authentic classics. In some other cases, the matter provided on these topics is quite new and interesting. Some such topics are given below :

1. *Nāḍi Parikṣā*

Even today, the current practice among the Āyurvedic physicians is to examine the pulse of the patient before embarking upon the treatment. But the description of *Nāḍi parikṣā* is not directly or indirectly available in any of the extant Āyurvedic classics like

Caraka saṁhitā, Suśruta saṁhitā, Aṣṭāṅga hṛdaya, Aṣṭāṅga saṁgraha, Bhela saṁhitā, Kāśyapa saṁhitā and *Hārita saṁhitā*. Reference to *Nāḍī parīkṣā* is available only in some more recent works like *Yoga ratnākara*. How such an important topic escaped the notice of the authors of Āyurvedic classics is a matter of hot debate among the Āyurvedic scholars. Some scholars have even gone to the extent of suggesting that pulse examination even though commonly resorted to at present by Āyurvedic physicians, is not an original contribution of Āyurveda. This popular practice, like many others, has come to this country during the exchange of scholarship in the medieval period either from China or from Tibet.

Ṭoḍara malla has provided in this work references which he claims to have compiled from *Caraka saṁhitā and Vṛddha hārita*. In this connection verse numbers 4 to 25 in the 6th *harṣa* may be perused. These verses unambiguously indicate that these references were compiled from the then available texts of *Caraka* and *Vṛddha hārita*. Unfortunately work of latter is not available now, and it is known per certain that the original *Agniveśa saṁhitā* which was subsequently redacted by Caraka was called *Caraka saṁhitā*. At a later stage this *Caraka saṁhitā* was not available in full. It was in mutilated condition. Therefore, Dṛḍhabala subsequently tried to replenish the work by compiling material from allied authentic sources and adding them to the original mutilated work. In this process, it is possible that the description of some important topics like pulse examination (*Nāḍī parīkṣā*) are left out and it was presumed subsequently that such topics were not available in the original text.

To elucidate the above view point the methods of pulse examination followed in Āyurveda and in Tibetan as well as Chinese medicine are given below :

Āyurvedic Method of Pulse Examination

It is carried out in the early morning when the patient is in empty stomach. It is prohibited immediately after bath, food and oil massage because the pulse then becomes erratic and does not indicate the correct condition of the patient. Similarly, a patient who is hungry and thirsty is not suitable for the purpose of pulse examination.

Pulse examination is carried out through the help of the radial artery. It is perceptible in the place about half an inch below the thumb. In the case of males the pulse of right hand and in the case of females that of the left hand is examined. For this purpose the arm should be stretched properly and the hand should be kept in slightly flexed position. Simultaneously, the fingers including the thumb should be in a stretched position. The physician should examine the pulse by the help of his right hand. Three fingers namely the index, the middle and the ring fingers are used for pulse examination. They are kept over the pulse, the index finger remaining near the thumb. Gentle and uniform pressure is applied through the tips of these fingers over the pulse and the pulsation of the artery is felt. The physician has to put pressure and release it repeatedly to correctly ascertain the exact finger on which the pulsation is more felt. If the pulsation is felt over the index finger then *vāyu* is dominant in the patient. Feeling in middle finger indicates the dominance of *pitta* and in ring finger indicates aggravation of *kapha* in the body of the patient.

Apart from this, the physician has also to ascertain the movement of the pulse. If the movement of the pulse is felt like the motion of a snake or a leech, then it indicates the dominance of *vāyu*. If there is dominance of *pitta* then the pulse moves like a crow or a sparrow or a frog. In the case of *kapha*, the movement of pulse is like that of a swan or a peacock or a cock. If the pulse at times moves like the snake and on some other times like a frog then there is dominance of both *vāyu* and *pitta*. In patients having predominance of *vāyu* and *kapha*, the pulse moves like a snake and a swan. Movement of the pulse like a frog and a swan indicates the dominance of *pitta* and *kapha*. When all the three *doṣas* are vitiated then the pulse moves like a wood-pecker bird.

If the pulse is regular continuously for thirty times then the patient is sure to survive. If there are interruptions then this indicates imminent death. Apart from what has been stated above, in āyurvedic texts, there is an elaborate description regarding the nature of pulse in different diseases, and this is very frequently used by the physicians as the means to probe the diseases.

Tibetan Method of Pulse Examination

There are many arteries in the human body, but the ones to be examined are those that pulsate, which originate in the heart and carry blood and air together. These arteries are like messengers between the doctor and the patient.

General rules for Doctors and Patients before Examination of the Pulse

In the evening, preceding the examination, the patient must refrain from having rich food such as meat and wine. Neither must he exert himself nor sit in the hot sun. He must be well rested and must have had light food so as to avoid disturbing the bile (*mkhris pa*), phlegm (*bad kan*) and air (*rlung*) in his constitution, to enable the doctor to make a clear diagnosis. The doctor in turn should be well prepared and relaxed before the examination in order to obtain good results.

If the disease comes suddenly necessitating an urgent examination, then both the doctor and the patient should try to relax just before the examination of the pulse takes place.

The pulse is examined at a spot one inch from the wrist joint. Pulsating arteries can be felt at other parts of the body as well, but the wrist is used because it is closest to the vital organs of the body. The reason why the pulsating artery in the neck is not used is that the comparative proximity of the heart and lungs has such an effect on the pulse as to mask the effect produced by other organs. The pulsating vein in the leg is also unsuitable for examination because it is too far from the vital organs of the body.

In examining the pulse one should use the index finger, middle finger and ring finger. (The first is called *mts'on,* the second *kan* and the third *chhag*). The fingers must be held in a line close to one another yet not touching each other. The index finger must not put too much pressure on the skin; more pressure should be applied by the middle and ring fingers.

Left hand of Patient Examined by the Right hand of the Doctor

When examining the pulse, (a) the tip of the index finger on the right side detects heart diseases and on the left intestinal diseases; (b) the tip of the middle finger on the right side detects diseases affecting the spleen, and on the left stomach diseases; and (c) the tip of the ring finger on the right side detects kidney diseases and on the left diseases affecting the seminal vesicle.

Right hand of Patient Examined by the Left hand of the Doctor

(a) the right tip of the index finger detects lung diseases, the left tip diseases affecting the guts; (b) the right tip of the middle finger detects liver diseases, the left tip diseases due to unbalanced bile; (c) the right tip of the ring finger detects kidney diseases, and the left tip diseases affecting the urinary bladder.

The right hand pulse should be examined first in the case of female patients, and the left hand in the case of males. The reason for this is that the tip of the female heart is titled towards the right and *vice versa* with males.

Chinese Method of Pulse Examination

In Chinese system of medicine the palpation of pulse and making a dignosis thereby, is indication of the perfection of the art of medicine. It is said about the pulse examination that it does not only give the present state of health but tells also of the diseases of the past and predicts those which may appear in the future (?). It is important to feel the right and the left pulse at the wrist. It is done by putting three fingers and with each finger the pulse is felt in the segment under that finger by light and deep touch respectively. Thus, there are six observations on each side and total of twelve pulses are felt on both sides.

The best time to feel the pulse is at 3 a.m. when the *Yin* and *Yang* are comparatively at rest and the stomach is empty. The distal deep pulse felt at the left wrist is the heart pulse, the middle deep is the liver pulse, the proximal deep is the kidney pulse. The superficial pulses in the same order are small intestine, gall bladder and urinary bladder pulses respectively. On the right wrist deep pulses in the same order are lung, spleen and circulation sex and superficially the large intestine, stomach and triple warmer. The deep pulses detect disorders of *Yin* organs and superficial pulse

Yang organs. The pulses identify the organs diseased and so the meridians affected. The meridians give the most effective acupuncture point to relieve pain and sufferings.

The basic fundamental normal pulse has to be judged by experience taking into consideration the age and constitution of an individual. Comparing with the expected norm the pulse in its abnormality may be plethoric. All the pulses in an ensemble may be plethoric in which case all the twelve basic pulses beat too strongly and feel overful. This is known as the total plethora of *Yin* and *Yang*. All the superficial pulses alone may be plethoric. This indicates total plethora of *Yang* alone. If all the deep pulses are plethoric it means total plethora of *Yin*. All pulses deep or superficial on both sides may be weak. This indicates weakness of both *Yin* and *Yang*. Weakness of deep pulses or superficial pulses will correspondingly mean weakness of *Yin* and *Yang* respectively. If pulses on the right side are stronger than those of left, there is excess of *Yang*. Converse is true of *Yin* when left pulses are strong. The plethoric or weak superficial or deep pulse also indicates the *Yang* or *Yin* state which reflects the quality of health and the meridian of the particular organ represented in the segment. Pulse is also said to inherit genetic characters. This is made use of when a person has lost an upper arm and the pulse of the arm is not available for palpation. If the pulse of any of his children is palpated in the arm right or left which is not available in the father, it will give the characters of the parents pulse. This become handy if an arm has been amputated or otherwise lost.

It will be seen from the above that the Tibetan and Chinese methods of pulse examination are radically different from the method followed by the Āyurvedic physician and described in the Āyurvedic texts including the references from *Caraka* and *Vṛddha Hārita* quoted in *Ṭoḍarānanda*. Therefore, it will perhaps be safe to presume that the method of pulse examination was originally available in Āyurvedic texts but subsequently got lost.

2. *Mūtra parikṣā*

Regarding *mūtra parikṣā*, there is no systematic description in any of the ancient Āyurvedic classics. Of course, its characteristic features in different diseases are described. This information is not comprehensive, and is scattered in different part of these books. Systematic description of urine examination is available only in much later work like *Yoga ratnākara* and *Cikitsā sār saṁgraha*. The latter work is popularly known, as *Vangasena*. They have introduced new techniques also to the methods of urine-examination; one of these worth mentioning is '*tailabindu parīkṣā*'. In the ancient Siddha System of Medicine, which is claimed to be very old, with its beginning in early centuries after Christ, and in the mediaeval Unani System of Medicine, *mūtra parikṣā* appears to have occupied a distinct and specific place in the diagnostic and prognostic methods of investigation of a disease.

From a perusal of available literature, one finds a gradual development of the methods of urine-examination. In the oldest literature available, namely, the *Ṛk veda*, there is hardly any reference to the description of the urine and its pathological changes, excepting a reference to the diseases of *gavinis*. Similar is the position of *Yajur veda*. In the literature which just follows the period of *Ṛk veda*, that is, in *Atharva veda* which is the main source of Āyurveda, there is no reference to urinary changes in different diseases though, it describes the symptomatology and treatment of number of diseases and also of the retention of urine.

From the Vaidika period to the *Saṁhitā* period, a gap of more than a thousand and odd years appears to have occurred. The oldest *Saṁhitā* which is available, at present, is that of Caraka, which is named after its redactor, though, the original writer of it is stated to be Agniveśa.

In *Caraka saṁhitā*, one finds references and evidence which point to the existence of many other *saṁhitās*, as well as different schools of thought, before and in his time. But all this literature is not available at present. Caraka has described many urinary changes in different diseases. But excepting the group of diseases known as urinary disease or *Vasti rogas* his descriptions pertain, mainly, to colour changes and that too, mostly with reference to the vitiated *doṣa*, in a disease. Thus, identical descriptions of colours appearing in urine are found in *vātika*, *paittika* and *ślaiṣmika* types of many diseases, namely, *jvara*, *gulma*, *arśas*, *pāṇḍu*, *udara* etc. While discussing *āyuḥ kṣaya lakṣaṇāni* (symptoms and signs of approaching cessation of life) in the *Indriya sthāna,* Caraka has described abnormal colours which may appear in various structures and substances of the body. Under these, he includes urine also. He also mentions, in this chapter, a special test for urine, for determining the imminence of death of a patient. Excepting the above two references, which are general, irrespective of any disease all other references in *Caraka saṁhitā* are found under the description of various diseases.

While describing the methodology of examination of diseases in general, Caraka states that, a disease is to be examined by *pratyakṣa, anumāna* and *āptopadeśa.* The *pratyakṣa* corresponds to the knowledge gathered through the instrumentality of the five sense organs. But out of these, he does not recommend *rasa parīkṣā* to be performed directly to determine the taste or *rasa* of various substances of the patient's body. Instead, he recommends that knowledge of *rasa* may be acquired by inference only. In the chapter in *Vimāna sthāna* which deals with examination of the patient, there is no separate mention of urine with reference to various pathological changes as may be seen in it, which might be gathered through these examinations.

Suśruta and *Vāgbhaṭa saṁhitās* have not furnished more data than are available in *Caraka saṁhitā,* as far as descriptions of pathological changes in urine are concerned. Suśruta has furnished a more vivid description of the urinary apparatus and its working, which of course is lying scattered in different places. One remarkable contribution of Suśruta, to the subject of urine-examination, is the description of normal urine, which he does while describing the *prameha mukta lakṣaṇās* i.e., the character of the urine of a patient who has become free from *prameha roga.* Such a description is lacking in other works.

Coming to the age of Bhāva Miśra, one finds that he has included urine also as one of the substances to be examined under the scheme of the examination of a patient. He says that the physician should examine the eyes, the tongue and the urine of every patient. He further describes various colours of urine and their significance in the determination of vitiated *doṣas* in disease states.

But, surprisingly enough, he has not furnished any description of the colour of normal urine. *Śāraṅgadhara* and *Mādhava kara* do not describe the examination of urine separately.

Yoga ratnākara, *Basava rajiyaṁ* and *Vaṅga sena* are the only works which deal with '*Mūtra parīkṣā*' as such methodically. These books furnish, in detail the methods of examination of urine as well as the mode of collection of specimens for such an examination. *Yoga ratnākara* lays great emphasis on the examination of urine by observing that, "A physician who is incapable of recording the changes in pulse, urine and tongue kills his patient." In the first verse on *Mūtra parīkṣā*, he emphasises its importance in the recognition of disease-states. In these works, a new method of urine-examination, is found to have been introduced. This new method is known as '*Taila bindu parīkṣā*', which is, particularly useful in determining the prognosis of a case. *Basava rajiyaṁ* furnishes one more test for determining the prognosis in patients suffering from *prameha*. This is done by evaporating a measured quantity of urine on fire and then, measuring the solid residue. Such a test is not found mentioned in any of the *saṁhitās* and other Āyurvedic literature available today.

Thus, one finds a gradual evolution of a recognition of the importance of *mūtra parīkṣā* in various diseases. There are some, who believe that urine-examination as such, is not an Āyurvedic *parīkṣā* and that it had crept into the Āyurvedic literature from the other systems of medicine. This assumption is not correct. It will be seen from the 6th *harṣa* of *Ṭoḍarānanda* that systematic urine-examination including *taila bindu parīkṣā* was available even in ancient classics like *Carpaṭi saṁhitā*, *Gopura saṁhitā* and *Hariścandra saṁhitā*. Unfortunately, these ancient classical works are no more extant. The references quoted in *Ṭoḍarānanda*, however convinces beyond any doubt about their antiquity and authenticity.

Dīpana and Pācana

The term *dīpana* means the "stimulation of the digestive enzymes" and *pācana* means "digestion". It appears *dīpana* is the cause and *pācana* is the effect. Thus, the distinction between these two terms is not very clear and it often causes confusion. There are drugs which are only *dīpana* and there are others which are only *pācana*. But there are many drugs which are both *dīpana* and *pācana*. Therefore, these terms are often the subject matter of hot debate among the scholars and physicians. In *Āyurveda saukhyaṁ* 3 : 26-43 an effort has been made to clarify this controversial point. In this connection the views of Kṛṣṇa Ātreya and Gopura have been quoted and an effort has been made to solve this problem by mentioning the probable queries and providing their appropriate replies.

Aṣṭāṅga or Eight Specialised Branches of Āyurveda

Āyurveda has eight specialised branches. These are as follows :

(1) *Kāya cikitsā* or Internal Medicine;

(2) *Śalya tantra* or Surgery;

(3) *Śālākya tantra* or the Treatment of diseases of head and the neck;

(4) *Agada tantra* or Toxicology;

(5) *Bhūta vidyā* or the management of seizures by evil spirits and other mental disorders;

(6) *Bāla tantra* or Paediatrics;

(7) *Rasāyana tantra* or Geriatrics including Rejuvenation therapy; and

(8) *Vāji karaṇa tantra* or science of Aphrodisiacs.

This division is accepted by the authors of all the Āyurvedic classics. There is only a little variation in the order of enumeration of these branches. At present, one āyurvedic text called *Hārita Saṁhitā* is also available. Hārīta was a sage of great antiquity and he was contemporary of Agniveśa the original author of *Caraka saṁhitā*. The extant text of *Hārīta saṁhitā* appears to be a much anterior work and the authorship of this work does not appear to have any relationship with *Hārīta*, the disciple of Punarvasu Ātreya. It is only in this *Hārīta saṁhitā*, these eight specialised branches of Āyurveda are described differently inasmuch as the branch '*Agada tantra*' has been interpreted to deal with five specialised therapies which taken together are called "*Pañca karma.*" In

Āyurvedic classics, this term, *Agada tantra* is interpreted as toxicology. *Pañca karma* therapy is not treated as a specialised branch but it is considered as a part of *Kāya cikitsā* or Internal medicine. In *Āyurveda saukhyaṁ* 1:37 the view of Atri in this connection has been quoted. Atri, it seems, has interpreted *Agada* as *Basti cikitsā* or medicated enema therapy. This view however is not acceptable to the author of *Āyurveda saukhyaṁ*. It has been made clear that *Basti* or enema therapy is a part of *Kāya cikitsā* or Internal medicine and it should not be treated either as a separate branch or as included in *Agada tantra*.

Formation of Tissue Elements

Rasa, *rakta*, *māṁsa*, *medas*, *asthi*, *majjā* and *śukra*, these are the seven *dhātus* or basic tissue elements. In the extant Āyurvedic classics and the authoritative commentaries on them, there is a great deal of controversy about the process of the synthesis of these *dhātus* or tissue elements. Whether one *dhātu* is nourished after the other, or all the *dhātus* are nourished simultaneously, is the problem for hot debates among the Āyurvedic scholars. Cakrapāṇi Dutta in his commentary on *Caraka saṁhitā*, has elaborated three basic concepts about this process of nourishment. These concepts were perhaps, prevalent in authoritative classics which were then available but subsequently lost. These three concepts are :

(1) *Kedāri kulyā Nyāya*;

(2) *Khale kapota Nyāya*; *and*

(3) *Kṣīra dadhi Nyāya*.

According to *Kedāri kulyā Nyāya*, the tissue elements (*dhātus*) get nourishment from the *poṣaka rasa* in succession. When some paddy fields are to be irrigated by a canal, then the water is made to enter one paddy field. When it is full of water, then the water is taken to the next field and thereafter, to the third field. In the same way, the *poṣaka rasa* nourishes the *poṣya rasa* and then *rakta*, *māṁsa*, *medas*, *asthi*, *majjā* and *śukra* consecutively.

According to *Khale kapota Nyāya*, the *poṣaka rasa* circulates over all the tissues (*dhātus*), and these *dhātus* draw the nourishment appropriate to them from this nourishing fluid. When grains are spread over the ground, different types of birds come to eat them. They, however, pick up the grain of their choice. Similarly, *dhātus* pick up nourishment of their own requirement.

According to the third concept, i.e. *Kṣīra dadhi Nyāya* the whole of the nourishing fluid is first transformed into *rasa*. Then the essence of *rasa* is transformed into *rakta*, and the essence of *rakta* is transformed into *māṁsa*, etc. This is on the analogy of the preparation of curd, cream, butter and ghee from the milk. The whole milk is transformed into curd, the essence of curd then becomes cream; from the cream the essence is butter and the essence of butter is ghee. Cakrapāṇi Dutta has advanced arguments in favour and against all these three concepts. This, however, is a matter of debate specially because there is no authentic text available now, in which this topic is discussed. In *Āyurveda saukhyaṁ*, Chapter 4, śloka Nos. 36-50, there is a discussion at great length on this topic. Along with Caraka and Agniveśa, they have quoted *Aupadhenava tantra*, *Cikitsā sāra saṁgraha*, *Videha saṁhitā*, *Suśruta*, *Vṛddhātreya*, *Vaśiṣṭha saṁhitā* etc., in this connection. Some references quoted in this work are also available in Vāgbhaṭa's *Aṣṭāṅga hṛdaya*. From these texts it appears that the controversy was inherent even in the authentic works and it was not the creation of Cakrapāṇi Dutta, as some scholars believe it to be.

In this chapter there is also a discussion on the nature of *ojas*, whether it is the essence of all the *dhātus* or it is an *upadhātu* of *śukra*, or it is a *mala* or waste product of *śukra*? In this text, while quoting the opinion of different scholars, the author himself gives his own opinion.

Tantra, Mantra and Cakras

The author of *Āyurveda saukhyaṁ* seems to have considerable faith upon *mantras*, *tantras*, *yantras* and *cakras*, for determining the nature of the disease, its curability and *ariṣṭa lakṣaṇas* or bad prognostic signs including the time of death. In Chapter 6:118-120, a *mantra* has been described which is to be written on a piece of *Bhūrja patra*. This has to be kept in a secret place and the next day it is to be taken out from the earthen pot and examined. The year, month and day in which the patient will die, can be determined on the basis of the number of the alphabet of the *mantra* which has disappeared.

Another interesting *tāntric* prediction is detailed in verse 6 : 121-122. In the finger digits of the patient the numbers of *tithis* (days of the fortnight) are to be written. Thereafter, the hands are to be smeared with the paint of lac. The number of digit in which the earlier writing will not be visible is the day on which the patient will die.

In this work, a text from *Rasārṇava tantra* has been quoted in which, following some tāntric rites, small children will be asked to see in a lamp the god or goddess who will predict the success or otherwise of the treatment.

From *Yoga ratnāvali*, *Vaikuṇṭha dvādaśākṣara mantra* has been extracted here from which, the span of life of the patient can be determined. There is a prescription of *Vaidika Mṛtyuñjaya mantra*, *Viṣṇu sahasra nāma*, *Mahākāla mantra* for saving the life of a patient in serious conditions.

Astrology

Occurrence of a disease in a partioular day, or *tithi* has some significance. In this connection, several references have been quoted from Astrological texts to determine the result of the treatment.

The names of the messenger and the patient are to be written on a rectangular house having 55 small houses to determine the prognosis of the disease. In this connection details are provided in Chapter 5 : 31-35.

Conclusion

From the information provided in Ṭoḍara malla's *Āyurveda saukhyaṁ*, it will be possible to ascertain the authenticity of various texts available in *Caraka saṁhitā*, *Suśruta saṁhitā* etc. Besides, the opinions of several scholars and texts of great antiquity on different Āyurvedic topics which are quoted in this work, will be of great value to research workers, students and teachers of Āyurveda. Certain topics like *Nāḍi parikṣā* which are now considered to be the contributions of other cultures and not of Indian origin, are of great interest to medical historians. They were originally āyurvedic. How they were lost and why they could not find a place in subsequent texts, like *Caraka saṁhitā*, *Suśruta saṁhitā*, Vāgbhaṭa's *Aṣṭāṅga hṛdaya* and *Aṣṭāṅga saṁgraha*, is a matter for research in future.

CHAPTER 1

मङ्गलाचरणम्

॥ श्री गणेशाय नमः ॥ ॥ श्री सरस्वत्यै नमः ॥

शिवं प्रणम्य वागीशं धन्वन्तरिमथाश्विनौ ।
क्रियते टोडरानन्दो ग्रन्थः सद्वैद्यसंमतः ॥१॥

Invocation

Obeisance to lord Gaṇeśa. Obeisance to goddess Sarasvati. Being instructed by the reputed physicians, the text on *Ṭoḍarānanda* is being composed, after paying obeisance to lord Śiva who is the master of all speeches and to Dhanvantari as well as the Aśvins.

दिशन्तु शं केशवशंकराद्याः देवाः सुदेव्योऽध्यग[1]सम्भवाद्याः ।
श्रीटोडरेन्द्रे नृपतौ सुमूर्तौ धर्मस्य भूमौ परिरक्षके च ॥२॥

Let the gods like Keśava and Śaṅkara and the goddess like Pārvati bestow peace on Śrī Ṭoḍarendra, the king having a beautiful physique and the protector of religion on this earth.

[उपक्रमः]

मान्धातृदुष्यन्तसुतादिभिर्या पूर्वं कृता पद्धतिरद्य येन ।[2]
मूर्धाभिषिक्तालिकभूषणेन समुद्धृता श्रीवरटोडरेण ॥३॥
भूदेवदेवान्भुविदानयज्ञैः संतोष्य साधूनथ सर्ववर्णान् ।
कामैरनेकैश्च विलोक्य रुग्णानाज्ञापयेद्रुग्विजये नरेन्द्रः ॥४॥

Introduction

The tradition which was created by Māndhātā and Bharata, the son of Duṣyanta etc., was revitalised by Śrī Ṭoḍara who was consecrated on his head with the ornament of virtue. He pleased the kings, the gods, the saints, and persons of all castes with charity, *yajña* (sacred oblation to fire) and different other achievements. Thereafter, seeing the ailing persons, the king ordered for a victory over the diseases.

प्राचीनशास्त्राणि सुदुर्गमाणि भिन्नप्रमेयानि निरीक्ष्य सम्यक् ।
एकत्र सर्वं भवतात् सुबोधं मतं कृतं टोडरमल्लभूपैः ॥५॥

The old texts are difficult to understand, they have different objectives. In view of this, the king Ṭoḍara malla decided to compile them in the form of an easily comprehensible text after careful examination of the old classics.

श्रीटोडरो नृपवरो रसालङ्कारसन्मणिः ।
गृहीतदेहो लोकस्य रक्षार्थमिति मे मतिः ॥६॥

The best of the kings Śrī Ṭoḍara is like a jewel in a beautiful ornament. I believe he has taken birth to protect human beings on this earth.

साधूनां रक्षिता नूनमसाधूनां विमर्दनः ।
तदाज्ञया सुश्रुतादिसारमुद्धृत्य सादरम् ॥७॥

निबध्यते हितं सर्वं विशदाक्षरनिर्मलम् ।
ग्रन्थेऽस्मिन् टोडरानन्दे सर्वार्थपरिबृंहिते ॥८॥

He is the protector of noble souls and destroyer of miscreants. By his order, with great respect, all the useful essence of Suśruta etc., have been extracted and utilised in the composition of this text called *Ṭodarānanda* in lucid and clear language. This text will comprise all the knowledge required by the physician.

[विषयप्रतिज्ञा]

इह खलु चतुर्वर्गसाधनं शरीरं, तच्चायुःपराधीनम्, तद्विकारकारिणो[3] रोगाः, तदभावहेतुचिकित्साप्रतिपादकतया तीसटाद्याचार्याणामायुर्वेदशास्त्रे प्रवृत्तिः । तद्ग्रन्थानामतिदुर्ज्ञेयतया इदानीन्तनानामप्रवृत्तेः[4] सुकरोपायेन ज्ञानार्थमेतस्मिन्ग्रन्थे[5] प्रयत्नः ॥९॥

Aims and Objects

In this world, body is the vehicle for the achievement of the four-fold objectives of human life, namely, *dharma* (religious virtue), *artha* (wealth and objects of senses), *kāma* (satisfaction of the worldly desires) and *mokṣa* (salvation). This body is controlled by *āyuḥ* (elan vital). Diseases bring about morbidity in this *āyuḥ*. To prevent and cure these diseases, treatment is necessary. It is with this in view that the great scholars like Tīsaṭa etc., have composed texts on āyurveda. These texts are, however, difficult of comprehension, because of which the present day physicians are not able to understand them. With a view to make āyurveda easily comprehensible to them, effort has been made for the composition of this text.

तदाह वाग्भटः

"आयुः कामयमानेन धर्मार्थसुखसाधनम् ।
आयुर्वेदोपदेशेषु विधेयः परमादरः ॥१०॥"

[अष्टाङ्गहृदय : सूत्र १:२]

According to Vāgbhaṭa

A person who desires longevity which is the suitable vehicle for the achievement of *dharma* (religious virtues), *artha* (wealth and satisfaction of the objects of senses) and *sukha* (happiness) should observe with great respect the instructions prescribed in āyurveda.

तदिदं शाश्वतं पुण्यं सौख्यं[6] वृत्तिकरं परम् ।

स्वर्ग्यं यशस्यमायुष्यं यदि सम्यक् प्रयोजितम् ॥११॥

This science is eternal, virtuous, promoter of happiness and an excellent profession. It leads to heaven and endows the person with fame and longevity if appropriately applied.

[आयुर्वेदलक्षणम्]

आयुर्हिताहितं व्याधिनिदानोपशयं[7] तथा ।

विद्यते यत्र विद्वद्भिः स चायुर्वेद[8] उच्यते ॥१२॥

ऋग्वेदस्योपवेदोऽयमायुर्वेद इति स्मृतः[9] ।

Definition of Āyurveda

The science through which scholars could ascertain the factors which are useful and harmful for life and the causative factors as well as the treatment of diseases is called āyurveda. Āyurveda is the *upa-veda* (subsidiary text) of the *Ṛk veda*.

[अष्टांगायुर्वेदः]

सृष्ट्युत्पादनचित्तेन स्मृतः पूर्वं स्वयंभुवा ॥१३॥

श्लोकानां शतसाहस्रं सहस्राध्यायसंयुतम् ।

ततोऽल्पायुदल्पमेधस्त्वं ज्ञात्वा नृणां सुनिश्चितम् ।

अष्टधा कारयामास भगवान्[10] कालमर्दनः॥१४॥

तद्यथा

शल्यं शालाक्यमगदं कुमारभरणं तथा ।
कायभूतक्रियावाजीकरणं च रसायनम्[11] ॥१५॥

Eight branches of Āyurveda

In the days of yore, lord Brahmā, desirous of creation of the universe brought to memory this science in one thousand chapters containing one lakh verses. Thereafter, lord Kāla mardana divided it into eight specialised branches, when he came to know for certain that human beings have low intellectual calibre. These eight branches are as follows :

1. *Śalya* or surgery;
2. *Śālākya* or the treatment of diseases of head and neck;
3. *Agada* or the treatment of poisoning;
4. *Kumāra bharana*, or maternity and paediatrics;
5. *Kāya cikitsā* or the treatment of internal diseases;
6. *Bhūta kriyā* or the treatment of afflictions by evil spirits;
7. *Vāji karaṇa* or the science of aphrodisiacs, and
8. *Rasāyana* or the science of rejuvenation.

[शल्यतन्त्रम्][12]

नाराचवाणभल्लीभिः[13] शक्तिकुन्तैश्च तोमरैः ।
खड्गैर्विभिन्नगात्रस्य तत्र स्याद् यदि शल्यकम् ॥
तस्य प्रतीकारकर्म यत्तच्छल्यचिकित्सितम् ॥१६॥
यन्त्रक्षाराग्निशस्त्राणि त्वौषधं पथ्यमेव च ।
तच्च शल्योद्धरणकं प्रोच्यते वैद्यकागमे ॥१७॥

Śalya tantra

Treatment of the wounds caused by the injury to the body

through weapons like *nārāca*, *vāṇa*, *bhallī*, *śakti*, *kunta*, *tomara* and *khaḍga* is called *Śalya cikitsā*.

In this specialised branch, *yantra* (blunt instruments), *kṣāra* (alkalies), *agni* (cauterization), *śastra* (sharp edged instruments), *auṣadha* (drugs) and *pathya* (wholesome diet) are used for the treatment. In the medical tradition this branch is called *Śalyoddharaṇaka* (removal of foreign bodies).

अथ सुश्रुतः

न केवलं काण्ठतृणादिशल्यमतिप्रवृद्धं मलदोषजं वा ।
यत्किञ्चिदाबाधकरं शरीरे तत्सर्वमेव प्रवदन्ति शल्यम् ॥१८॥

According to Suśruta

Not only injury by wood, grass etc., but also the painful ailments of the body caused by the vitiated *malas* (waste products) and *doṣas* are called *śalya* (foreign body).

[14]
[शालाक्यतन्त्रम्]

ऊर्ध्वजत्रुषु ये रोगाः श्रवणादिषु संश्रिताः[15] ।
तेषां यत्क्रियते कर्म शालाक्यं तत्[16] प्रकीर्तितम् ॥१९॥
यस्मात्तत्क्रियते कर्म प्रायशस्तु शलाकया ।
तस्माच्छालाक्यमित्युक्तमृषिभिः[17] शौनकादिभिः ॥२०॥

Śālākya tantra

The treatment of diseases of head and neck located in ear etc., are called *śālākya*.

Treatment of these diseases is generally done through the help of *śalākā* (probes). Therefore, according to sages like Śaunaka etc., this specialised branch is called *Śālākya*.

[18]
[अगदतन्त्रम्]

स्थावराणां जङ्गमानां तथा संयोगजन्मनाम् ।
विषाणां व्यञ्जनार्थाय तथोपशमनाय च ॥
प्रोच्यते या क्रिया तस्या अगदं नाम कथ्यते ॥२१॥

Agada tantra

The branch which deals with the identification and treatment of various types of poisons, namely, *sthāvara* (poisons of vegetable and mineral origin), *jāṅgama* (poisons of animal origin) and *saṁyogaja* (poisons prepared by combination of different drugs) is called *Agada.*

[19]
[कौमारभृत्यम्]

गर्भोपक्रमविज्ञानं कुमारभरणं तथा ।
धात्रीणां लक्षणं क्षीरदोषसंशोधनौषधम् ॥२२॥
योगिनीनां ग्रहाणां च लक्षणं तन्निवारणम् ।
सूतिकारोगशमनं क्रिया बालचिकित्सितम् ॥२३॥

Kaumāra bhṛtya

The branch which deals with the management of pregnancy and child after delivery, the selection of wet-nurse (*dhātri*), defects in the breast milk and their corrections, signs and symptoms of afflictions by *yoginis* and evil planets and their treatment and treatment of diseases during sūtikā (ailments of women after delivery) is called *Bāla cikitsā.*

[20]
[कायचिकित्सा]

[21]
कायशब्देनात्र जाठरोऽग्निः ॥२४॥

Kāya cikitsā

The term '*kāya*' in the present context means '*jāṭharāgni*'.

उक्तं च वृद्धभोजेन

जाठरः प्राणिनामग्निः[22] काय इत्यभिधीयते ।

यस्तं चिकित्सेत्सीदन्तं विषमं चापि देहिनाम् ॥

आयुर्वेदाभियोगेन स वै कायचिकित्सकः ॥२५॥

It has been stated by Vṛddha Bhoja

"*Jāṭharāgni* of living beings is called *kāya*. The physician who treats diseases caused by the suppression or irregularity of this *agni* according to the principles of āyurveda is called *Kāya cikitsaka*."

अथ[23] विदेहः

"चतुर्णां भिषगादीनां शस्तानां धातुवैकृते[24] ।

प्रवृत्तिर्धातुसाम्यार्था[25] चिकित्सेत्यभिधीयते ॥२६॥"

[चरक संहिता : सूत्र९:५]

Accarding to Videha

"All the efforts of the four categories, viz., physician, medicament, attendant and patient, possessing requisite qualities for the revival of the equilibrium of *dhātus* in the event of their equilibrium being disturbed, is known as *cikitsā* (therapy)".

अतएवोच्यते

ज्वरोन्मादप्रमेहेषु वातरक्तास्रपित्तयोः[26] ।

कुष्ठातिसारशोफादौ[27] शोषेपाण्ड्वामयेऽरुचौ ॥२७॥

मेदोऽर्शः शूलोदरिषु योनिलिङ्गामयेषु च ।

विशेषतः सर्वगात्रप्रसरेषु गदेषु च ।

निवारणं यत्क्रियते तद्धि कायचिकित्सितम् ॥२८॥

Therefore, it is said, "the prevention and treatment of diseases which pervade the entire body specially those like *jvara* (fever), *unmāda* (insanity), *prameha* (obstinate urinary disorders including diabetes), *vāta rakta* (gout), *asra pitta* (a condition characterised by bleeding from different parts of the body), *kuṣṭha* (obstinate skin diseases including leprosy), *atisāra* (diarrhoea), *śopha* (oedema) etc., *śoṣa* (consumption), *pāṇḍu* (anemia), *aruci* (anorexia), *medas* (adiposity), *arśas* (piles), *śūla* (colic pain), *udara* (obstinate abdominal diseases including ascitis), *yoni-liṅgāmaya* (diseases of female and male genital organs) is called *kāya cikitsā*."

[भूतविद्या[28]]

देवासुरगन्धर्वग्रहराक्षसपितृपिशाचयक्षाद्यैः व्याप्तं शरीरं
शान्तिकर्मबलिकर्महोमदानाद्यैः कृत्वा शान्तिमुपयान्ति
डाकिन्यादयश्च सा भूतचिकित्सा ॥२९॥

Bhūta vidyā

Performance of *śānti karma* (propitious rituals), *bali karma* (sacrificing rituals), *homa* (oblation to fire), *dāna* (charity) etc., to propitiate *devas* (the gods), *asuras* (demons), *gandharvas*, *grahas* (planets), *rākṣasas*, *pitṛs* (dead ancestors), *piśācas*, *yakṣas*, *ḍākinis* etc., when they afflict the body, is called *Bhūta cikitsā*.

तदाह

बन्धावेशनताडननस्याञ्जनधूमयोजनं[29] चापि तस्य ज्ञेया ।
संज्ञा भूतचिकित्सेति सद्वैद्यैरिति ॥३०॥

As it is said

"The treatment given in the form of *bandha* (tieing by ropes), *āveśana* (controlling measures), *tāḍana* (beating), *nasya* (inhalation therapy), *añjana* (collyrium) and *dhūma* (fumigation) is called *Bhūta cikitsā* by the expert physicians."

[वाजीकरणतन्त्रम्][30]

अल्पं दुष्टं तथा क्षीणं यच्छुक्रं शुष्कतां गतम् ।

तस्यैवाप्यायनं चैव प्रसादोपचयस्तथा

जनकं तर्प्पणं यच्च तद्धि वाजीकरं मतम् ॥३१॥

[31]वाजोऽन्नं तस्य सम्यक् परिणतस्य यो भागस्तच्छुक्रं,

तद्वाजी इत्युच्यते, तस्य करणं वाजीकरणमिति श्रुतिः ॥३२॥

Vāji karaṇa tantra

Factors which are responsible for the *āpyāyana* (increase in quantity), *prasāda* (purification), *upacaya* (accumulation), *janana* (ejaculation) and *tarpaṇa* (nourishment) of the semen which has become *alpa* (less in quantity), *duṣṭa* (vitiated), *kṣiṇa* (diminished) and *śuṣka* (dried), are called *Vāji kara.*

The term '*vāja*' means '*anna*' (food). *Śukra* arises as final product of its proper transformation. Therefore, *Śukra* is called *vāji.* Factors which help in the manifestation (*karaṇa*) of its excellence in quality and quantity are called *vāji karaṇa* in the *Vedas* (*śruti*).

अथवा

वाजीशब्देन शुक्रमभिधीयते, येन शुक्ररहितस्य

शुक्रं क्रियते तद्वाजीकरणमिति ॥३३॥

Another derivation

The term '*vāji*' means *śukra.* Factors which help in the production of *śukra* in a person who is devoid of it are called *Vāji karaṇa.*

[रसायनतन्त्रम्][32]

देहस्येन्द्रियदन्तानां दृढीकरणमेव च ।

वलीपलितखालित्यवर्जनेऽपि च या क्रिया ॥
मेधायुःस्थापनार्थाय या क्रिया तद्रसायनम् ॥३४॥
च कारादारोग्यार्थम् ।

Rasāyana tantra

The therapy that is administered for producing sturdiness of the body, the sense organs and teeth, which prevents wrinkles in the skin, greying of hair and baldness and which promotes intellect as well as longevity is called *rasāyana.*

This therapy helps in maintenance of positive health. This has been indicated by the use of the term "*ca*" in the above verse.

रसरक्तादीनामयनमाप्यायनं रसायनं वा ॥३५॥

Other definitions

The *āpyāyana* or the nourishment of the *ayanas* or the channels of circulation of *rasa* (plasma), *rakta* (hemoglobin fraction of the blood) etc., is called *rasāyana*.

रसादीनामायुःप्रभृतिकारणानामयनं विशिष्टलाभोपायो रसायनम् ॥३६॥

The word '*rasāyana*' is composed of two terms viz., '*rasa*' and '*ayana*'. *Rasa* and other *dhātus* are responsible for sustenance of life etc. The term '*ayana*' means "specific measures for obtaining". Thus, the specific measures used for obtaining *rasa* etc., which are responsible for longevity etc., are called *rasāyana.*

[अगदक्रिया अथवा बस्तिचिकित्सा]

अत्रिमते नवप्रकारिका चिकित्सा। चरकसुश्रुतादिभिर्विषोपशमनार्थं[33]
या अगदा[34] नाम क्रिया प्रोक्ता सैवात्रिणा बस्तिचिकित्सा कृता ॥३७॥

Agada kriyā or Basti cikitsā

According to Atri there are nine types of *cikitsā* (therapies). *Agada kriyā*, according to Caraka and Suśruta, means the treatment of poisoning. This *agada kriyā* is called *basti cikitsā* by Atri.

तद्यथा

गुदामयानां या बस्तिः शमनं च निरूहकम् ।

आस्थापनानुवासश्च अगदं नाम कथ्यते ॥३८॥

Definition

Administration of different types of *bastis* (medicated enemas) viz., *śamana*, *nirūhaka*, *āsthāpana* and *anuvāsana*, for the treatment of the diseases located in the anus, is called *agada*.

सुश्रुतादीनां मते बस्तिचिकित्सा कायचिकित्सान्तर्भूतैव ॥३९॥

According to Suśruta etc., *basti cikitsā* (treatment by medicated enema) is included under the branch *kāya cikitsā* (internal medicine).

आयुर्वेदस्तु अष्टाङ्ग एव सर्वत्र श्रूयते ।

यदा बस्तिचिकित्सा पृथग् लिख्यते[35] तदा नवधा[36] भवति ॥

अतोऽत्र[37] मया न अंगीकारः कृतः । इति अष्ट चिकित्सा ॥४०॥

Everywhere, āyurveda is described as having eight specialised branches. If *basti cikitsā* is accepted as a special branch, then in total there will be nine branches and this is not in conformity with the tradition of āyurvedic classics. Therefore, I (the author of *Ṭoḍarānanda*) have not accepted it (*basti cikitsā*) as a separate branch.

Thus, ends the eight specialised branches of *cikitsā* (therapeutics).

[चिकित्सापादाः[38]]

वैद्यो व्याध्युपसृष्टश्च भेषजं परिचारकः ।

एते पादाश्चिकित्सायाः कर्मसाधनहेतवः ॥४१॥

Limbs of Treatment

The four limbs which are responsible for the accomplishment of treatment are as follows :

1. *Vaidya* or the physician;
2. *Vyādhyupaśṛṣṭa* or the patient;
3. *Bheṣaja* or the drugs and medicines; and
4. *Paricāraka* or the attendant including nurses.

39
[वैद्यगुणाः]

"तत्त्वाधिगतशास्त्रार्थो दृष्टकर्मा स्वयंकृती ।
लघुहस्तः शुचिः शूरः सज्जोपस्करभेषजः ॥४२॥
प्रत्युत्पन्नमतिर्धीमान् व्यवसायी कृतोद्यमः ।
सत्यधर्मपरो यश्च भिषक्पादः स उच्यते ॥४३॥"

[सुश्रुत : सूत्र ३४:१९-२१]

Attributes of the Physician

The following are the attributes of the physician :

(1) Acquaintance with the meanings and essence of the medical texts;

(2) Experience of observations of the administration of the therapeutics;

(3) Experience of the administration of therapeutics by himself;

(4) *Laghu hasta*, that is, who is very swift in the administration of therapeutics;

(5) Purity;

(6) Bravery;

(7) Possession of all the implements and drugs;

(8) Presence of mind;

(9) Intelligence;

(10) Enterprising nature;

(11) Sincerity in efforts ; and

(12) Observance of the path of truth and virtue.

[औषधगुणाः] 40

"बहुकल्पं बहुगुणं सम्पन्नं योग्यमौषधम् ।" 41

[अष्टाङ्गहृदय : सूत्र१:२८]

Attributes of Drug

The following are the attributes of the drug :

(1) *Bahu kalpa* or the administerability through several pharmaceutical processes ;

(2) Possession of several qualities ;

(3) Saturation with therapeutic qualities ; and

(4) Suitability for the administration to the patient.

[परिचारकगुणाः] 42

"अनुरक्तः शुचिर्दक्षो बुद्धिमान् परिचारकः ॥४४॥"

[अष्टाङ्गहृदय : सूत्र१:२९]

Qualities of Nurse

Attachment, purity, expertise and intelligence—these are the qualities of *paricārakas* (nurses and attendants).

[रोगिगुणाः] 43

"आढ्योरोगी भिषग्वश्यो ज्ञापकः सत्त्ववानपि ।

सर्वौषधक्षमे देहे यूनः पुंसो जितात्मनः ॥४५॥"

[अष्टाङ्गहृदय : सूत्र१:२९-३०]

Qualities of Patients

Possession of wealth, obedience to the physician, ability to express the complaints, strong will power, having a suitable body for different types of therapies prescribed for the disease, young age, male sex, self-control—these are the qualities of the patient.

44
[रोगसाध्यता]

"अमर्मगोऽल्पहेत्वग्ररूपरूपोऽनुपद्रवः ।
45
अतुल्यदूष्यदेशर्तुप्रकृतिः पादसम्पदि ।
ग्रहेष्वनुगुणेष्वेकदोषमार्गो नवः सुखः ॥४६॥"
[अष्टाङ्गहृदय : सूत्र १:३०-३१]

ज्वरे तुल्यर्त्तुदोषत्वं प्रमेहे तुल्यदूष्यता ।
रक्तगुल्मे पुराणत्वं सुखसाध्यस्य लक्षणम् ॥४७॥

Curability of the Disease

The following are the characteristic features of diseases which are curable :

1. Non-involvement of *marmas* (vital organs) in the manifestation of the disease ;
2. Diseases which are caused by less number of etiological factors ;
3. Diseases having less of *pūrva rūpa* (premonitory signs and symptoms) ;
4. Diseases which have less of *rūpa* (manifested signs and symptoms) ;
5. Absence of complications ;
6. Dissimilarity among the *dūṣya* (afflicted tissue elements), *deśa* (locality), *ṛtu* (nature of the season) and the *prakṛti* (physical constitution of the patient);
7. Availability of the excellence of the *pādas* (the physician, the drug, the nurse and the patient);
8. Favourable disposition of the planets;
9. Involvement of only one *doṣa* in the manifestation of the disease;
10. Involvement of only one *mārga* (channel) in the pathogenesis of the disease; and
11. Disease which has occurred recently.

In the case of certain diseases, there are exceptions to these rules, and their curability is determined on the basis of the following :

(1) *Jvara* (fever) is curable when the nature of the *doṣas* and the season are similar;

(2) *Prameha* (obstinate urinary disorders including diabetes) is curable if the *doṣas* are similar in nature to that of the *dūṣyas* (afflicted tissue elements); and

(3) *Rakta gulma* becomes curable in its chronic stage.

[वैद्यमहत्त्वम्]

"मृद्दण्डचक्रसूत्राद्याः कुम्भकारादृते यथा ।
नावहन्ति गुणं[46] वैद्यादृते पादत्रयं तथा[47] ॥४८॥"

[चरक : सूत्र९:१३]

Importance of Vaidya

A pot cannot be manufactured in the absence of a pot-maker even though other subsidiary elements like mud, *daṇḍa* (the rod of the wheel), *cakra* (wheel on which the pot is manufactured), *sūtra* (thread) etc., are present. Similarly, in the absence of a physician, the other three *pādas*, namely, excellence of the drug, the nurse and the patient do not produce the desired effect.

[प्राणाभिसरवैद्यलक्षणम्]

"तस्माच्छास्त्रेऽर्थविज्ञाने प्रवृत्तौ कर्मदर्शने ।
भिषक् चतुष्टये युक्तः प्राणाभिसर उच्यते ॥४९॥"

[चरक : सूत्र९:१८]

Characteristics of Prāṇābhisara Physician

A physician who is acquainted with four factors, namely, the medical texts, the implied meaning of the textual prescriptions, *pravṛtti* (sincerity) and *karma darśana* (practical knowledge) is called *prāṇābhisara* or giver of life.

अथ अग्निवेशात्

हेतौ लिङ्गे प्रशमने रोगाणामपुनर्भवे ।
ज्ञानं चतुर्विधं यस्य स विज्ञेयो भिषक्तमः[48] ॥५०॥

[चरक : सूत्र९:१९ परिवर्त्तितं किंचित्]

According to Agniveśa

The physician who is well versed in the four categories of knowledge viz., (1) the etiology of diseases (2) the signs and symptoms of diseases (3) method of curing diseases and (4) measures to prevent the recurrence of the diseases, is known as *bhiṣaktama* (physician par excellence).

गां दृष्ट्वा पङ्कनिर्मग्नां ब्राह्मणं रोगपीडितम् ।
उद्धरन्ति नरा ये वै तेषां लोकोऽश्वमेधिनाम्[49] ॥५१॥

॥ पद्मात् ॥

According to Padma purāṇa

An individual, who saves the life of a cow when she is immersed in mud and the life of a Brahmin who is suffering from diseases, gets the virtues of *aśvamedha yajñas* (a type of vedic ritual in which a horse is sacrificed).

धर्मस्यार्थस्य कामस्य नृलोकस्याभयस्य च ।
दाता स उच्यते वैद्यो दानाद्देहसुखायुषाम् ॥५२॥

The physician gives the happiness of the body and longevity. Therefore, he is called the giver of *dharma* (religious virtue), *artha* (wealth), *kāma* (worldly desires) and *abhaya* (fearlessness) in this human world.

अकालमृत्युं प्रति[हन्ति][50] जीवितं ददाति यो देहसुखं च देहिनाम् ।

न तेन दातास्ति समः कुतोऽधिको न जीवितो दानमिहातिरिच्यते ॥५३॥

A physician prevents untimely death, gives life and happiness of the body to human-beings. Therefore, there is no other *dātā* (giver or donor) who is equal, much less more, than a physician, because nothing excells the gift of life.

[जीवितदानमहत्त्वम्]

फलं शुभं जीवितदानजन्मं विहाय सौख्यार्थधनं य ईप्सति ।

श्रमेण गत्वा महता महागिरिं विहाय हेमं स मृदं जिघृक्षति ॥५४॥

Importance of Saving Life

A person (physician) who desires wealth for his own happiness in lieu of the auspicious fruits which accrue to him as a result of the gift of the life, is like a person who is in search of mud by giving up gold after going to a high mountain with a great deal of efforts.

यथेक्षुहेतोः सलिलं प्रसेचितं तृणानि वल्लीरपि तं निषिञ्चति ।

तथा क्रिया धर्मनिमित्तमर्जिता सुखार्थलाभेऽपि न धर्महापिका ॥५५॥

When a field is irrigated with water for growing sugar-cane, the grass and creepers in that field also get irrigated. Similarly, a physician, who practises his profession for *dharma* (religious virtues), do not commit an error if through that he earns wealth as well as happiness. This does not come in the way of his acquiring *dharma* (religious virtues).

[त्रिविधाः भिषजः]

अथ चरकात् त्रिविधा[51] भिषज इति—

भिषक्छद्मचराः[52] सन्ति सन्त्येके सिद्धसाधिनः[53] ।

सन्ति वैद्यगुणैर्युक्तास्त्रिविधा भिषजो भुवि ॥५६॥

[चरक : सूत्र११:५०]

Categories of Physician

According to Caraka, there are three categories of physicians namely, pseudo-physicians, feigned physicians and genuine physicians endowed with the requisite qualities.

[छद्मचरवैद्यः]

तद्यथा

वैद्यभाण्डौषधैः पुस्तैः पल्लवैरवलोकनैः ।

लभन्ते ये भिषक्शब्दं[54] ज्ञेयास्ते प्रातिरूपिकाः[55] ॥५७॥

Pseudo-physician

Those, who come to be known as physicians simply by virtue of the exhibitions of the physician's box containing certain drugs and medical books, by bluffing and posing as a physician, are pseudo-physicians. They are ignorant of the science of medicine. They are simply counterfeits.

[सिद्धसाधितवैद्यः]

श्रीयशोज्ञानसिद्धानां व्यपदेशादतद्विधाः ।

वैद्यशब्दं लभन्ते ये ज्ञेयास्ते सिद्धिसाधिनः[56] ॥५८॥

[चरक : सूत्र ११:५१-५२]

Feigned Physician

Some persons, because of their association with persons accomplished in wealth, fame and knowledge come to be known as physicians even though they are not so. Persons of this category are to be regarded as feigned physicians.

[प्राणाभिसरवैद्यः[57]]

प्रयोगज्ञानविज्ञानसिद्धिसिद्धाः सुखप्रदाः ।

जीविताभिसरा ये स्युर्वैद्यत्वं तेष्ववस्थितम् ॥५९॥

[चरक : सूत्र ११:५३]

Genuine Physician

Those, who are accomplished in the administration of therapy, insight and the knowledge of therapeutics, who are endowed with infalliable success and who can give happiness to the patient are called saviers of life. Such persons come under the category of genuine physicians.

[कुवैद्यः]

अथ खरनादात्

कुवैद्यैः श्लाघितं वैद्यं तं वैद्यं नैव विश्वसेत् ।
पशुः पशूनां दौर्बल्यात्कश्चिन्मध्य वृकायते ।
स सत्यं वृकमालोक्य[58] प्रकृतिं भजते पशुः[59] ॥६०॥

[चरक : सूत्र३०:७५ परिवर्त्तितं किंचित्]

तद्वदज्ञोऽज्ञमध्यस्थो मुखरश्चातिसाहसात् ।
विश्वास्य रोगिणं पश्चान्मारयेन्नात्र संशयः ॥६१॥

Description of a Pseudo-physician

According to Kharanāda, a physician who is praised by a pseudo-physician should never be believed. Taking advantage of the weakness of others, any animal may play the role of an wolf. But when it comes across a real wolf, its true nature is exposed. Similarly, an ignorant individual, because of his garrulous nature, tries to deceive the ignorant ones. He takes the patient into confidence, and thereafter, kills him. There is no doubt about it.

[तद्विद्यसंभाषा]

अतः कुर्याद्भिषक्कर्म सद्वैद्यैर्बहुभिः सह ।
निःसंशयकरणपटुर्वैद्यसमुहो[60] भवेदवश्यं हि[61] ।
तस्माद्भिषक्तमैः सह गोष्ठीं कुर्याद्विहाय तस्करान् पशुवत्[62] ॥६२॥

Scholarly Debate

Therefore, a physician should carry out his profession in association with many other noble physicians. The assembly of noble physicians undoubtedly helps in the removal of doubts. Therefore, a good physician should always have association with other good physicians and give up the association of pseudo-physicians. The latter are like animals who believe in robbing others.

[प्रशस्तवैद्यलक्षणम्]

शास्त्रं गुरुमुखोद्गीर्णमादायोपास्य चाऽसकृत् ।
यः कर्म कुरुते वैद्यः स वैद्योऽन्ये [63] तु तस्कराः ॥६३॥

Characteristics of an Excellent Physician

A person who has studied medical classics from the mouth of his preceptors and who has practised the preceptors instructions severally before entering into the possession, is a genuine physician. All others are bandits.

[दण्डपात्रकुवैद्याः]

त्यक्तह्रीधर्ममर्यादः केवले साहसे रतः ।
[64] मृषाप्रगल्भसारम्भः पौरुषाक्लिष्टभाषणः ॥६४॥

पक्षाद्द्रविणभूयस्त्वादज्ञानाद्वापि गर्वितः ।
यदृच्छाकर्मसिद्धया वा [65] केषांचिन्नियतायुषाम् ॥६५॥

मुहुरात्मगुणश्लाघी पराभिभवभाषिणः ।
एष एव महाव्याधिरन्येषां बलवत्तरः ॥६६॥

निर्जितः किं पुनरयं काचिदास्थाऽस्ति चात्र मे ।
ददाति चौषधं दम्भात् सर्वं प्रच्छाद्य नामतः ॥६७॥

66 लुब्धः कुचेलः क्रूरश्च मद्यपः शास्त्रवर्जितः ।

देशे तस्मिन् रतिस्तस्य प्रमत्तो यत्र पार्थिवः ।

67 ते तु वर्जनीया मृत्योर्ये चरन्त्यनुचरा भुवि ॥६८॥

पञ्च वा सप्त वा वैद्यो यो न वेत्तीह संहिताः ।

राज्ञा दुर्भिषजस्तस्य छेत्तव्यो दक्षिणः करः ॥६९॥

Punishment for Pseudo-physician

Pseudo-physicians are devoid of the limit of *hri* (humility) and *dharma* (religious virtues). They only indulge in adventurous enterprises. They initiate treatment by false and garrulous statements. Their speech is harsh and unintelligible. They are proud, partially of the abundance of their wealth or because of their ignorance. Sometimes, they achieve success in treating a patient who is otherwise destined to be cured because of *niyatāyuḥ* (predetermined period of life). They often praise their own achievements and speak ill of others. "This is a serious type of disease and it is more dangerous than others. I shall be able to cure it if the patient has confidence in me." By making such statements, he administers medicine in an adventurous spirit and he gives false names to his medicines. He is greedy, ill-mannered, wrathful, drunkard and devoid of the knowledge of medical classics. Such people thrive in countries where the King is mad. These so called physicians are the lieutenants of the God of Death. They should not be permitted to practise medical profession. A physician who is not acquainted with five or seven medical classics is a pseudo-physician. The king should punish such people by cutting their right hand.

उद्ध्रियते च अथ सुश्रुतात्

यस्तु केवलशास्त्रज्ञः कर्मस्वपरिनिष्ठितः ।

स मुह्यत्यातुरं प्राप्य प्राप्य भीरुरिवाहवम् ॥७०॥

यस्तु कर्मसु निष्णातो धाष्ट्र्याच्छास्त्रबहिष्कृतः ।

स सत्सु पूजां नाप्नोति वधं चार्हति राजतः ॥७१॥

यस्तूभयज्ञो मतिमान् स समर्थोऽर्थसाधने ।

आहवे कर्मनिर्वोढुं[68] द्विचक्रः स्यन्दनो यथा ॥७२।

[सुश्रुत : सूत्र३:४८-४९, ५३]

Reference from· Suśruta

The physician who is only acquainted with medical classics and who is not well-versed in medical practice, gets confused when he comes across a patient, like a coward when he faces a war. A person who is well versed in medical practice, but out of ego, who is deprived of the knowledge of medical classics, is not respected by noble persons. Such pseudo-physicians are entitled to death sentence by the King. On the other hand, an intelligent physician who is well-acquainted with the knowledge of medical classics as well as the practical knowledge is capable of accomplishing the objectives. He is capable of successful fighting in the war. He is like a cart with two wheels which is capable of smooth movement with heavy loads.

[शिष्यलक्षणम्]

अथ आत्रेयात्[69]

आयुर्वेदो ह्ययं सम्यङ् न देयो यस्य कस्यचित् ।

नाभक्तायाप्यशान्ताय[70] न मूर्खाय न चाधमे ।

शान्ते देयं न देयं स्यात् सर्वथा नाधमेऽधने[71] ॥७३॥

[हारीतसंहिता१:२०]

Characteristics of a Disciple, according to Ātreya

The knowledge of āyurveda should not be imparted to any ordinary person. It should not be given to a person who is not obedient, who has no tranquility of mind, who is an idiot and who is involved in evil acts. It should be imparted only to a person who has tranquility of mind. It should never be given to a person who is involved in evil acts and who is in want of wealth.

[गुरुचर्या]

शिष्यो गुरुं परिचरेदग्निवत् परिचर्यया ।
धर्मतो देववद् भक्त्या पितृवद् राजवद् भयात् ॥७४॥
प्रेषिताप्रेषितः कुर्यात् कार्यं यद्गुरवे हितम् ।
प्राणाहितं नृपे दुष्टं धर्मघ्नं च विना त्रयात् ॥७५॥
यत् कृतं पर्शुरामेण पितुरादेशकारणात् ।
तन्नरेण [72] न कर्तव्यं न देवचरितं चरेत् ॥७६॥

Respect for Preceptor

The disciple should render service to the preceptor like *agni*. The preceptor should be treated as God from religious point of view, as father with devotion and as a king with humility (fear). Whether instructed or not, the disciple should perform such actions as are beneficial to the preceptor except in such three circumstances when his (of disciple) life is in danger, or when his action is likely to go against the king, or the religion. The action of Parśurāma (killing his mother by the instruction of his father) is befitting only to the gods and such actions should not be performed by human-beings.

अथ वाग्भटात्

सर्वतेजोनिधानं हि नृप इत्युच्यते भुवि ।
अदूषयन्मनस्तस्माद् भक्तिमान् समुपाचरेत् ॥७७॥
पर्यंस्तिकोपाशयकोपहासविवादनिष्ठीवनजृम्भणानि ।
सर्वाः प्रकृत्याल्पाधिकाश्च चेष्टास्तत्सन्निधाने परिवर्जयेच्च ॥७८॥

According to Vāgbhaṭa

King is the reservoir of all *tejas* (energy) in this world. Therefore, he should not be made hostile, and all actions should be performed paying due regard to him. In his presence, one should avoid *paryastika* (wrong posture), *upāśaya* (enjoyment), *kopa* (anger), *hāsa* (joke), *vivāda* (quarrel), *niṣṭhīvana* (spitting), *jṛmbhaṇa* (yawning) and such acts which are more or less of similar nature.

स्मृत्वा ह्यवस्था विविधाश्च तास्तास्सम्यक् परीक्ष्यात्महितं विदध्यात् ।

अन्योऽपि यः कश्चिदिहास्ति मार्गो हितोपदेशेषु भजेत तं च ॥७९॥

Keeping in memory the various conditions, and after carefully examining each one of them, one should initiate actions which are useful for the person himself. One should also follow in this world the other instructions provided in *hitopadeśa* (useful sayings).

73

अधोमुखो रोगिगृहं प्रविशेच्चोपविश्य च ।

नान्यत्र चारयेद् दृष्टिं कर्मातुरहितं विना ॥८०॥

वृत्तान्तमातुरगृहान्न कदाचित् प्रकाशयेत् ।

परस्त्रीद्रव्यभोगांश्च मनसापि न कामयेत् ॥८१॥

स्त्रीभिः सहास्यं संवादं परिहासं च वर्जयेत् ।

दत्तं ताभिर्न गृह्णीयाद्वैद्यो बन्धुजनादृते ॥८२॥

The physician should enter into the patient's house keeping his face downwards, and after sitting there, should not look to different directions unless the same is required for the benefit of the patient. The information collected from the patient's house should not be divulged. Indulgence with another man's wife, or his wealth, should not be thought of even in mind. Secret discussions with women and jokes with them should be avoided. The physician should not accept any gift from the women unless they are related.

तपस्विनां श्रोत्रियाणां रोगगोपकिनां तथा ।

बालानां राजसान्निध्यं सन्ततस्थायिनामपि ॥८३॥

साध्यरोगा न सिध्यन्ति तस्माद् यत्नेन साधयेत् ।

Curable diseases of the following types of persons do not get cured :

(1) *Tapasvis* or persons engaged in penance;

(2) *Śrotriyas* (persons engaged in vedic rituals);

(3) Persons who hide their diseases;

(4) Young children; and

(5) Persons who constantly remain by the side of the king. Therefore, the diseases of these persons should be treated with great care.

बन्धुभूतेन भूतानां चरेन्नित्यं सदैव हि ॥८४॥

उपकारप्रधानः स्यावपकारपरेऽप्यरौ ।

74

संपद्विपत्स्वेकमना हेतावीर्ष्येत् फले न तु ॥८५॥

[अष्टांगहृदय : सूत्र२:२५]

The physician should always have friendly feelings for all types of creatures. He should always make efforts to benefit others—even to his own enemy. One should treat happiness and sorrow, similarly. One should not be envious of the result (of others achievements) but should be so for the cause of these results.

त्रिवर्गशून्यं नारम्भं भजेत् तं चाविरोधयन् ।

[अष्टांगहृदय : सूत्र२:३०]

One should not make effort which is devoid of *tri varga* (namely, *dharma* or religious virtues, *artha* or acquirement of wealth and *kāma* or the satisfaction of the worldly desires). One should perform such acts as would not go against the *tri varga*.

मातरं पितरं पुत्रान् बान्धवानपि चातुरः ॥८६॥
अप्येतानभिशङ्केत वैद्ये विश्वासमेति च ।
विसृजत्यात्मनात्मानं न चैनं परिशङ्कते ॥८७॥

तस्मात् पुत्रवदेनं हि पालयेच्चातुरं भिषक् ।
न प्रकुर्वीत लोभेन चिकित्सापण्यविक्रयम् ॥८८॥ [75]

The patient does not believe even the mother, the father, his sons and the relatives, but he puts full confidence upon the physician. He keeps himself completely at the disposal of the physician and then never nourish any doubt about him. Therefore, the physician should treat the patient as his own son.

Out of greediness the physician should not sale his medical profession.

ईश्वराणां वसुमतां लिप्सेतार्थं स्ववृत्तये [76] ।
कुर्वन्ति ये तु वृत्त्यर्थं चिकित्सापण्यविक्रयम् [77] ॥८९॥
ते हित्वा काञ्चनं राशिं पांशुराशिमुपासते ।
[चरक : चिकित्सा १:४:५६]

Physicians who sale the medical profession with a view to acquiring wealth from persons in power and from wealthy persons, they are like persons who run after a heap of ash by giving up a heap of gold.

न प्राणिरहितो देशो नहि प्राणी निरामयः ॥९०॥
तस्मात् सर्वत्र भिषजा कल्पिता एव वृत्तयः ।
तस्मात् सर्वप्रयत्नेन लोभं त्यक्त्वा भिषक्तमः ॥९१॥
असाध्यस्यापिसाध्येत [78] प्रोक्तं कुर्यात्क्रियाक्रमम् ।

There is not a country which is not inhabited by living beings and there is not a living being who does not suffer from diseases. Therefore, for a physician, professional possibilities are available everywhere. In view of this, the excellent physician should not be greedy and with all his efforts should try to cure even incurable diseases.

यावन्निःश्वसते जन्तुस्तावत् कार्या प्रतिक्रिया ।

कदाचिद् दैवयोगेन दृष्टारिष्टोऽपि जीवति ॥६२॥

79

॥ इति वैद्यलक्षणपरीक्षा ॥

At times, by providential grace, the patient is likely to live even after the *ariṣṭa* (signs of imminent death) has appeared. Therefore, the physician should treat a patient till there is breath in him.

Thus, ends the examination and characteristics of a physician.

ज्ञात्वाल्पकोऽपि भिषजैरपि चिन्तनीयो ।

नोपेक्षणीय इति रोगगणो ह्यसह्यः ॥६३॥

Diseases are intolerable. Therefore, they should not be neglected. The physician should treat the disease even if it is of a minor nature.

उक्तं च

स्वल्पोऽपि शत्रुविषवह्निसमानरूप ।

प्राप्त्वा बलं न च शमं ह्युपयाति काले ॥६४॥

Thus it is said

Diseases are like an enemy or a poison or a fire. In the beginning they may be of minor nature, but slowly they gain strength, and after some time, they become incurable.

यस्तु रोगमविज्ञाय कर्माण्यारभते भिषक् ।

न स सिद्धिमवाप्नोति न सुखं न परां गतिम् ॥६५॥

A physician who initiates treatment without proper knowledge of the disease, does not achieve success in profession, and therefore, he does not get happiness or *parāṅgati* (excellent path or salvation).

कर्मप्रकोपेण कदाचिदेके दोषप्रकोपेण भवन्ति चान्ये ।
तथाऽपरे प्राणिषु कर्मदोषप्रकोपजाः कायमनोविकाराः ॥६६॥

The physical and psychic diseases are of the following three categories :

(1) Those which occur as a result of the past actions ;
(2) Those occurring as a result of the aggravation of *doṣas*; and
(3) Those occurring as a result of the past actions and also the aggravation of the *doṣas*.

कर्मक्षयात् कर्मकृतो दोषजः स्वयमौषधैः ।
कर्मदोषोद्भवो याति कर्मदोषक्षयात् क्षयम् ॥६७॥

The diseases of the first category get cured when the *karma* (result of past actions) is over. The diseases of the second category get cured when the aggravated *doṣas* are alleviated. The diseases of the third category get cured at the end of the *karma* (result of the past actions) and by alleviation of the aggravated *doṣas*.

दानैर्दयाभिरपि च द्विजदेवतागोगुर्वर्चनैः प्रणतिभिश्च जपैस्तपोभिः ।
इत्युक्तपुण्यनिचयैरपचीयमानाः प्राक्पापजा यदि रुजः प्रशमं प्रयान्ति ॥६८॥

If a disease occurs as a result of the sinful acts of the past, then it gets cured by the extinction of these signs as a result of the accumulation of *puṇya* (virtuous acts). One can acquire *puṇya* by the following means :

(1) By charity and compassion ;
(2) By offering prayer and bowing before *dvijas* (twice born), *devatā* (the gods), cows and preceptors;
(3) By *japa* (recitation of incantation); and
(4) By *tapa* (practice of penance).

कुष्ठमेहोदरश्वित्रज्वरोन्मादभगन्दराः ।

अन्येऽपि दुर्निवारास्तु क्षयाद्या ये प्रकीर्तिताः ॥९९॥

अविशुद्धशरीराणां देहिनां च भवान्तरे ।

80
सर्वथा हि प्रसर्पन्ति तस्माच्छोधनमाचरेत् । १००॥

अशोधनादन्वयेऽपि प्रसरन्ति न चान्यथा ।

In a living being whose body is not cleansed, the following diseases transmigrate from one life to the other;

1. *Kuṣṭha* (obstinate skin diseases including leprosy);
2. *Meha* (obstinate urinary diseases including diabetes) ;
3. *Udara* (obstinate abdominal diseases including ascitis);
4. *Śvitra* (leucoderma) ;
5. *Jvara* (obstinate type of fever);
6. *Unmāda* (insanity);
7. *Bhagandara* (fistula-in-ano); and
8. Other incurable diseases like *kṣaya* (tuberculosis).

Therefore, the body of these patients should be cleansed by the administration of elimination therapies. If the body is not cleansed completely, these diseases transmigrate even if they are suppressed. This transmigration does not take place if the body is cleansed.

यथा शास्त्रेषु निर्णीतस्तथा व्याधिः चिकित्सतः ॥१०१॥

न शमं याति यो व्याधिः स ज्ञेयः कर्मजो बुधैः ।

स्वल्पदोषो गरीयान् यः स ज्ञेयः कर्मजो बुधैः ॥१०२॥

The physician should treat diseases according to instructions provided in the medical classics. If, inspite of that treatment, the disease does not get cured then it should be determined by a wise physician as *karmaja* (caused as a result of evil actions of the past).

In such diseases the *doṣas* are not much aggravated, and inspite of it, the diseases become very serious. These are the characteristic features of a *karmaja* disease (caused by the evil acts of the past).

[व्याधिप्रकारः]

ते वातपित्तकफजास्त्रिविधा द्विधा च ।
काये मनस्यपि च सन्त्यपरे नराणाम्[81] ॥१०३॥
साध्याः क्वचित्क्वचिदपि प्रभवन्ति याप्याः ।
केचित्क्वचित्पुनरसाध्यतमाः प्रदिष्टाः ॥१०४॥
कृच्छ्रोपायः सुखोपायो द्विविधः साध्य उच्यते ।
असाध्यो द्विविधो ज्ञेयो याप्यो यश्चाप्रतिक्रियः ॥१०५॥

Classification of Diseases

Diseases are classified into various categories on the basis of the following :

1. Depending upon the aggravation of *doṣas*, these are classified into three categories namely, (1) *vātika* (2) *paittika* and (3) *kaphaja;*
2. Depending upon the location, namely, the body and the mind, diseases in human beings are of two types ; and
3. Depending upon the amenability to treatment, they are of three types, namely (1) curable, (2) palliable and (3) incurable. Curables are again of two types, namely, easily curable and curable with difficulties. The incurable diseases again are of two types namely *yāpya* (palliable) and *apratikriya* (which are absolutely incurable).

एकैकदोषजनिता निरुपद्रवाश्च दीप्तानलस्य च सदात्मवतश्च जन्तोः ।
वित्तान्वितस्य[82] च रुजः सदुपक्रमेण[83] साध्या भवन्ति भिषजामचिरोद्गताश्च ॥१०६॥

ये यावदेव भिषजामगदप्रयोगास्तावत् प्रशान्तिमुपयान्त्यगदैर्विना ये ।
प्रादुर्भवन्ति च पुनः सहसा द्विदोषास्तादृग्विधाः स्युरिति याप्यतमा गदास्ते ॥१०७॥

The following are the characteristic features of curable diseases:

1. Those caused by the aggravation of only one *doṣa*;
2. Those which are free from complications;
3. If the patient has a strong power of digestion and metabolism;
4. If the patient has a strong will power, or self-confidence;
5. If the patient is wealthy;
6. If proper treatment is administered; and
7. If the disease is not chronic.

Some diseases are relieved and remain in a suppressed stage till medicines are administered. At times these diseases get alleviated even without any medicine, but suddenly they recur, because of the aggravation of the *doṣas*. This type of diseases are *yāpyatama* (exceedingly palliable).

ये कर्मजाः सह भवन्ति शरीरिणां ये ये च त्रिदोषचयजाश्चिरकालजा ये ।
सोपद्रवाश्च्युतधनस्य च वै गताग्ने-स्त्रागदा गदवतामगदैरगम्याः ॥१०८॥

The following diseases are not amenable to the treatment of the physician :

1. Diseases which are *karmaja* (caused as a result of past evil acts);
2. Diseases which are caused by the aggravation of all the three *doṣas*;
3. Chronic diseases;
4. Diseases associated with complications;
5. Diseases of a patient who has exhausted all his wealth;
6. If there is absence of the *agni*, or power of digestion and metabolism in the patient; and
7. If the disease is of very acute nature.

याप्याः केचित् प्रकृत्यैव, साध्या याप्या उपेक्षिताः।

स्वाभावाद् व्याधयोऽसाध्याः केचिद् याप्या[84] उपेक्षिताः ॥१०९॥

Some diseases, by nature, are palliable. Some curable diseases, if neglected, become palliable. There are some diseases which are by nature incurable. Sometimes, palliable diseases, if neglected, become incurable.

[उपद्रवः]

एक एवामयः कश्चित् स्वावस्थः सम्प्रवर्तते।

स्वतन्त्रो लिङ्गभूतश्च तेष्वन्योपद्रवाय[85] च ॥११०॥

Complication

Sometimes a disease remains within its own self (within the *doṣas* and *dūṣyas* already vitiated). In such cases, the signs and symptoms of the particular disease are only manifested. Those which do not stand to these criteria are called complications.

अथ अग्निवेशात्

व्याधेरुपरि यो व्याधिर्भवत्युत्तरकालजः ।

उपक्रमाभिघाती च स उपद्रव उच्यते ॥१११॥

संजातोपद्रव इति दुःखस्त्याज्यो न जायते।

वैद्य[86] [स्त्व]यं कुशलतापूर्वं चोपद्रवं जयेत् ॥११२॥

According to Agniveśa

Another disease which occurs subsequently after the original disease is manifested and which is not amenable to the treatment of the original disease, is called *upadrava* or complication. The physician should not leave the patient because of the appearance of a complication. No doubt, such conditions are very difficult for treatment; but the proficiency of the physician lies in handling such complications with efficiency.

उपद्रवेषु बहषु प्रागजयेदाशुकारिणम् ।
निवृत्तोपद्रवं ज्ञात्वा तं रोगं त्वरया जयेत् ॥११३॥
मूलव्याधौ क्रियां वापि कुर्याद्यो वा भवेद्बली ।
अविरोधेन वा कुर्यादुभयोस्तत्त्वधीर्द्विजः ॥११४॥

If there are many complications, then, in the beginning, the acute ones should be treated. When the patient is free from complications, the physician should make effort to cure the original disease. If, however, the original disease becomes very strong, then a wise physician should first of all treat it by administering the therapies to simultaneously cure the original disease as well as its complications.

[अत्वरितचिकित्सादुष्परिणामः]

साध्या याप्यत्वमायान्ति याप्याश्चासाध्यतां तथा ।
घ्नन्ति प्राणानसाध्याश्च नराणामक्रियावताम् ॥११५॥

87

लोभान्मोहात्प्रमादाद्वा प्रागुपेक्ष्याल्पमामयं ।
पश्चात्प्राप्तबले व्याधौ भवेदत्यन्तपीडितः ॥११६॥
ततः पुत्रांश्च दारांश्च ज्ञातींश्चाहूय भाषते ।
सर्वस्वेनापिमे कश्चिद्भिषगानीयतामिति ॥११७॥
न मूढो लभते प्रज्ञां तावद्यावन्न पीड्यते ।
पीडितस्तु मतिं पश्चात् कुरुते रोगनिग्रहे ॥११८॥
तथाविधं च कः शक्तस्त्रातुं च मरणोन्मुखम् ।
क्षीणमांसबलोत्साहं प्रवृद्धोपद्रवामयम् ॥११९॥

[चरक : सूत्र ११:५८-६१ परिवर्तितं किंचित्]

Adverse effects of Negligence

If the treatment is neglected, then curable diseases become palliable and the palliable diseases become incurable. If the treatment of incurable diseases is neglected then it leads to sudden death. If because of greediness, ignorance or by mistake, the patient neglects a minor disease in the beginning, then the disease gains strength and considerably afflicts him. Thereafter, he calls his sons, wives and relatives and requests them to call a physician to treat him and agrees to spend all his wealth for the treatment. An ignorant person does not get wisdom unless he is seriously afflicted by the disease. When he is seriously ill, only then, he makes up his mind for the treatment of the disease. Such a patient loses his muscle tissue, strength and enthusiasm. The disease is aggravated and complications appear in him. He is facing towards death. Who is capable of curing such a patient ?

आयासं कर्मनैष्फल्यं विद्यासिद्धि यशःक्षयम् ।

विद्वेषं च भिषक् प्राप्नोत्यसाध्यव्याध्युपक्रमात् ॥१२०॥

By initiating treatment of an incurable disease the physician wastes much of his energy. The result of his treatment becomes disappointing. His knowledge, ability to achieve success and fame get reduced, and he becomes the object of the anger of others.

तरिष्यति सुरापिश्च[88] ब्रह्महाऽपि तरिष्यति ।

आतुरस्य प्रतिग्राही कथं तात तरिष्यति ॥१२१॥

A drunkard can get salvation and a criminal who killed a Brahmin may also get salvation. But a physician has no salvation if he takes money from the patient, but does not endow him with the requisite benefits.

चिकित्सितं शरीरं यो न निष्क्रीणाति दुर्मतिः ।

स यत् करोति सुकृतं तत्सर्वं भिषगश्नुते[89] ॥१२२॥

A patient who does not reciprocate the treatment of his ailment is a devil. Whatever virtuous acts he performs, the results of these acts are enjoyed by the physicians.

तस्माद्यत्नात्सुखोपायं कष्टोपायं च साधयेत् ।
यथोक्तं यापयेद्याप्यं वर्जयेत् त्वप्रतिक्रियम् ॥१२३॥

Therefore, with due care, the physician should treat diseases which are easily curable and which can be cured with difficulty. The palliable diseases are to be palliated and the diseases which are absolutely incurable should be given up.

सद्वैद्यास्ते न ये[90][ऽ]साध्यान् आरभन्ते चिकित्सितुम् ।
अवैद्यजीविका सिद्धिः स्याद्घुणाक्षरवत् क्वचित् ॥१२४॥
माषान्नं विट्क्षये मेहे[91] पानं मद्यं मदात्यये ।
अबुद्धिपूर्वमप्याशु सेवितं भेषजं भवेत् ॥१२५॥
एवं सिद्धिसमुत्पन्ने यः करोति पुनः पुनः ।
अन्यत्रापि स दण्ड्यः स्याद्ब्रह्महा दुष्टधीः शठः ॥१२६॥

Efficient physicians are those who do not attempt any treatment of incurable diseases. Sometimes, accidentally (*ghuṇākṣara nyāya*) he may be able to cure an incurable disease. But this accomplishment is quackery. Administration of *māṣa*, if there is *viṭ kṣaya* (diminution of stool) in a patient suffering from *meha* (obstinate urinary disorders including diabetes) and administration of alcohol to a patient suffering from *madātyaya* (alcoholism) without proper understanding, may work as therapeutic agents. Banking upon such accidental achievements, if the physician repeats them again and again in other cases, he should be punished. He is like a criminal who has killed a Brahmin. He is a devil and he is a cheat.

[परीक्षाक्रमम्]

आदौ रोगं परीक्षेत ततो[ऽ]नन्तरमौषधम् ।
ततः कर्म भिषक् पश्चात् ज्ञानपूर्वं समाचरेत् ॥१२७॥
यस्तु रोगमविज्ञाय कर्माण्यारभते भिषक् ।
न स सिद्धिमवाप्नोति न सुखं न परां गतिम् ॥१२८॥

[चरक : सूत्र२०:२०-२२ किंचित् परिवर्तितम्]

Method of Examination of Patient

The physician should first of all, examine the disease, and thereafter, start the treatment. After having full knowledge of the disease, the physician should administer therapies. A physician who starts the treatment without having full knowledge of the disease, does not accomplish his objective. As a result of this, he neither gets happiness, nor *parāṁgati* (excellent path or salvation).

विकारनामाकुशलो न जिह्रीयात् कदाचन ।
न हि सर्वविकाराणां नामतोऽस्ति ध्रुवा[92] स्थितिः ॥१२९॥

[चरक : सूत्र१८:४४]

If a physician is not able to name a particular disease, he should not feel ashamed on that account because it is not always possible to name all types of diseases in definite terms.

[त्रिविधा परीक्षा]

अग्निवेशात्

आप्तोपदेशः प्रत्यक्षमनुमानं तथैव च ।
परीक्षा त्रिविधा लोके रोगाणां शृणु[93] तत्त्वतः ॥१३०॥

Three types of Examination According to Agniveśa

The examination of diseases in this world is of three types, namely :

1. *Āptopadeśa* or scriptural testimony including the words of sages;
2. *Pratyakṣa* or perception including direct observation; and
3. *Anumāna* or inference including reasoning.

[आप्तोपदेशः]

वीतरागभयद्वेषमोहमानमदभ्रमाः ।
ध्यानयोगतपोधर्मविमलज्ञानदर्शनात् ॥१३१॥
आप्ताः शिष्टाश्च मन्तव्याः संततं ज्ञानचिन्तनात् ।
वेदवद्वचनं तेषां ध्रुवं सत्यं महात्मनाम् ॥१३२॥

[चरक : सूत्र ११:१८-१९ किंचित् परिवर्तितम्]

Āptopadeśa

Āptas (sages) are free from attachments, fear, envy, ignorance, ego, illusion and doubts. They are engaged in meditation, *yoga*, penance and religious activities. They have the perception of pure knowledge. They are gentle in nature. They are the constant seekers of pure knowledge. Therefore, the words of these great souls are eternally true like the statements in the Vedas.

अप्रमाणां पुनर्मत्तप्रमत्तोन्मत्तभाषितम् ।
94
बालबालिशपापिष्ठरागद्वेषवतामपि ॥१३३॥

The statements of persons who are intoxicated, delinquent and insane, and the statements of children (ignorant ones), *bāliśa* (persons having childish habits), persons involved in evil acts and of persons who have attachment and jealousy are not authentic.

[प्रत्यक्षम्]

यदक्षणा वीक्ष्यते रूपं प्रत्यक्षं तदिहेष्यते[95] ।

Pratyakṣa or Direct Observation

Things which are directly seen by the eyes are called '*pratyakṣa*' in the present context.

[अनुमानपरीक्षा]

अग्निं जरणशक्त्या च बलं व्यायामशक्तितः ॥१३४॥
विज्ञानं व्यवसायेन[96] क्रोधं द्रोहेण लक्षयेत् ।
शोकं दैन्येन विज्ञेयं श्रद्धामाश्वा[द?स]नेन च ॥१३५॥
हर्षमाचारयोगेन स्मरणेन स्मृतिं तथा ।
अपत्रपेण तु ह्रीयं धृतिं लौल्यवतस्तथा ॥१३६॥
उपशयानुपशयाभ्यां गूढलिङ्गामयं बुधः ।
एवं सदानुमानेन परीक्षां कारयेद्द्विजः ॥१३७॥
मिथ्यादृष्टा विकारा हि दुराख्यातास्तथैव च ।
तथा दुष्परिपृष्टाश्च मोहयेयुश्चिकित्सकान् ॥१३८॥

[सुश्रुत : सूत्र१०:७]

Anumāna or Inference

Determination of the *agni* by the power of digestion as well as metabolism, and the strength by one's capacity to perform exercise is done by inference. Similarly, by enterprising activities, "the knowledge" can be inferred. By malicious acts, the anger can be inferred. By sorrowful appeals, the grief can be inferred. By the relishing, the liking of a person can be inferred. By initiating, the excitement (*harṣa*) of a person can be inferred. By the capacity to remember, the memory of a person can be inferred. By timidity, the sinful disposition can be inferred; and by repeated attempts, the courage of a person can be inferred. A wise person can infer the exact nature of a disease whose signs and symptoms are not properly manifested by *upaśaya* (things which are wholesome) and *anupaśaya* (things which are harmful). In the same manner, a physician should always examine the disease of the patient by inference. If the disease is not properly examined, if the disease is not properly expressed and if the patient is not properly put questions about his disease, then these lead to the confusion of the physician to determine the exact nature of the disease.

[षड्विधपरीक्षा][97]

षड्विधं चार्थविज्ञानं[98] गदानां लिख्यतेऽधुना ।
पञ्चबुद्धीन्द्रियैः[99] प्रश्नैः कृष्णात्रेयेण भाषितम् ॥१३९॥

Six types of Examination of the Patient

We shall now explain six methods by which the exact nature of the disease could be properly ascertained.

According to *Kṛṣṇātreya*, the six methods are, the examination by five senses, viz., eyes, ears, tongue, nose and skin and by putting questions.

[श्रवणपरीक्षा][100]

हिक्काश्वासादिनिर्घोषं वाक्चेष्टं चान्त्रकूजनम् ।
स्फोटांश्चाङ्गुलिपर्वाणां भिषक् श्रोत्रेण लक्षयेत् ॥१४०॥

Examination by Ears

The sounds produced by hic-cup or during the attack of asthma, the voice of the patient, the gugling sound of the intestine, the cracking sound of the phalanges in the fingers are to be examined by the physician by his ears.

[स्पर्शपरीक्षा][101]

शीतमुष्णं खरं श्लक्ष्णं कठिनं मृदु चापि यत् ।

शोफगुल्माश्मरीणां च भिषक् स्पर्शेन लक्षयेत् ॥१४१॥

Examination by Touch

Cold, heat, roughness, smoothness, hardness and softness of *gulma* (phantum tumor) and *aśmari* (stone in the urinary tract) are to be examined by the physician by touch.

[दर्शनपरीक्षा][102]

वर्णप्रमाणं संस्थानमायुर्वक्त्राङ्गवैकृतम् ।

चेष्टां नेत्रद्युतिं छायां पुष्टिं कार्श्यं च दर्शनात् ॥१४२॥

Examination by Eyes

The colour, the size, the signs, the span of life, the mouth, morbidity in the limbs, activities of the bodily organs, the glaze of the eyes, the aura, nourishment and emaciation are to be examined by eyes.

[रसनापरीक्षा]

अम्लपित्तं रक्तपित्तं प्रमेहं सामदोषजम् ।

निरामं च रसं[103] किं च रसनायां सुलभ्यते ॥१४३॥

स्वादुगात्ररसं विद्याद् भृशं षट्पदसेवनैः ।

यूकादीनां सेवनाच्च कषायमधुरं वदेत् ॥१४४॥

तद्वर्जनैश्च कटुकं शोणितेप्ययेव संविधिः ।

श्वकाकभक्षणाद्धारिलोहितं तदभक्षणात् ।

104

निःसंशयं रक्तपित्तं विजानीयाच्चिकित्सकः ॥१४५॥

Examination by Tongue

Amla pitta, rakta pitta, prameha, sāmatva as well as *nirāmatva* of *doṣas* and the tastes can be examined by tongue. If ants are exceedingly attracted towards the body, then this indicates the presence of sweetness in it. If *yūkā* (lice) are found in the body, then this indicates the presence of astringent and sweet tastes in it. If they leave the body, then this indicates the presence of pungent taste. The same rule will be applicable towards the taste of the blood. If dogs and crows eat the blood then the physician should infer that it is the unpolluted blood of the patient If they do not eat it, then the physician should determine that the blood is that of *rakta pitta* (vitiated by *pitta*).

[आघ्राणपरीक्षा]

परीक्ष्य गात्रगं गन्धं गन्धं व्रणगतं तथा ।

105

कुणपादिकगन्धं च भिषग् घ्राणेन लक्षयेत् ॥१४६॥

Examination by Nose

The physician should examine by his nose the smell of the body of the patient and different types of smell of the ulcer which are like *kuṇapa* (smell of a dead body) etc.

[प्रश्नपरीक्षा]

106 107 108

व्याध्युत्थानं रुजास्थानं [कालं वृद्धिक्षयौ] बलम् ।

109

व्याध्यातुरोपदेशेन रसं मुखगतं तथा ॥१४७॥

Examination by Interrogation

The cause of the disease, the location of the pain, the time of increase and decrease of the disease, the strength of the disease and the taste in the mouth of the patient, are to be ascertained by interrogating him.

अथ सुश्रुतात्

चतुर्विधास्ते विज्ञेयाः शारीरागन्तुमानसाः ।

स्वाभाविकाश्च ते सप्तभेदभिन्ना भवन्ति च [110] ॥१४८॥

तद्यथा

आदि-जन्म-दोष-काल-संघात-दैव-स्वाभावबलप्रवृत्ताः [111] ॥१४९॥

Classification of Diseases According to Suśruta

Diseases are of four types, viz., *śārira* (physical), *āgantu* (caused by extraneous objects), *mānasa* (mental) and *svābhāvika* (natural). These diseases are again divided into seven categories as follows :

1. *Ādibala pravṛtta* or inherited diseases;
2. *Janmabala pravṛtta* or congenital diseases;
3. *Doṣabala pravṛtta* or diseases caused by the aggravation of the *doṣas*;
4. *Kālabala pravṛtta* or diseases caused by the vagaries of time including seasonal changes ;
5. *Sanghātabala pravṛtta* or diseases caused by injuries;
6. *Daivabala pravṛtta* or diseases caused by providential factors; and
7. *Svabhāvabala pravṛtta* or natural diseases.

अथ कोऽयं रोगो नाम? पुरुषस्य दुःखसम्बन्धः [112] ॥१५०॥

What is a disease ? Association of misery in an individual is called a disease.

तथा चोक्तं सुश्रुतेन

तद्दुःखसंयोगविशेषा व्याधय इत्युच्यन्ते[113, 114] ।१५१।।

According to Suśruta

The specific association of miseries with the individual soul is called a disease.

तथान्यैरप्युक्तं

विकृतदोषदूष्यसमवायो विकारः[115] ।।१५२।।

It is stated elsewhere

The inter-action between the morbid *doṣas* and *dūṣyas* (tissue elements) is called a disease.

[यदाह][116] चरकः

रोगः पाप्मा ज्वरो व्याधिर्विकारो दुःखमामयः ।

यक्ष्मातंको गदाबाधा शब्दाः पर्यायवाचकाः[117] ।।१५३।।

According to Caraka

Roga, pāpmā, jvara, vyādhi, vikāra, duḥkha. āmaya, yakṣmā, gada and *ābādhā*—these are the synonymous terms indicating the disease.

ननु किमर्थं व्याधीनां साध्याद्यनेकभेदकथनम् ?

उच्यते, शिष्यमतिविकासार्थम् ।।१५४।।

What is the purpose of describing the several (types of) classifications of diseases, like curable diseases and incurable diseases ?

These are described with a view to developing the power of understanding in the mind of the disciple.

[त्रिविधदुःख]

तद् दुःखं त्रिविधम्, आध्यात्मिकमाधिभौतिकमाधिदैविकमिति ॥१५५॥

[सुश्रुत : सूत्र२४:४]

Categories of Diseases

Duḥkha or diseases are of three categories, namely,

1. *Ādhyātmika* (arising out of one's own self);
2. *Ādhibhautika* (arising out of external objects); and
3. *Ādhidaivika* (arising out of providential causes).

तत्रादिबलजाः रोगाः शुक्रशोणितदोषजाः ।

कुष्ठार्शाद्यास्तद्द्विधा हि पितृमातृविभेदतः ॥१५६॥

(1) The *Ādhyātmika* type of diseases are again of three varieties as follows :

(i) *Ādibalaja* or hereditary : these diseases occur as a result of the vitiation of the sperm and the ovum of the parents, *Kuṣṭha* (obstinate skin diseases including leprosy), *arśas* (piles) and similar diseases belong to this category.

This is again divided into two types namely, (a) those arising out of the father; and (b) those arising out of the mother.

जन्मजास्तेहि विज्ञेया ये मातुरपचारतः ।

जात्यन्धपङ्गुमूकादि-षण्ढ-मिन्मिन-वामनाः ॥१५७॥

(ii) *Janmabalaja* or congenital—this type of diseases occur as a result of improper diet, and regimen of the mother during the period of gestation. *Jātyandha* (congenital blindness), *paṅgu* (immobility of limbs), *mūka* (dumbness), *ṣaṇḍha* (impotency), *minmina* (lulling speech or stammering) *vāmana* (dwarfism) etc., belong to this category.

[118]
ते द्विधा रसजाश्चाथ दोहृदस्यावमाननात् ।
ये दोषबलजा रोगा मिथ्याहारविहारतः।
ते द्विधा[ऽऽ]माशयोत्थाश्च तथा पक्वाशयोत्थिताः ॥१५८॥

These are again of two types as follows :

(a) *rasaja* caused by the vitiation of the chyle or plasma of the mother ; and

(b) *dauhṛda apacāraja* (improper management of the mother during bi-cardiac stage of the pregnancy).

(iii) *Doṣabalaja*—this type of diseases occur as a result of the wrong diet and regimen of the individual.

These are again of two types as follows :

(a) *āmāśayottha* (diseases arising out of the stomach and the upper portion of the small intestine); and

(b) *pakvāśayottha* (diseases arising out of the large intestine).

[119]
दोषो वातादिः, रजस्तमसी च ॥१५९॥

[120]
[एते आध्यात्मिकाः]

बलं शक्तिः ॥१६०॥

Vāyu etc. are called *doṣas* of the body. *Rajas* and *tamas* are the *doṣas* of the mind.

The term *bala* means strength or power.

121
संघातबलजा ये च ते स्युरागन्तवो नृणाम् ।
दुर्बलानां प्राणिनां च बलवद्विग्रहाच्च ये ।
रोगास्ते द्विविधा ज्ञेया व्यालशस्त्रादिभेदतः ॥१६१॥

122
॥ एते आधिभौतिकाः ॥

(2) The *Ādhibhautika* diseases are as follows :

(i) *saṅghāta balaja* (diseases caused by the affliction by external objects). In human beings these diseases are called *āgantu* (extraneous) and these are caused in weak animals when they are attacked by the stronger ones.

These are again of two types as follows :

(a) *vyālaja* (diseases caused by wild animals); and

(b) *śastraja* (diseases caused by weapons etc.)

ये कालबलजास्ते हि वर्षाशीतोष्णसंभवाः ।
वातातपप्रभृतिभिस्ते चापि द्विविधा मताः ॥१६२॥

123
व्यापन्नऋतुजाश्चैके अव्यापन्नेषु चापरे ।

124
व्यापन्नऋतुजानां च भिषक्पूर्वोपसञ्चितः ॥१६३॥
तपसामौषधीनां च सेवनं देवतार्चनम् ।
अव्यापन्नकृतानां च यथाकालस्तथा क्रमः ॥१६४॥

(3) The *Ādhidaivika* diseases are divided into the following types :

(i) *Kālabalaja* (seasonal)—These diseases occur as a result of rain, cold or the heat in different seasons.

They are again divided into two types as follows :

(a) *vātaja* (diseases arising out of wind); and

(b) *ātapaja* (diseases arising out of sunray).

These diseases are again divided into two types as follows :

(a) *vyāpanna ṛtuja* (diseases arising as a result of the vagaries of the seasons); and

(b) *avyāpanna ṛtuja* (diseases arising out of normal seasons).

When diseases are caused by abnormality of seasons, then the physician should treat such patients by drugs which are collected earlier. Such diseases can also be treated by *tapas* (penance), *auṣadhi* (drugs or talisman) and *devatārcana* (offering prayer to the gods). Diseases which occur during the normal seasons should be treated according to the nature of the season.

ये [125]दैवबलसम्भूता [126]देवद्रोहा[127]भिशस्तकाः ।

उपसर्गा[128]थर्वकृतास्ते द्विधा संभवन्ति हि ॥१६५॥

विद्युदग्निकृताश्चापि पिशाचादिकृतस्तथा ।

संसर्गजाकस्मिकाश्च द्विधा भेदेन लक्षयेत् ॥१६६॥

(ii) *Daivabala saṁbhūta* (diseases caused by the displeasure of the gods)—This type of diseases are caused by the anger of the gods and by their curse. These are of two types as follows :

(a) *upasargaja* (contageous); and

(b) *atharva kṛta* (diseases caused by evil tantric rites).

These are again of two types as follows :

(a) diseases caused by lightening and fire; and

(b) diseases caused by *piśāca* (evil spirits) etc.

These are also classified into two categories as follows :

(a) *sansargaja* (contageous or epidemic diseases); and

(b) *ākasmika* (accidental).

अभिशस्तकाः[129] मुनीश्वरादीनामाक्रोशजाः । उपसर्गाः उपसृज्यन्त इत्युपसर्गाः[130], देव द्रोहादिजनसम्पर्कात्[131] । आकस्मिकाः[132] पूर्वकर्मनिपीडितत्वेन जाताः ॥१६७॥

The diseases which occur as a result of anger of great saints are called *abhisaptaka.* The term *upasarga* means transmission. A person suffers from such diseases when he is afflicted with anger etc., of the gods. *Ākasmika* or accidental diseases are manifested as a result of the maturity of the evil *karmas* of the past.

स्वभावबलजाश्चैव क्षुत्पिपासाजरास्तथा ।
निद्राहंकारकामादिः विज्ञेयाः कुशलैरिह ॥१६८॥

॥ एते आधिदैविकाः[133] ॥

(iii) *Svabhāvabalaja* (natural diseases)—Hunger, thirst, old age, sleep, ego, passion etc., are the natural diseases.

॥ इति व्याधिपरीक्षा ॥

Thus, ends the description of examination of diseases.

इति श्रीमहाराजाधिराजटोडरमल्लविरचिते टोडरानन्दे आयुर्वेदसौख्ये आयुर्वेदप्रयोजनाष्टचिकित्सालक्षणवैद्यावैद्यप्रतिरूपिका[134]वैद्यलक्षणदीक्षारोगलक्षणकथनं नाम प्रथमो हर्षः ॥

Thus, ends the first Chapter of *Āyurveda saukhyaṁ* in *Ṭoḍarānanda* composed by the great king Ṭoḍara malla which deals with the following topics :

(1) Objects of āyurveda;

(2) Eight specialised branches of āyurveda;

(3) Characteristic features of genuine physician, pseudo-physician and faigned physician;

(4) *Dikṣā* or initiation of training; and

(5) Classification of diseases.

NOTES AND REFERENCES

1. सुदेवाऽध्यगसंभवाद्याः इति षष्ठपुस्तके पाठः ।
2. मांधातृद्रुःकुन्त इति षष्ठपुस्तके पाठः ।
3. विघ्नकारिणो इति द्वितीयपुस्तके पाठः ।
4. इदानींतयानामप्रवृत्ते इति षष्ठपुस्तके पाठः ।
5. ज्ञानार्थमेतत् तस्मिन्ग्रन्थे इति षष्ठपुस्तके पाठः ।
6. द्रष्टव्यम् सुश्रुत : सूत्र १:१६ ।
7. द्रष्टव्यम्—आयुर्हिताहितं रोगनिदानं शमनं तथा।
   विद्यन्ते यत्र विद्वद्भिः स आयुर्वेद उच्यते ।।
   (शब्दकल्पद्रुमः)
8. इयं पङ्क्तः द्वितीयपुस्तके नास्ति ।
9. (क) इह खल्वायुर्वेदं नामोपाङ्गमथर्ववेदस्य ।
   (द्रष्टव्यम् सुश्रुत : सूत्र १:६)

   (ख) चतुर्णामृक्सामयजुरथर्ववेदानामातमनोऽथर्ववेदे भक्तिरादेश्या ।
   (चरक : सूत्र ३०:२१)

   (ग) उपवेदाः...ऋग्वेदस्य आयुर्वेदः ।
   (चरणव्युहः)
10. द्रष्टव्यम्—सुश्रुत : सूत्र १:६ ।
11. (क) दशमश्लोकादारभ्य पंचदशश्लोकपर्यन्तं पाठोऽयं पञ्चमपुस्तके नोपलभ्यते ।

    (ख) द्रष्टव्यम्—

    १. शल्यं, शालाक्यं, कायचिकित्सा, भूतविद्या, कौमारभृत्यम्, अगदतन्त्रं, रसायनं तन्त्रं, वाजीकरणतन्त्रमिति ।।
    (सुश्रुत : सूत्र १:७)

    २. कायचिकित्सा, शालाक्यं, शल्यापहर्तृकं, विषगरवैरोधिकप्रशमनं, भूतविद्या, कौमारभृत्यकं, रसायनं, वाजीकरणमिति ।।
    (चरक : सूत्र ३०:२८)

    ३. कायबालग्रहोर्ध्वाङ्गशल्यदंष्ट्राजरावृषान् ।।
    (अष्टाङ्गहृदय : सूत्र १:५)

४. शरीर-नेत्र-व्रणरोपणानि विषाणि भूतानि च बालतन्त्रम् ।

रसायनं पञ्चविधं च कर्म अष्टाङ्गम् आयुः कथयन्ति वैद्याः ।।

(योगशतक : ५)

५. शल्यशालाक्यकायाश्च तथा बालचिकित्सितम् ।

अगदं विषतन्त्राख्यं भूतविद्या रसायनम् ।।

(हारीतसंहिता २:५)

12. द्रष्टव्यम्—सुश्रुत : सूत्र २६:५, सुश्रुत : सूत्र १:८ (१) ।
तथा हारीतसंहिता २:६ ।

13. नाराचवह्निवल्लिभिः इति पाठः षष्ठपुस्तके उपलभ्यते ।

14. द्रष्टव्यम्– सुश्रुत : सूत्र १:८ (२) ।

55. संस्थिताः इति द्वितीयपुस्तके पाठः ।

16. तेषां यत्क्रियते कर्म प्रायशस्तु शलाकया ।

तस्माच्छालाक्यमित्युक्तमृषिभिः शौनकादिभिः ।।

इति द्वितीयषष्पुठस्तकयोः पाठः ।

17. द्रष्टव्यम्—हारीतसंहिता २:१३-१४ ।

18. द्रष्टव्यम्– (क) सुश्रुत : सूत्र १:८ (६) ।

(ख) हारीतसंहितायाम् अगदतन्त्रात् विषतन्त्रं पृथक् पठितम् ।

तत्र अगदतन्त्रलक्षणम्

गुदामयबस्तिरुजं शमनं बस्तिरूहकम्

आस्थापनानुवासन्तु अगदं नाम एव च ।।

टोडरमलस्य स्वमतं अस्मिन् विषये अस्य अध्यायस्य

३७-४० पाठे द्रष्टव्यम् ।

हारीतसंहितायां विषतन्त्रलक्षणम्

सर्पवृश्चिकलूतानां विषोपशमनी तु या ।

सा क्रिया विषतन्त्रञ्च नाम प्रोक्तं मनीषिभिः ।।

19. द्रष्टव्यम्—सुश्रुत : सूत्र १:८ (५) ।

20. द्रष्टव्यम्—सुश्रुत : सूत्र १:८ (३) ।

21. कायशब्देन जाठरोऽग्निः इति प्रथमपुस्तके पाठः ।

22. जाठरस्याग्निः कायाग्निः इति द्वितीयषष्ठपुस्तकयोः पाठः ।
23. सीदन्ति इति षष्ठपुस्तके पाठः ।
24. विदितः इति द्वितीयपुस्तके पाठः तथा विदिह्ः इति पञ्चमपुस्तके पाठः ।
25. वैकृतौ इति प्रथमपञ्चमषष्ठपुस्तकेषु पाठः ।
26. प्रवृत्तिर्द्धातु इति प्रथमपञ्चमपुस्तकयोः पाठः ।
27. वातरक्तास्रपित्तिनाम् इति द्वितीयपुस्तके पाठः ।
28. कुष्ठातीसारशोफादि इति प्रथमपञ्चमषष्ठपुस्तकेषु पाठः ।
29. द्रष्टव्यम्—सुश्रुत : सूत्र १:८ (४) ।
30. वापि इति द्वितीयपुस्तके पाठः ।
31. द्रष्टव्यम्—सुश्रुत : सूत्र १:८ (८) तथा चरक : चिकित्सा १(१) : ९-१२।
32. यतो इति द्वितीयषष्ठपुस्तकयोः पाठः ।
33. द्रष्टव्यम्—सुश्रुत : सूत्र १:८ (७) तथा चरक : चिकित्सा १ (१) : ७-८।
34. विशेष इति षष्ठपुस्तके पाठः ।
35. आगदा इति द्वितीयपुस्तके पाठः ।
36. पृथगिष्यते इति षष्ठपुस्तके पाठः ।
37. नवभागा भवन्ति इति प्रथमपंचमपुस्तकयोः पाठः ।
58. अतोऽत्र सा च न अङ्गीकारः कृतः इति षष्ठपुस्तके पाठः ।
39. द्रष्टव्यम्—(क) चरक : सूत्र ६:५ ।

    (ख) अष्टाङ्गहृदय : सूत्र १:२७ ।
40. द्रष्टव्यम्—चरक : सूत्र ६:६ तथा अष्टाङ्गहृदय : सूत्र १:२८ ।
41. द्रष्टव्यम्—चरक : सूत्र ६:७ तथा सुश्रुत : सूत्र ३४:२२-२३ ।
42. बल्यम् इति द्वितीयपुस्तके पाठः ।
43. द्रष्टव्यम्—चरक : सूत्र ६:८ तथा सुश्रुत : सूत्र ३४:२८ ।
44. द्रष्टव्यम्—चरक : सूत्र ६:९ तथा सुश्रुत : सूत्र ३८:२१-२२।
45. द्रष्टव्यम्—चरक : सूत्र १०:११-१३ ।
46. (क) अनल्पदूष्यदेशर्त्तुः इति षष्ठपुस्तके पाठः ।

    (ख) अतुल्यदोषदूष्यर्तु इति प्रथमद्वितीयपुस्तकयोः पाठः ।
47. न चार्हन्ति इति प्रथमद्वितीयपञ्चमपुस्तकेषु पाठः ।

48. यथा इति द्वितीयषष्ठपुस्तकयोः पाठः ।
49. स ज्ञेयो भिषगुत्तमः इति षष्ठपुस्तके पाठः ।
50. अत्र षष्ठपुस्तके श्लोकोऽयमधिकः ।
51. प्रतिहन्त्यजीवितं इति आदर्शपुस्तकेषु पाठः ।
52. विविधा इति द्वितीयषष्ठपुस्तकयोः पाठः ।
53. छन्द इति पञ्चमपुस्तके पाठः ।
54. अत्र चरकधृतः 'सिद्धसाधित्ताः' इति पाठस्तु साधीयान् ।
55. अज्ञास्ते इति चरकसम्मतपाठः ।
56. अत्र चरकधृतः 'प्रतिरूपकाः' साधीयान् ।
57. सिद्ध साधिताः इति चरकसम्मतपाठः ।
58. द्रष्टव्यम्—चरक : सूत्र २९:७ ।
59. वृकमासाद्य इति चरकसम्मतपाठः ।
60. द्रष्टव्यम्—चरक : सूत्र २९:८-९ ।
61. ०कर्म० इति द्वितीयपुस्तके पाठः ।
62. ...स वैद्योन्यो तु तस्कराः इति षष्ठपुस्तके पाठः ।
63. पाठोऽयं षष्ठपुस्तके नोपलभ्यते ।
64. श्लोकोऽयं षष्ठपुस्तके नोपलभ्यते ।
65. मृषा प्रगल्भं सारंभः इति षष्ठपुस्तके पाठः ।
66. विनियतायुषां इति पाठः षष्ठपुस्तके उपलभ्यते ।
67. लुचब्धः कुचीलः इति प्रथमद्वितीयपुस्तकयोः पाठः ।
68. ते वर्जनीया मृत्योस्ते चरन्त्यनुचरा भुवि इति प्रथमपञ्चमषष्ठपुस्तकेषु पाठः ।
69. निर्वोढुं इति पञ्चमवर्जपुस्तकेषु पाठः ।
70. हारीतात् इति पञ्चमपुस्तके पाठः ।
71. नाभक्तायाथ शान्ताय इति द्वितीयपुस्तकपाठो न समीचीनः ।
72. अत्र पञ्चमपुस्तकेऽयमधिकः पाठः ।
73. च इति प्रथमपुस्तके पाठः ।
74. प्रविश्योच्चोपविश्य च इति पञ्चमपुस्तके पाठः ।
75. हेतावीर्षेत्फलेषु इति पञ्चमपुस्तके पाठः ।

76. ०पुण्य इति पञ्चमपुस्तके पाठः ।
77. तु इति प्रथमद्वितीयपुस्तकयोः पाठः ।
78. ०पुण्य इति षष्ठपुस्तके पाठः ।
79. असाध्यस्याप्यसाध्योऽयं इति द्वितीयषष्ठपुस्तकयोः पाठः ;
असाध्यस्याप्यसाध्येत इति प्रथमपुस्तके पाठः ।
80. ०दीक्षा इति प्रथमपञ्चमपुस्तकयोः पाठः ।
81. भवान्तरे इति प्रथमपुस्तके पाठः ।
82. यान्त्यपरे इति षष्ठपुस्तके पाठः ।
83. चिन्तान्वितस्य इति षष्ठपुस्तके पाठः ।
84. च स रुजः इति प्रथमपुस्तके पाठः ।
85. अपेक्षिताः इति प्रथमपुस्तके पाठः ।
86. ०मयः इति षष्ठपुस्तके पाठः ।
87. वैद्यस्येयं इति आदर्शपुस्तकेषु पाठः ।
88. प्रागुपेक्ष्याल्पमायुषः इति द्वितीयपुस्तके पाठः ।
89. सुरापी इति प्रथमपुस्तके पाठः ।
90. अस्तु ते पञ्चमवर्जसर्वपुस्तकपाठः ।
91. (क) अर्थसङ्गतयेऽवग्रप्रश्लेषः कृतः ।
(ख) साध्यान्नारभन्ते इति द्वितीयपुस्तके पाठः ।
92. देहे इति द्वितीयपुस्तके पाठः ।
93. व्यवस्थितिः इति द्वितीयषष्ठपुस्तकपाठः; व्यवस्थितेः इति प्रथमपुस्तकपाठः।
94. द्रष्टव्यम्—चरक : सूत्र ११:१७; चरक : विमान ४:३,६;
चरक : विमान ८:८३ ।
95. द्रष्टव्यम्—चरकः विमोन ४:४ ।
96. द्रष्टव्यम्—चरक : सूत्र ११:२०; चरक : विमान ८:३६;
चरक : विमान ४:७ ।
97. अत्र प्रथमपञ्चमपुस्तकयोः बलमिति अधिकः पाठः ।
98. द्रष्टव्यम्—सुश्रुत : सूत्र १०:४.
99. चाथ इति प्रथमद्वितीयषष्ठपुस्केषु पाठः ।
100. कृत्वात्रेयेण इति प्रथमपञ्चमपुस्तकयोः पाठः ।

101. द्रष्टव्यम्—चरक : विमान ४:७; सुश्रुत : सूत्र १०:५।
102. द्रष्टव्यम्—चरक : विमान ४:७; सुश्रुत : सूत्र १०:५।
103. द्रष्टव्यम्—चरक : विमान ४:७; सुश्रुत : सूत्र १०:५।
104. निरामयं इति प्रथमपञ्चमपुस्तकयोः पाठः।
105 द्रष्टव्यम्—चरक : विमान ४:७; सुश्रुत : सूत्र १०:५।
106. अयं श्लोकार्धः प्रथमपञ्चमपुस्तकयोः नास्ति।
107. रजोत्थानं इति षष्ठपुस्तके पाठः।
108. कालवृद्धिक्षयो इति उपलब्धः पाठः स त्वसमीचीनः प्रतिभाति।
109. अयं श्लोकार्धः प्रथमपञ्चमपुस्तकयोः नास्ति।
110. अयं श्लोकार्धः प्रथमषष्ठपुस्तकयोः दृश्यते।
111. द्रष्टव्यम्—सुश्रुत : सूत्र १:२४-२६।
112. द्रष्टव्यम्—सुश्रुत : सूत्र २४:४-७।
113. द्रष्टव्यम्—सुश्रुत : सूत्र १:२३।
114. तद्दुःखसंयोगा व्याधय उच्यन्ते इति मूलसुश्रुतपाठः।

[सुश्रुत : सूत्र १:२३]

115. अयं पाठः प्रथमपुस्तके नोपलभ्यते।
116. अयं पाठः प्रथमपञ्चमपुस्तकयोर्नोपलभ्यते।
117. तथा च इति षष्ठपुस्तके पाठः।
118. तत्र व्याधिरामयो गद आतङ्को यक्ष्मा ज्वरो विकारो रोग इत्यनर्थान्तरम् इति मूलचरकवचनम्। [चरक : निदान १:५]

ज्वरो विकारो रोगश्च व्याधिरातङ्क एव च।
एकोऽर्थो नामपर्यायैर्विधैरभिधीयते॥

इत्यपि। [चरक : चिकित्सा ३:११]

119. दौहृदस्यापमाननात् इति द्वितीयपुस्तके पाठः।
120. वासादिः इति षष्ठपुस्तके पाठः।
121. यद्यपि कस्मिन्नपि पुस्तके इयानंशो नोपलभ्यते तथाऽपि बोधसौकर्याय उत्तरग्रन्थदृष्टया चास्माभिः विन्यस्तः। द्रष्टव्यम्—सुश्रुत : सूत्र २४:५।

122. ज्ञेयागन्तवो इति प्रथमद्वितीयषष्ठपुस्तकेषु पाठः ।

123. द्रष्टव्यम्—सुश्रुत : सूत्र २४:६ ।

124. अथापन्नेषु इति षष्ठपुस्तके पाठः ।

125. सञ्चिताः इति प्रथमद्वितीयपुस्तकयोः पाठः ।

126. यद्दैव० इति द्वितीयपुस्तके पाठः ।

127. द्रव० इति पञ्चमपुस्तकपाठः ।

128. ०सप्तकाः इति षष्ठपुस्तके पाठः ।

129. उपसर्गार्थवत्कृताः इति षष्ठपुस्तके पाठः ।

130. तत्र इति द्वितीयपुस्तकेऽधिकः पाठः ।

131. इति इति द्वितीयपुस्तके पाठः, कोऽर्थ इति प्रथमपञ्चमपुस्तकयोरधिकः ।

132. सम्पर्काः इति द्वितीयपुस्तके पाठः ।

133. तावत इति द्वितीयपुस्तकेऽधिकः पाठः ।

134. द्रष्टव्यम्—सुश्रुत : सूत्र २४:७ ।

135. परीक्षा इति द्वितीयषष्ठपुस्तकयोः पाठः ।

CHAPTER 2

विश्वम्भराभारमपि प्रहर्तुं ब्रह्माण्डराशौ [1]नहिमाति कर्तुम् ।

मनोरथान्भक्तजनस्य गर्भं प्राप्तः प्रपायाद् [2]भुवि भूपवर्यम् ॥१॥

Invocation

God, who has entered into the heart of his retinues by satisfying their desires with a view to reducing the weight of the universe, by killing the demons and by not permitting the manifestation of any excess in this universe, may bless the great king (Ṭodara malla) of this world.

[3][षट्क्रियाकालः]

संचयं च प्रकोपं च प्रसरं स्थानसंश्रयम् ।

व्यक्तिं भेदं च यो वेत्ति दोषाणां स भवेद्भिषक् ॥२॥

[सुश्रुत : सूत्र २१:३६]

Six kriyākālas, or the Stages of Manifestation of a Disease

A person who is well versed with the *sañcaya* (accumulation) *prakopa* (aggravation), *prasara* (over flowing), *sthāna saṁśraya* (lodgement in a particular place), *vyakti* (manifestation) and *bheda* (classification or dissolution) of the *doṣas* is a genuine physician.

स्त्यान[गत]स्य[4] सर्पिषः क्वाथ्यमानस्य[5] प्रथमं संचयनमात्रमेव प्रकोपः । तस्य चातिक्वाथ्यमानस्य फेनमण्डलेनोपसर्पतो देशान्तरप्रसरणमिव प्रसरेति डल्हणः[6] ॥३॥

According to Ḍalhaṇa

When heat is applied to condensed ghee, it melts. A similar condition of the *doṣas* is called *prakopa* (aggravation). When the ghee is further heated, foam comes out of it, and it overflows out of the vessel to get accumulated in another place. A similar conditions of the *doṣas* is called *prasara* (overflowing).

[त्रयो दोषाः]

वायुः पित्तं कफश्चेति त्रयो दोषाः समासतः ।
प्रत्येकं ते त्रिधा वृद्धिक्षयसाम्येति[7] भेदतः ॥४॥

Three doṣas

Vāyu, *pitta* and *kapha*—these three in brief, are the *doṣas*. Each one of them has three states, namely, *vṛddhi* (aggravation), *kṣaya* (diminution) and *sāmya* (remaining in the state of equilibrium).

उत्कृष्टमध्याल्पतया त्रिधा वृद्धिक्षयावपि[8] ।
विकृताविकृता देहं घ्नन्ति[9] ते वर्तयन्ति च ॥५॥

Vṛddhi (aggravation) and *kṣaya* (diminution) are again of three types, namely (1) *utkṛṣṭa* (excessive aggravation or diminution); (2) *madhya* (moderate aggravation or diminution); and (3) *alpa* (less aggravation or diminution). When in abnormal condition, they destroy the body, and in their normal condition, they sustain it.

[दोषाणां स्थानं वृद्धिकालं च]

ते व्यापिनोऽपि हृन्नाभ्योरधोमध्योर्ध्वसंश्रिताः[10] ।
वयोऽहोरात्रिभुक्तानां तेऽन्तमध्यादिगाः क्रमात् ॥६॥

[अष्टाङ्गहृदय : सूत्र १:७-८]

Location and Time of Aggravation of Doṣas

These *doṣas* pervade all over the body. Even then they are mainly located above the cardiac region (*kapha*), between the cardiac and umbilical region (*pitta*) and below the umbilical region (*vāyu*). *Vāyu, pitta* and *kapha* get aggravated respectively during the end, middle and beginning of day time, night and digestion.

[वायोः स्थानानि]

मलाशयेचरेत् कोष्ठे वह्निस्थाने तथा हृदि ।
कण्ठे सर्वाङ्गदेशेषु वायुः पञ्चप्रकारतः ॥७॥

Location of Vāyu

Vāyu is of five types and they are located in *malāśaya* (rectum including anus), *koṣṭha* (viscera), *vahni sthāna* (site of digestion), *hṛdaya* (heart) and *kaṇṭha* (*throat*). One variety of it is located in all the organs of the body.

अथ विवेकमार्तण्डात् [प्राणवायुः]

हंसरूपस्थितः प्राणः प्राणस्तेन प्रकीर्तितः ।

According to Viveka mārtaṇḍa

The location of different types of *vāyu* are as follows :

1. *Prāṇa vāyu*—In this *vāyu*, the *prāṇa* (or *elan vital*) is located in the form of a swan. Therefore, it is called *prāṇa vāyu.*

[अपानवायुः]

मलं मूत्रं वहेद्वायुरपानस्तेन कथ्यते ॥८॥

2. *Apāna vāyu*—It eliminates stool and urine, for which it is called *apāna vāyu.*

[समानवायुः]

पीतं भक्षितमाघ्रातं रक्तपित्तकफादिकं ।

समं नयति गात्राणि समानस्तेन मारुतः ॥९॥

3. *Samāna vāyu*—In the body, *pīta* (things taken by drinking), *bhakṣita* (eatables), or *āghrāta* (things taken inside the body by smell), *rakta* (blood), *pitta*, *kapha* etc., are maintained by this *vāyu* in a state of equilibrium (*sama*) for which it is called *samāna vāyu*.

[उदानवायुः]

स्पन्दनं चाधरं चोर्ध्वं नेत्रवक्त्रादिकम्पनम् ।

ऊर्ध्वं नयति कार्येण उदानो नाम मारुतः ॥१०॥

4. *Udāna vāyu*—The *vāyu* which is responsible for *spandana* (pulsation) above and below, fluttering of eyes, mouth etc., and which by its action takes things above (*ūrdhva*) is called *udāna vāyu*.

[व्यानवायुः]

व्यानो विनाशयेदङ्गं[11] व्यानो रोगप्रकोपकः ।

प्रीतिं नाशयते वायुस्तेनैव व्यान उच्यते ॥११॥

5. *Vyāna vāyu*—The *vāyu* which destroys the organs of the body, which aggravates the diseases and which anihilates the sense of pleasure is called *vyāna vāyu.*

[पञ्चवायोः रूपलक्षणम्]

द्रुततारनिभं रक्तं[12] इन्द्रगोपसमप्रभम् ।
क्षीराभं स्फटिकाभं च पञ्चानां रूपलक्षणम् ॥१२॥

Colours of five Vāyus

The colours of the five *vāyus* are like the *druta tāra* or molten silver (*prāṇa*), *rakta* or red (*apāna*), *indra gopa* or reddish (*samāna*), *kṣira* or milk (*udāna*) and *sphaṭika* or crystal (*vyāna*).

[पञ्चपित्तानि]

पाचकं भ्राजकं चैव रञ्जकालोचके तथा ।
साधक[[13]ञ्चे]ति पञ्चानां पित्तानां नाम संज्ञितम् ॥१३॥

Five Varieties of Pitta

Pācaka, bhrājaka, rañjaka, ālocaka and *sādhaka*—these are the five varieties of *pitta.*

[पाचकपित्तम्]

चतुर्विधान्नपानं च पचत्याशु विवेचति ।
स्वशक्त्या पाचकं नाम पक्वामाशयमध्यगम् ॥१४॥

Pācaka pitta

Pācaka pitta is located between *pakvāśaya* (colon) and *āmāśaya* (stomach). It helps by its own power in the immediate digestion and disintegration of four types of food and drinks.

[रञ्जकपित्तम्]

यकृत्प्लीह्नोः स्थितं पित्तं रञ्जकं रसरञ्जनात् ॥१५॥

Rañjaka pitta

It is located in liver and spleen, and it imparts colour (*rañjana*) to *rasa* (chyle or plasma) because of which it is called *rañjaka pitta.*

[साधकपित्तम्]

हृदयस्थं तमोरूपं[14] कफं भित्त्वा ददाति यत् ।
धर्मार्थविभिमानादिं[15] तस्मात् तत् साधकाग्निकम् ॥१६॥

Sādhaka pitta

It is located in the heart. It penetrates the *kapha* which is lodged in the heart in the form of *tamas*, and by doing so, it helps in the accomplishment (*sādhana*) of *dharma* (religious virtues), *artha* (satisfaction of desires), *abhimāna* (ego) etc. Therefore, it is called *sādhakāgni.*

[आलोचकपित्तम्]

दृष्टिस्थरूपग्रहणादालोचकमिति[16] स्मृतम् ॥१७॥

Ālocaka pitta

It is located in the eyes. It helps in the perception (*ālocana*) of vision for which it is called *ālocaka pitta.*

[भ्राजकपित्तम्]

अभ्यङ्गपरिषेकादीन् यः पचेत् स्वबलेन[17] च ।
छायां प्रभां द्योतयति भ्राजकोऽग्निरिति स्मृतः ॥१८॥

Bhrājaka Pitta

The *pitta* which by its own power helps in the assimilation of drugs that are used in the form of *abhyaṅga* (massage), *pariṣeka* (sprinkling) etc., and which helps in the manifestation of *chāyā* (complexion) and *prabhā* (aura) is called *bhrājakāgni*.

[कफस्थानानि]

कफ आमाशये मूर्ध्नि कण्ठे हृदि च सन्धिषु ।

तिष्ठन् करोति देहस्य स्थैर्यं सर्वाङ्गपाटवम् ॥१९॥

Location of Kapha

Kapha, being located in *āmāśaya* (stomach), *mūrdhā* (chest), *kaṇṭha* (throat), *hṛdaya* (heart) and all *sandhis* (joints), gives sturdiness and compactness to the whole body.

[अवलम्बककफः]

कफधाम्नां च शेषाणां यः करोत्यवलम्बनम्[18] ।

अतो[ऽ]वलम्बकः श्लेष्मा यश्चामाशयगश्च सः ॥२०॥

Avalambaka Kapha

Being located in *āmāśaya* (stomach), it supports (*avalambana*) the locations of the remaining *kaphas* for which it is called *avalambaka kapha.*

[क्लेदक-बोधक-तर्पक-श्लेषक कफाः]

क्लेदकः[19] सोऽन्नसंघातक्लेदनात्[20], रसबोधनात् ।

बोधको रसनास्थायी, शिरःसंस्थोऽक्षितर्पणात् ॥२१॥

तर्पकः, संधि संश्लेषात् श्लेषकः संधिषु स्थितः[21] ।

Kledaka Kapha

It causes disintegration and *kledana* (paste form) of food for which it is called *kledaka kapha.*

Bodhaka Kapha

It is located in the tongue. It helps in the perception (*bodhana*) of tastes for which it is called *bodhaka kapha.*

Tarpaka Kapha

It is located in the head. It causes *tarpaṇa* (nourishment) of the eyes for which it is called *tarpaka kapha.*

Śleṣaka Kapha

It is located in the joints. It helps in the cohesiveness (*śleṣaṇa*) of the joints for which it is called *śleṣaka kapha.*

इति प्रायेण दोषाणां स्थानान्यविकृतात्मनाम् ।

व्यापिनामपि जानीयात्स्थानानि विविधानि च ॥२२॥

Thus, ends the description of the general locations of the normal *doṣas*. These *doṣas* are no doubt, all pervading. Even then, the physician should know their various important locations as described above.

[वायोः गुणाः]

लघू रूक्षश्चरः शीतो व्यवायी विशदः खरः ।

22

सूक्ष्मः शीघ्रचरः स्तम्भी वेगवान् मारुतो बली ॥२३॥

Attributes of Vāyu

Vāyu is *laghu* (light), *rūkṣa* (ununctuous), *cara* (mobile), *śita* (cooling), *vyavāyi* (which gets digested after it pervades the entire body), *viśada* (non-slimy), *khara* (rough), *sūkṣma* (subtle), *śighra cara* (which moves very fast), *stambhī* (which restricts the normal movement of stool, urine etc.), *vegavān* (which has the power to move with speed) and *balī* (which is very powerful).

[पित्तस्य गुणाः]

सूक्ष्माम्लकटुतिक्तोष्णं सस्नेहं दारूणं द्रवम् ।
सरं पीतं हरिद्रक्तं पित्तं तीक्ष्णं विकाशी च ॥२४॥

Attributes of Pitta

Pitta is *sūkṣma* (subtle), *amla* (sour), *kaṭu* (pungent), *tikta* (bitter), *ūṣṇa* (hot), *sasneha* (which has the association of unctuousness), *dāruṇa* (which has acute performances), *drava* (liquid), *sara* (which has the ability to spread), *pīta* (yellow), *harita* (green), *rakta* (red), *tīkṣṇa* (sharp) and *vikāśi* (which causes looseness of joints).

[कफस्य गुणाः]

स्वादुः स्निग्धो मृदुः शीतः स्थिरः श्लक्ष्णोऽथ[23] पिच्छिलः[24] ।
गुरुः सान्द्रश्च मन्दश्च श्लेष्मा शुक्लः[25] स्वभावतः[26] ।
मधुरस्त्वविदग्धः स्याद्विदग्धो लवणः स्मृतः ॥२५॥

Attributes of Kapha

Kapha is *svādu* (sweet), *snigdha* (unctuous), *mṛdu* (soft), *śita* (cold), *sthira* (stable), *ślakṣṇa* (smooth), *picchila* (slime), *guru* (heavy), *sāndra* (dense), *manda* (sluggish) and *śukla* (white) by nature. When in the state of *avidagdha* (proper digestion) it is sweet in taste. In the state of *vidagdha* (improper digestion), it has saline taste.

[दोषाणां वैशेषिकगुणाः]

वातपित्तकफानां च त्रयो वैशेषिका गुणाः ।

रौक्ष्यं वातस्य पित्तस्य तैक्ष्ण्यं स्नैग्ध्यं कफस्य तु ॥२६॥

Specific Attributes of Doṣas

There are three specific attributes of three *doṣas*, namely, *vāyu*, *pitta* and *kapha*. The specific attribute of *vāyu* is roughness; that of *pitta* is sharpness and that of *kapha* is unctuousness.

[दोषाणां देहधारकत्वम्]

27
विसर्गादानविक्षपैः सोमसूर्यानिला यथा ।

धारयन्ति जगद्देहं कफपित्तानिलास्तथा ॥२७॥

[सुश्रुत : सूत्र२१:८]

॥ इत्यविकृतदोषलक्षणम् ॥

Sustenance of the Body by Doṣas

Soma (moon), *sūrya* (sun) and *anila* (wind) sustain the universe by *visarga* (elimination of energy), *ādāna* (absorption of energy) and *vikṣepa* (movement of energy), respectively. In the same manner, *kapha*, *pitta* and *vāyu* help in the sustenance of the human body by *visarga*, *ādāna* and *vikṣepa*.

Thus, ends the description of the characteristics of normal *doṣas*.

[दोषाणां संचयप्रकोपप्रशमकराः गुणाः]

उष्णेन युक्ता रूक्षाद्या वायोः कुर्वन्ति सञ्चयम् ।

शीतेन कोपमुष्णेन शमं स्निग्धादयो गुणाः ॥२८॥

Attributes for Accumulation etc., of Doṣas

Ununctuousness etc., associated with *uṣṇa* (heat) cause the accumulation of *vāyu*. This gets aggravated by cold and alleviated by attributes like unctuousness etc.

शीतेन युक्तस्तीक्ष्णाद्याश्चयं पित्तस्य कुर्वते ।

उष्णेन कोपं, मन्दाद्याः शमं शीतोपसंहिताः ॥२९॥

Pitta gets accumulated when sharpness etc., are associated with cold. It gets aggravated by heat and alleviated by *manda* (sluggishness) etc., associated with *śita* (cold).

शीतेन युक्ताः स्निग्धाद्याः कुर्वते श्लेष्मणश्चयम् ।

उष्णेन कोपं, तेनैव गुणा रूक्षादयः शमम् ॥३०॥

[अष्टाङ्गहृदय : सूत्र१२:१९-२२]

Kapha gets accumulated by unctuousness etc., when they are associated with cold. It gets aggravated by heat and alleviated by attributes like ununctuousness etc.

[दोषाणां चयलक्षणम्]

स्तब्धत्वं पूर्णता कोष्ठे मन्दोष्मा पीतता तनौ ।

आलस्यं गौरवत्वं च द्वेषो निष्कारणं गुणे ॥३१॥

चये ह्येतानि लिङ्गान्याहाराचारचारणात्[28] ।

चयादीन् यान्ति सद्योऽपि दोषाः[29] कालेन वा तनुम्[30] ॥३२॥

Signs and Symptoms of Accumulated Doṣas

By *āhāra* (improper food) and *ācāra* (improper regimens) *doṣas* undergo the process of *caya* (accumulation) etc. This may happen instantaneously or gradually, in appropriate time. The signs and symptoms of the accumulation of *doṣas* are as follows :

1. *Stabdha koṣṭha* (absence of any peristaltic movement of the intestines);

2. *Pūrṇa koṣṭha* (a feeling as if the intestines are filled up with something);
3. Reduction in the temperature;
4. Yellowishness of the body;
5. Laziness and heaviness in the body; and
6. Finding fault, without any reason, in a thing which is not faulty.

[दोषाणां कोपलक्षणम्]

व्याप्नोति सहसा देहमापादतलमस्तकम् ।

[निवर्तते तु][31] कुपितो मलो[ऽ]ल्पाल्पजलौघवत् ॥३३॥

[अष्टाङ्गहृदय : सूत्र १२:२९-३०]

नानारूपैरसंख्येयैर्विकारैः कुपिता मलाः ।

तापयन्ति तनुं तस्मात् तद्धेत्वाकृतिसाधनम् ॥३४॥

[शक्यं नैकैकशो वक्तुमतः सामान्यमुच्यते ।

दोषा एव हि सर्वेषां रोगाणामेककारणम्[32] ॥३५॥]

[अष्टाङ्गहृदय : सूत्र १२:३०-३२]

Signs and Symptoms of the Aggravation of Doṣas

The aggravated *doṣas* instantaneously spread all over the body right from the sole of the feet upto the head. Like a cloud with moisture, it gradually settles down. These aggravated *doṣas* produce innumerable diseases of different characteristics, depending upon the etiological factors and the nature of the manifestation. Thus, they afflict the body. It is impossible to describe each one of their manifestations. Therefore, in the medical classics, they are described only in general. *Doṣas* are the exclusive causative factors of all the diseases.

वाग्भटात्

यथा पक्षी परिपतन् सर्वतः सर्वमप्यहः ।
छायामन्वेति[33] चात्मीयां[34] यथावत्कृत्स्नमप्यदः ॥३६॥

[अष्टाङ्गहृदय : सूत्र१२:३२-३३]

According to Vāgbhaṭa

As a bird moving all over the sky, for the entire day, cannot overcome its own shadow, similarly, the diseases in their entirety cannot get manifested away from their ownself, i.e. without the aggravated *doṣas* specific to each one of them.

[त्रिविधा गतिः]

स्थानं वृद्धिः क्षयश्चेति दोषाणां त्रिविधा गतिः[35] ।

तत्स्थानकृतमारोग्यं रोगो वृद्धिक्षयात्मकः ॥३७॥

Three States of Doṣas

Sthāna (location in their normal sites), *vṛddhi* (aggravation) and *kṣaya* (diminution)—these are the three different states of the *doṣas*. When they are in their own sites or in their normal condition, they maintain positive health of the individual. Their aggravation or diminution is responsible for the manifestation of diseases.

अग्निवेशात्

ऊर्ध्वं चाधश्च तिर्यक् च विज्ञेयास्त्रिविधाः पुनः ।

[चरक : सूत्र१७:११२]

प्रायस्तिर्यग्गता दोषाः क्लेशयन्त्यातुरं बहु[36] ॥३८॥

According to Agniveśa

The other three states of *doṣas* are *ūrdhva* (upward movement), *adhaḥ* (downward movement) and *tiryak* (sideward movement). Generally, *doṣas* in their sideward movement exceedingly afflict the patient.

[दोषोपक्रमविधिः]

शमयेत् तान् प्रयत्नेन सुखं वा कोष्ठमानयेत् ।

ज्ञात्वा कोष्ठप्रपन्नांश्च [यथासन्नं] विनिर्हरेत् ॥३६॥

[अष्टाङ्गहृदय : सूत्र १३:२२-२३]

Line of Treatment

The aggravated *doṣas* should be alleviated or gently brought to the *koṣṭha* (gastro-intestinal tract). After ascertaining their arrival in the *koṣṭha*, they should be suitably eliminated.

[त्रिविधमार्गः]

त्रिविधाश्चापराः शाखाकोष्ठमर्मादयस्तथा ।

शाखा रक्तादयस्त्वक् च बाह्यरोगायणं हि तत् ॥४०॥

तत्राश्रितामया व्यङ्गगण्डालज्यर्बुदादयः ।

बहिर्भागाश्च पाण्ड्वर्शोगुल्मशोफादयो गदाः ॥४१॥

Three Channels

The three channels for the spread of *doṣas* are *śākhā*, *koṣṭha*, *marma* etc. Tissue elements namely, *rakta* (hemoglobin fraction of the blood), etc., and the skin constitute *śākhā* (periphery). This is the channel of the external diseases. The diseases which are located in the *śākhā* are *vyaṅga* (black or white spots in the skin), *gaṇḍa* (goitre), *alaji* (pimple like growth in the skin), *arbuda* (tumour), etc. Some other diseases like *pāṇḍu* (anemia), *arśas* (piles), *gulma* (phantom tumour), *śopha* (oedema) etc., also spread through the external channel.

42

अन्तःकोष्ठो महास्रोत आमपक्वाशयाश्रयः ।

तत्स्थानाच्छर्द्यतीसारकासश्वासोदरज्वराः ॥४२॥

The *koṣṭha* (gastro-intestinal tract) is also called *mahā srotas* and it comprises *āmāśaya* (stomach including small intestine) and *pakvāśaya* (colon including rectum). The diseases located in the *koṣṭha* are *chardi* (vomiting), *atisāra* (diarrhoea), *kāsa* (bronchitis), *śvāsa* (asthma), *udara* (obstinate abdominal diseases including ascites) and *jvara* (fever).

शिरोहृदयबस्त्यादिमर्मण्यस्थ्नां च सन्धयः ।

43

रोगमार्गस्थितास्तत्र कम्पपक्षवधार्दिताः ॥४३॥

शिरोरुजादयश्च ।

The third channel of diseases is constituted of vital organs like the brain, the heart, the urinary bladder etc., and the joints of bones. The diseases manifested in this channel are *kaṁpa vāta* (trembling of the body), *pakṣa vadha* (paralysis) and *ardita* (facial paralysis). Headache etc., are also manifested in this channel.

44

अथ दोषदुष्टिश्च लिख्यते

वातस्य पित्तस्य कफस्य चापि विकारिणः कायवतो हि काये ।

प्रकोपहेतुः कुपितस्य लिङ्गं चिकित्सितं चेति निरूपणीयम् ॥४४॥

Vitiation of Doṣas

It is necessary for the physician to be acquainted with the

cause of aggravation, the signs and symptoms manifested by aggravation, and the treatment of the aggravated *doṣas*, namely *vāyu*, *pitta* and *kapha* in the afflicted body of the individual.

[दोषप्रकोपविधिः]

45

न केवलं चयं प्राप्य दोषाः कुप्यन्ति देहिनाम् ।
अन्यतोऽपि हि कुप्यन्ति हेतुबाहुल्यतो बलात् ॥४५॥

Mode of Aggravation

It is not necessary that *doṣas* in the body of the individual get aggravated only after their state of *caya* (accumulation). They also get aggravated otherwise, if the etiological factors are multiple in number and if they are very strong.

सुश्रुतात्

तत्र बलवद्विग्रहातिव्यायामव्यवायाध्ययनप्रपतनप्रधावनप्रपीडनाभिघातलङ्घनप्लवनप्रतरणरात्रिजागरण-भारहरणगजतुरगरथपदातिचर्याकटुकषायतिक्तरूक्षलघुशीतवीर्यशुष्कशाकवल्लूर-वरकोद्दालककोरदूषश्यामाकनीवारमुद्गमसूराढकीहरेणुकलायनिष्पावानशनविषमाशनाध्यशनवातमूत्रपुरीषशुक्रच्छर्दिक्षवथूद्गारबाष्पवेगविघातादिभिर्विशेषैर्वायुः प्रकोपमापद्यते ॥४६॥

[सुश्रुत : सूत्र २१:१९]

According to Suśruta

Vāyu gets aggravated by fighting with a stronger person, excessive physical exercise, excessive indulgence in sex, excessive study in loud voice, fall, running, pressure or injury to the body, fasting, floating, swimming, remaining awake at night, carrying heavy weight, travelling long distances on elephants, horses, *ratha* (car or cart), intake of food and drinks which are pungent, astringent, bitter, ununctuous, light and of *śita virya* (cold in potency), intake of dried vegetables, dried fish, *varaka*, *uddālaka*, *kora dūṣa*, *śyāmāka*, *nivāra*, *mudga*, *masūra*, *āḍhakī*, *hareṇu*, *kalāya* and *niṣpāva*, fasting, irregularity in taking food, taking food before the previous meal is digested, suppression of the urge for passing flatus, micturition, defecation, sexual intercourse, vomiting, sneezing, eructation and tear and such other factors.

स शीताभ्रप्रवातेषु घर्मान्ते च विशेषतः ।
प्रत्यूषस्यपराह्णे च जीर्णेऽन्ने च प्रकुप्यति ॥४७॥

[सुश्रुत : सूत्र२१:२०]

It gets specially aggravated by cold, onset of cloud, wind, at the end of the summer season, in the late night, in the afternoon and after the digestion of the food.

क्रोधशोकभयायासोपवासविदग्धमैथुनोपगमनकट्वम्ललवणतीक्ष्णोष्णलघुविदाहितिलतैलपिण्याककुलत्थसर्षपातसीहरितकशाकगोधामत्स्याजाविकमांसदधितक्रकूर्चिकामस्तुसौवीरकसुराविकाराम्लफलकट्वरप्रभृतिभिः पित्तं प्रकोपमापद्यते ॥४८॥

[सुश्रुत : सूत्र२१:२१]

Pitta gets aggravated by anger, grief, fear, exertion, fasting, *vidagdha* (indigestion leading to acid formation), sexual intercourse, intake of pungent, sour, saline, sharp, hot, light, *vidāhi* (food-ingredients which lead to indigestion and acid formation), til oil, *piṇyāka* (oil cake), *kulattha*, *sarṣapa*, *atasī*, green vegetables, flesh of iguana, fish, meat of goat and sheep, curd, butter milk, *kūrcikā*, *mastu*, *sauvīra*, alcoholic preparations, sour fruit, *kaṭvara* etc.

तदुष्णैरुष्णकाले च घनान्ते च विशेषतः ।
मध्याह्ने चार्धरात्रे च जीर्यत्यन्ने च कुप्यति ॥४९॥

[सुश्रुत : सूत्र२१:२२]

It gets specifically aggravated by heat, during summer season, at the end of the rainy season, during mid-day and mid-night and at the time of digestion of food.

दिवास्वप्राव्यायामालस्यमधुराम्ललवणशीतस्निग्धगुरुपिच्छिलाभिष्यन्दिहायनकयव-कनैषधेत्कटमाषमहामाषगोधूमतिलपिष्टविकृतिदधिदुग्धकृशरापायसेक्षुविकारानू-पौदकमांसवसाविसमृणालकसेरुकशृङ्गाटकमधुरवल्लीफलसमशनाध्यशनप्रभृतिभिः श्लेष्माप्रकोपमापद्यते ॥५०॥

Kapha gets aggravated by sleep during day time, lack of exercise, lazy habits, intake of sweet, sour, saline, cold, unctuous, heavy, slimy and *abhiṣyandi* (which obstructs the channels of circulation) type of food, intake of *hāyanaka*, *yavaka*, *naiṣadha*, *itkaṭa*, *māṣa*, *mahā māṣa*, *godhūma*, *tila*, pastry prepared out of *tila* and its other preparations, curd, milk, *kṛśarā*, *pāyasa*, preparations of sugarcane juice, meat of marshy and aquatic animals, *vasā* (muscle fat), *visa*, *mṛṇāla*, *kaseruka*, *sṛṅgāṭaka*, *madhura phala*, *valli phala*, intake of more food, intake of food before the previous meal is digested and such other food and regimens.

स शीतैः शीतकाले च वसन्ते च विशेषतः ।

पूर्वाह्ने च प्रदोषे च भुक्तमात्रे प्रकुप्यति ॥५१॥

[सुश्रुत : सूत्र२१:२३-२४]

It gets specifically aggravated by cold, in winter season, in spring season, in the forenoon, in the evenings and immediately after taking food.

अथ चिकित्साकलिकातः

दृशि शिरसि च शङ्खश्रोत्रनेत्रान्तरेषु,

भ्रुवि[46] हृदि[47] हनुमन्यास्कन्धमूर्धादिसन्धौ ।

रुगति निशि दिवाऽल्पा स्यादकस्मात्[48] प्रशान्ति-

र्भवति हि भुजजङ्घास्तब्धसङ्कोचता च ॥५२॥

कटिविटपयकृत्सु क्लोम्नि च प्लीह्नि पृष्ठे,
जठरवृषणवक्षः – कुक्षिकक्षान्तरेषु ।
प्रसरति गुरुशूलं नाभिवस्तिस्तनेषु,
त्रिकगुदवलिगुह्योपान्तपक्षद्वयेषु ॥५३॥
वदनविरसता स्याद्वर्चसः कर्कशत्वं,
भवति वपुषि कार्श्यं रात्रिनिद्रानिवृत्तिः ।
त्वचि च परुषता स्यात् स्याच्च वैषम्यमग्ने-
रिति पवनविकारे लक्षणं प्रोक्तमेतत् ॥५४॥

[चिकित्साकलिका : ३४-३६]

According to Cikitsā Kalikā

The following signs nnd symptoms are manifested in diseases caused by the aggravation of *vāyu* :

1. Excessive pain in eyes, head, temporal region, ears, the space in between eyes, eye brows, cardiac region, jaw bone, sterno-mastoid region, shoulder, chest and such other joints. It gets aggravated during night and is reduced during day time. There is instantaneous remission of the pain;

2. Rigidity and contraction of hands and legs;

3. Spread of acute pain to *kaṭi* (lumber region), *viṭapa* (pelvic region), liver, *kloman*, spleen, back of the chest, abdomen, testicles, chest, lower abdomen, axillary region, umbilical region, region of the bladder, breasts, *trika* (lumbosacral joints), sphincters of the anus, sides of the anus, and both the sides of the chest;

4. Bad taste in mouth;

5. Dryness of the stool;

6. Emaciation of the body;
7. Sleeplessness during night;
8. Roughness of the skin; and
9. Irregularity of *agni* (power of digestion).

रुद्रकौतुकात्

शोषयित्वा रसादीनां सारं वायुर्महाबली[49] ।
दुष्टः श्लेष्मान्वितो वापि श्यावतां जनयेत् तनौ[50] ।
कषायत्वं मुखे कुर्यात् कृष्णत्वं च नखादिषु ॥५५॥

According to Rudra Kautuka

Vāyu which is very powerful, dries up the essence of *dhātus*, namely, rasa etc. Being vitiated and at times being associated with *kapha*, it produces *śyāvatā* (bluish stains along with roughness) in the body. There is astringent taste in the mouth and black colouration in nails etc.

भ्रम-मद-मुखशोष-स्वेद-संताप-मूर्छा-
मुख-नख-नयन-त्वक्-मूत्रविट्पीतताश्च ।
प्रलपनमतिसारश्चारुचिश्च ज्वरश्च
तृडतिशिशिरतेच्छा[51] पित्तरोगस्य चिह्नम् ॥५६॥

The signs and symptoms manifested in diseases caused by *pitta* are *bhrama* (giddiness), *mada* (feeling of intoxication), dryness of mouth, sweating, excessive heat in the body, fainting, yellow colouration of the face, nails, eyes, skin, urine and stool, delirium diarrhoea, anorexia, fever, excessive thirst and liking for cooling things.

अङ्गस्य गौरवमपाटवमन्तराग्ने-

रुत्क्लेशता च हृदयस्य मुखप्रसेकः

आलस्यमास्यमधुरत्वमकाण्डकण्डू-

रापाण्डुतानयनयोरतिलोमहर्षः ॥५७॥

52

प्रज्ञाप्लुतिर्वमथुपीनसकासनिद्रातन्द्रादयश्चुलुचुलायनमुल्वणं च ।

स्यादोष्ठकण्ठरसनारदमूलतालुघ्राणेक्षणश्रवणसष्कुलिकान्तरेषु ।

श्लेष्मोद्भवे भवति लिङ्गमिदंविकारे, संसर्गजेषु च गदेषु भवेद्द्विदोषम् ॥५८॥

[चिकित्साकलिका : ३७-४०]

The signs and symptoms that are manifested in diseases caused by *kapha* are heaviness of the body, suppression of the power of digestion, nausca, cardiac diseases, salivation, laziness, appearance of sweet taste in the mouth, itching over the body, paleness in the eyes, excessive horripilation, ineffectiveness of wisdom, vomiting, *pinasa* (chronic rhinitis), bronchitis, excessive sleep, drowsiness and tingling sensation in lips, throat, tongue, gums, pallet, nose, eyes, ears and ear-lobes.

In diseases caused by the vitiation of two *doṣas* (*saṁsargaja*), signs and symptoms of both the *doṣas* are manifested.

सुश्रुतः

सर्वैर्भावैस्त्रिभिर्वापि द्वाभ्यामेकेन वा[53] पुनः ।

संसर्गे कुपितः क्रुधं दोषं दोषोऽनुधावति[54] ॥५९॥

संसर्गे यो गरीयान् स्यादुपक्रम्यः स वै भवेत् ।

शेषदोषाविरोधेन सन्निपातेस्त्वयं विधिः[55] ॥६०॥

[सुश्रुत : सूत्र२१:३८-३९]

According to Suśruta

In *sannipātika* type of diseases, either of the three *doṣas* or two of them, or only one of them gets excessively aggravated. Other aggravated *doṣas* only play a secondary role. Therefore, in such diseases, the physician should take necessary steps for the alleviation of the excessively aggravated *doṣa* or *doṣas*. However, care should be taken so that the administered therapies do not further aggravate the remaining *doṣas*.

नास्ति रोगो विना दोषैर्यस्मात्तस्माद्विचक्षणः ।

अनुक्तमपि दोषाणां लिङ्गैर्व्याधिमुपाचरेत् ॥६१॥

[सुश्रुत : सूत्र३५:१९]

There is no disease in which aggravated *doṣas* do not play their role. Therefore, when the name of a disease is not described, the wise physician should treat it keeping in view the signs and symptoms manifested by these aggravated *doṣas*.

यत्र[56] दोषपरिज्ञानं[57] रोगः सम्यक् न दृश्यते ।

साधारणीं क्रियां तत्र भिषक् सम्यक्प्रयोजयेत् ॥६२॥

When the physician experiences any difficulty to clearly ascertain the disease and the *doṣas* which are aggravated, then he should appropriately administer moderate type of therapies.

अग्निवेशात्

रूक्षं शीतं लघु वायुं तैलं स्निग्धोष्णगौरवात् ।

शमयेत्, च तथा सर्पिः पित्तं तद्वच्च योजितम् ॥६३॥

According to Agniveśa

Vāyu is ununctuous, cold and light. *Taila* (gingili oil) is unctuous, hot and heavy for which it alleviates *vāyu*.

उष्णमस्वादु तीक्ष्णं च शैत्यमाधुर्यमार्दवात्,

स्निग्धं हि मधुरं मन्दं कफं तद्वज्जयेन्मधु ।

रौक्ष्यात् कषायभावाच्च तैक्ष्ण्यात्तद्वत् प्रयोजितम्[59] ॥६४॥

Pitta is hot, *asvādu* (not sweet in taste) and sharp. Ghee is cooling, sweet and soft, because of which it alleviates *pitta* when used.

Kapha is unctuous, sweet and *manda* (sluggish). Honey is ununctuous, astringent and sharp, because of which it alleviates *kapha*, when used.

[वातस्योपक्रमः]

वातस्योपक्रमः स्वेदः स्नेहः संशोधनं मृदु ।

स्वाद्वम्ललवणोष्णानि भेषजान्नानि[60] मर्दनम् ।

वेष्टनं त्रासनं सेको मद्यं पैष्टिकगौडिकम् ॥६५॥

[अष्टाङ्गहृदय : सूत्र१३:१-२]

स्निग्धोष्णा बस्तयो बस्तिनियमः सुखशीलता ।

दीपनैः पाचनैः सिद्धा स्नेहाश्चानेकयोनयः[61] ॥६६॥

विशेषान्मेद्यपिशितरसतैलानुवासनम्[62] ।

[अष्टाङ्गहृदय : सूत्र१३:२-३]

उपनाहावगाहश्च मांसं मांसरसं पयः ॥६७॥

Line of Treatment of Vāyu

For the treatment of *vāyu*, the following therapies should be administered :

1. Fomentation and oleation therapies;

2. Mild *saṁśodhana* (elimination) therapy;
3. Drugs and diet which are sweet, sour and saline in taste and which are hot;
4. Massage;
5. *Veṣṭana* (binding), *trāsana* (terrorising) and *seka* (sprinkling) therapies;
6. Alcohol prepared of *piṣṭa* (pastries) and *guḍa* (molasses);
7. Medicated enema, prepared of unctuous and hot drugs;
8. Regular intake of medicated enema;
9. Leisurely living;
10. Oil, ghee etc., collected from different sources and boiled with drugs which are *dīpana* (digestive stimulant) and *pācana* (carminative);
11. *Anuvāsana* type of medicated enema which is specifically prepared of oil and the soup of meat of animals which are fatty;
12. *Upanāha* (application of hot ointment) and *avagāha* (hot medicated bath); and
13. Meat, meat soup and milk.

[पित्तस्योपक्रमः]

पित्तस्य सर्पिषः पानं स्वादुशीतैर्विरेचनम् ।
स्वादुतिक्तकषायाणि भोजनान्यौषधानि च ॥६८॥

[अष्टाङ्गहृदय : सूत्र १३:४]

सुगन्धामलकैः स्नानं चन्द्रचन्दनलेपनम् ।
कण्ठे मुक्तादिरचितो हारिहारस्तथाधृतिः ॥६९॥

प्रदोषे चन्द्रमाः सौधं द्राक्षाखर्जूरसेवनम् ।
अयन्त्रणसुखं[63] मित्रं पुत्रः सस्निग्धमुग्धवाक् ॥७०॥
[64]स्वच्छन्दावर्तिनो दाराः कर्पूराभरणान्विताः ।
शीताम्बुधारागर्भाणि गृहाण्युद्यानदीर्घिकाः ॥७१॥
सुतीर्थविपुलस्वच्छसलिलाशयसैकते[65] ।
स्थितं पित्तविनाशार्थं कारयेत्सिद्धिवाञ्छया[66] ॥७२॥

Line of Treatment of Pitta

For the treatment of *pitta*, the following therapies should be administered:

1. Intake of ghee;
2. Purgation by drugs which are sweet and cooling;
3. Drugs and diet which are sweet, bitter and astringent;
4. Bath in *sugandhāmalaka*;
5. External application of camphor and sandalwood paste;
6. Wearing of ornaments in the neck prepared of pearl etc;
7. Patience;
8. Exposure in the early hours of the night to the moonrays on the roof of a building;
9. Intake of *drākṣā* and *kharjūra*;
10. Association with friends who are free and informal;
11. Talking to the son whose speech is pleasing and sweet;
12. Association with ladies who are informal and who have used camphor and ornaments;
13. Residence in cold house, house below the water, house

through which the stream of water flows and underground cellars;

14. Walk in parks and on the banks of lakes; and

15. Sitting in the sand by the side of a big pond which has well-formed banks and clean water.

साम्भोजजलतीरान्ते कायमाने द्रुमाकुले ।

67

सौम्या भावाः पयः सर्पिर्विरेकश्च विशेषतः ॥७३॥

[अष्टाङ्गहृदय : सूत्र१३:६]

The following regimens are specifically useful for the alleviation of *pitta* :

1. The bank of a lotus pond;
2. A park full of trees;
3. Pleasing gestures;
4. Milk and ghee; and
5. Purgation therapy.

[कफस्योपक्रमः]

तीक्ष्णैर्वमननस्याद्यैः लघुरूक्षैश्च भोजनैः ।

व्यायामोद्वर्त्तनाघातैर्धूमगण्डूषसेवनैः ॥७४॥

मेदोघ्नभेषजैः स्वेदैर्जयेत् श्लेष्माणमुल्वणं ।

पुराणयवगोधूमक्षौद्रजाङ्गलशाल्यभुक् ।

मद्यं पुरातनं सेव्यं दिवानिद्रां विवर्जयेत् ॥७५॥

Line of Treatment of Kapha

The following therapies are useful for the alleviation of *kapha* :

1. Administration of emetic and inhalation therapies with sharp drugs;
2. Intake of light and ununctuous food;
3. Exercise, unction, kneading, smoking, *gaṇḍūṣa* (medicated gargles);
4. Drugs which reduce fat;
5. Fomentation therapy;
6. Intake of old *yava*, *godhūma*, honey and meat of *jāṅgala* animals;
7. *Śalya* type of meat preparation;
8. Old alcoholic drinks; and
9. To avoid day sleep.

अथ चिकित्साकलिकायाम्[68]

स्निग्धोष्णस्थिर-बल्य-वृष्य-लवण-स्वाद्वम्ल-तैलातप-
स्नानाभ्यञ्जन-बस्ति-मांसमदिरा-संवाहनोन्मर्दनम् ।
स्नेह-स्वेद-निरुहणानि[59] शयन-स्थानोपनाहादिकं ।
पानाहार-विहार-भेषजमिदं वातं प्रशान्तिं नयेत् ॥७६॥

[योगशतक ११५]

According to Cikitsā kalikā

Drinks, diet, regimens and medicines which are unctuous, hot, subtle, aphrodisiac, strength promoting, saline, sweet and sour, oils, exposure to sun, bath, massage, enema, meat, wine, *saṁvāhana* (kneading the body), *unmardana* (unction), oleation, sudation, *nirūha* type of enema, inhalation therapy, sleep, taking rest, application of hot ointments etc., alleviate *vāta*.

अत्र बस्तिः स्नेहबस्तिः । स्थानं स्थितिः ॥७७॥

The term *basti* in the present context, implies unctuous type of medicated enema. The term *sthāna* means residence.

तिक्त-स्वादु-कषाय-शीतपवन-च्छाया-निशा-वीजनं[70] ।

ज्योत्स्ना-भूगृह-यन्त्रवारि-जलदस्त्रीगात्रसंस्पर्शनम् ॥७८॥

सर्पिः[71]-क्षीर-विरेक-सेक-रुधिरस्राव-प्रलेपादिकं ।

पानाहार-विहार-भेषजमिदं पित्तं प्रशान्तिं नयेत्[72] ॥७९॥

[योगशतक ११६]

Drinks, diet, regimens and medicines which are bitter, sweet and astringent, cold wind, shade, night, water, moon rays, underground residence, fountain, lotus, embracing (touch) of the body of females, ghee, milk, purgation, sprinkling of water, blood letting anointment etc., alleviate *pitta*.

रूक्ष-क्षार-कषाय-तिक्त-कटुक-व्यायाम-निष्ठीवनं ।

स्त्री-सेवाध्वनियुद्ध[73]-जागर-जलक्रीडा-पदाघातनम् ॥८०॥

धूमात्युष्ण[74]-शिरोविरेक-वमनं स्वेदोपवासादिकं[75] ।

पानाहार-विहार-भेषजमिदं श्लेष्माणमुग्रं जयेत् ॥८१॥

[योगशतक ११७]

Drinks, diet, regimens, and medicines which are rough, alkaline, astringent, bitter and pungent, exercise, spitting (therapy), sexual indulgence, walking, fighting, remaining awake, aquatic games, *pādāghāta* (putting pressure on different parts of the body through feet), smoking, exposure to heat (sun rays), errhine therapy, emetic therapy, fomentation, *upanāha* (application of hot ointments) etc., alleviate the aggravated *kapha*.

वाग्भटात्

तत्राद्या मारुतं घ्नन्ति त्रयस्तिक्तादयः कफम् ।
कषायतिक्तमधुराः पित्तमन्ये च कुर्वते[76] ॥८२॥

[अष्टाङ्गहृदय : सूत्र१:१५-१६]

According to Vāgbhaṭa

Drugs which are sweet, sour and saline, alleviate *vāyu*. Drugs which are bitter, pungent and astringent alleviate *kapha*. *Pitta* gets alleviated by drugs which are astringent, bitter and sweet in taste. Remaining tastes (which are not alleviaters) aggravate the concerned *doṣas*.

[77] संसृष्टदोषेषु सदा ज्ञात्वा तरतमं बुधः ।
चिकित्सां कारयेद्वैद्यः कालावस्थादिभागवित् ॥८३॥

When there is a combination of vitiated *doṣas*, the physician should first of all determine which one is more aggravated and which one is less. Thereafter, he should initiate treatment keeping in view the time, as well as the state of the *doṣas* (including the stage of the disease).

खरनादात्

विशेषविधिः रोगाणां दोषास्तरतमात्मकाः ।
तरो द्वन्द्वप्रकर्षेषु तमो बहुषु चोच्यते ॥८४॥

According to Kharanāda

In a disease when many *doṣas* are vitiated, then the one more vitiated among the two, is called *vṛddhatara*. When there are three *doṣas* involved, then the one which is most vitiated among the three is called *vṛddhatama.*

जैज्जटः

कफपित्तप्रकोपे नस्य-वमन-विरेचनानि

पित्तवातप्रकोपे तु रेचनं बस्तिकर्म च[78] ॥८५॥

कफवातप्रकोपे हि वमननस्यबस्तयः ।

सन्निपातेऽमूनि[79] सर्वाणि यथा योग्यं प्रयोजयेत् ॥८६॥

According to Jejjaṭa

If there is aggravation of *kapha* and *pitta*, then the patient should be given inhalation, emetic and purgation therapies. If both *pitta* and *vāta* are aggravated, then purgation and medicated enema therapies should be administered. If, however, both *kapha* and *vāta* are aggravated, then emetic, inhalation and medicated enema therapies should be administered to the patient. In *sannipāta* when all the three *doṣas* are aggravated, all these therapies can be appropriately administered.

[सामनिरामलक्षणानि]

तत्र, अवस्था द्विविधा लोके प्रोक्ता तत्त्वार्थवेदिभिः ।

निरामा वाथ सामा च तयोर्लक्षणमुच्यते ॥८७॥

Sāma and Nirāma

Physicians who are proficient in the science of medicine describe two stages of the disease, namely, *nirāma* (free from *āma*) and *sāma* (association with *āma*). Their signs and symptoms are described below.

[निराममलरुजा]

भुक्ते जीर्यति जीर्णेऽन्ने जीर्णे भुक्ते तु जीर्यति ।

जीर्णे जीर्यति भुक्ते च दोषैर्नाल्पातिरुक् क्रमात् ॥८८॥

एवं क्रमेण विज्ञेया निराममलजारुजा ।

80
एतस्मिन्विपरीते तु सामा ज्ञेया रुजा बुधैः ॥८९॥

Signs and Symptoms of Nirāma Mala

If there is no association of *āma* along with aggravated *vāyu*, then there will be no pain at the time of intake of food; there will be less of pain at the time of digestion of food, and there will be more of pain after the digestion of food. If there is no association of *āma* along with vitiated *pitta*, then there will be no pain after the digestion of food; there will be less of pain at the time of intake of food, and there will be more of pain during the digestion of food. If there is no association of *āma*, along with vitiated *kapha*, then there will be no pain after digestion of food; there will be less of pain at the time of digestion of food and there will be more of pain immediately after taking food. If pain occurs in the reverse order, then the wise physician should know that it is caused because of the association of *āma*.

[आमलक्षणम्]

ऊष्मणोऽल्पबलत्वेन धातुमाद्यमपाचितम् ।

दुष्टमामाशयगतं रसमामं प्रचक्षते ॥९०॥

Description of āma

If the power of *ūṣmā* (factors responsible for digestion and metabolism) is subdued then the first *dhātu* namely, *rasa* (plasma and chyle) does not get properly digested. Being vitiated, this *rasa* enters into *āmāśaya* (stomach including small intestine) which is called *āma*.

81
अन्ये दोषेभ्य एवातिदुष्टेभ्योऽन्योन्यमूर्च्छनात् ।

कोद्रवेभ्यो विषस्येव वदन्त्यामस्य सम्भवम् ॥९१॥

According to some other scholars, *āma* is produced as a result of *mūrchanā* (inter-action) among the excessively vitiated *doṣas* (one with the other). This is on the analogy of the production of poison by (fermented) *kodrava*.

आमेन तेन सम्पृक्ता दोषा दूष्याश्च दूषिताः ।

सामा इत्युपदिश्यन्ते ये च रोगास्तदुद्भवाः ॥६२॥

[अष्टाङ्गहृदय : सूत्र१३:२५-२७]

When the vitiated *doṣas* and *dūṣyas* (tissue elements) get associated with this *āma*, they are called *sāma* (associated with *āma*) The diseases produced by such vitiated *doṣas* and *dūṣyas* having association with *āma* are also called *sāma*.

स्रोतोरोधो बलभ्रंशगौरवारुचिमूढताः[82] ।

आलस्यापक्ति-निष्ठीव-मलसङ्गारुचिक्लमाः. ॥६३॥

विण्मूत्रनखदन्तानां[83] नेत्रयोः पीतता भवेत्[84] ।

[रक्तत्वमथ कृष्णत्वं पृष्ठास्थिकटिसन्धिरुक् ॥६४॥][85]

शिरोरुग्जायते तन्द्रा पृष्ठास्थिकटिसन्धिरुक् ।

[क्वचिच्च श्वयथुर्गात्रे ज्वरातीसारहर्षणम् ॥६५॥][86]

वैवर्ण्यं मुखवैरस्यं क्षवथुर्जायते क्वचित् ।

लिङ्गं मलानां सामानां, निरामाणां विपर्ययः ॥६६॥

[अष्टाङ्गहृदय : सूत्र१३:२३-२४]

Signs and Symptoms of Sāma doṣa

If *āma* is associated with the *malas* (*doṣas*) then the following signs and symptoms are manifested :

1. *Sroto rodha* (obstruction to the channels of circulation);

2. *Bala bhraṁśa* (diminution of strength);
3. Heaviness, anorexia, dumbness, *mūḍhatā* (absence of any movement of the *vāyu*) and laziness;
4. Indigestion and spitting (salivation);
5. Obstruction to the passage of stool and urine;
6. *Aruci* (anorexia);
7. *Klama* (a feeling of fatigue without effort;
8. Yellow colouration of stool, urine, nail, teeth and eyes;
9. Red or black colouration of the above organs;
10. Headache;
11. Drowsiness;
12. Pain in back, bone, lumber region and joints;
13. Occasional appearance of oedema in the body;
14. Fever and diarrhoea;
15. Tingling sensation;
16. Discolouration;
17. Absence of any taste in the mouth; and
18. Sneezing.

If the above symptoms are not manifested, then the physician should know that the *doṣas* are not associated with *āma*.

आलस्य-तन्द्रा-हृदय-अविशुद्धि-दोष-अप्रवृत्ति[87]-आकुल[88]-मूत्रताभिः ।
गुरु[89]-उदरत्व-अरुचि-सुप्तताभिरामान्वितं व्याधिं उदाहरन्ति ॥९७॥

[योगशतक ११४]

Laziness, drowsiness, *hṛdaya aviśuddhi* (a subjective feeling as if there is an impairment in the functioning of the heart), non-excretion of *doṣas*, changes in the colour (muddy colour) of the urine, heaviness in the stomach, anorexia and numbness are the examples of the association of *āma* with the disease.

दोषः पुरीषम्, आकुलमूत्रता अप्रसन्नमूत्रता ॥९८॥

The term '*doṣa*' used in the above paragraph implies in the present context, 'stool'. When the urine is not transparent, it is called *ākula mūtra*.

[सामवायुलक्षणम्]

90

वायुः सामो विबन्धाग्निसादतन्द्रान्त्रकूजनैः ।

वेदनाशोफनिस्तोदैः क्रमशोऽङ्गानि पीडयेत् ॥९९॥

[अष्टाङ्गहृदय : सूत्र १३:२७]

विचरेद्युगपच्चापि गृह्णाति कुपितो भृशम् ।

91

स्नेहाद्यैर्वृद्धिमायाति मेघ सूर्योदये निशि ॥१००॥

Signs and Symptoms of Sāma Vāyu

When *vāyu* is associated with *āma*, it causes *vibandha* (constipation), *agni sāda* (suppression of the power of digestion), *tandrā* (drowsiness), *antra kūjana* (gargling sound in the intestines), *vedanā* (pain), *śopha* (oedema) and *nistoda* (excruciating pain). Thus, it gradually afflicts all the organs of the body. It moves all over the body, and being aggravated, afflicts the entire body. This condition gets aggravated by the administration of ghee etc. It is also aggravated during the onset of cloud, rising of the sun and at night.

निरामवायुलक्षणम्

निरामो विशदो रूक्षो निर्विबन्धोऽल्पवेदनः ।

विपरीतगुणैः शान्ति स्निग्धैर्याति विशेषतः ॥१०१॥

Signs and Symptoms of Nirāma vāyu

When the vitiated *vāyu* is not associated with *āma* then it is *viśada* (non-slimy) and ununctuous. It does not cause any obstruction. It produces less of pain. It gets alleviated by substances having properties opposite to it. It gets alleviated specially by the administration of *sneha* (unctuous substances like oil, ghee, muscle fat and bone marrow).

[सामपित्तलक्षणम्]

दुर्गन्धि हरितं श्यावं पित्तमम्लं घनं गुरु ।
अम्लीकाकण्ठहृद्दाहकरं सामं[92] विनिर्दिशेत् ॥१०२॥

Signs and Symptoms of Sāma Pitta

When vitiated *pitta* is associated with *āma*, it produces foul smell. It is green or *śyāva* (greenish grey) in colour. It becomes sour, dense and heavy. It produces acidity and burning sensation in the throat and cardiac region.

[निरामपित्तलक्षणम्]

आताम्रपीतमत्युष्णं रसे कटुकमस्थिरम् ।
पक्वं विगन्धि विज्ञेयं रुचिपक्तिबलप्रदम् ॥१०३॥

Signs and Symptoms of Nirāma Pitta

When the *pitta* is not associated with *āma*, it is coppery or yellow in colour. It is excessively hot and pungent in taste. It is unstable. When it undergoes *pāka* (reaction by enzymes), it produces foul smell. It causes *ruci* (relish or appetite), *pakti* (digestion) and *bala* (strength).

[सामकफलक्षणम्]

आविलस्तन्तुलः स्त्यानः कण्ठदेशे[93] प्रतिष्ठते ।
सामो बलासो दुर्गन्धक्षुधोद्गारविघातकृत्[94] ॥१०४॥

Signs and Symptoms of Sāma Kapha

When *kapha* is associated with *āma*, it is turbid, thready and dense. It remains in the throat region. It produces foul smell. It suppresses appetite and eructation.

[निरामकफलक्षणम्]

फेनवान् पिण्डितः पाण्डुनिःसारोऽगन्ध एव च ।

[95]

पक्वः कफः स विज्ञेयः क्लेदवान् वक्त्रशुद्धिकृत् ॥१०५॥

[अष्टाङ्गहृदय : सूत्र१३:२७]

Signs and Symptoms of Nirāma Kapha

Kapha which is not associated with *āma* is foamy, compact, yellowish-white in colour and *niḥsāra* (without any sticky material). It is free from any bad smell. If it is moist and if it produces cleanliness in the mouth then it should be determined that it has undergone *pāka* (enzymatic action).

[सामदोषचिकित्सोपक्रमम्]

पाचनैर्दीपनैर्द्रव्यै — रुक्षस्वेदैर्विरेचनैः ।

[96]

वमनैः प्रतिमर्शैश्च लङ्घनैश्चोपचारयेत् ॥१०६॥

Line of Treatment of Sāma Doṣa

When *doṣas* are associated with *āma*, then the following therapies should be administered :

1. Drugs which are *pācana* (carminative) and *dipana* (digestive stimulants);
2. Ununctuous fomentation;
3. Purgation by ununctuous drugs;
4. *Vamana* (emetic therapy);

5. *Pratimarśa* (a type of inhalation therapy); and

6. *Laṅghana* (fasting).

[रोगाधिष्ठानम्]

कुपितानां च[97] दोषाणां शरीरे परिधावताम् ।

यत्र सङ्गः खवैगुण्याद्[98] व्याधिस्तत्रैव जायते[99] ॥१०७॥

[सुश्रुत : सूत्र२४:१०]

Site of Manifestation of the Disease

The vitiated *doṣas* while circulating all over the body, get obstructed (lodged) in a particular place because of the vitiation of the channel of circulation in that particular organ. This is the site of manifestation of the disease.

कृत्स्नेऽर्धेऽवयवे चापि[100] यत्राङ्गे[101] कुपितो भृशम् ।

दोषो विकारं नभसि मेघवत्तत्र वर्षति ॥१०८॥

[सुश्रुत : सूत्र२१:२६]

The excessively aggravated *doṣas* may get lodged either in the whole body or in half of it, and there, they cause the disease on the analogy of the rain in a particular place by the cloud in the sky.

यत्रस्थमामं विरुजेत्तमेव देशं विशेषेण विकारजातैः ।

दोषेण येनावततं शरीरं[102] तल्लक्षणैरामसमुद्भवैश्च ॥१०९॥

[सुश्रुत : उत्तरतन्त्र५६:१०]

The vitiated *doṣas* afflict a particular organ in which there is *āma* formation, and then, in this organ the diseases are manifested. By the signs and symptoms of these vitiated *doṣas* along with those of *āma*, that part of the body gets afflicted.

[दोषाणां व्याधिकारकत्वम्]

वाग्भटः

रसादिस्थेषु दोषेषु व्याधयः संभवन्ति ये ।
तज्जानित्युपचारेण तानाहुर्घृतदग्धवत् ॥११०॥

[अष्टाङ्गसंग्रह : सूत्र१:३२]

Doṣas as the Causative Factors of Disease

According to Vāgbhaṭa

The aggravated *doṣas* cause disease by afflicting the tissue element namely, *rasa* etc. Such diseases are at times described as *rasaja* etc. only in a secondary sense. This is on the analogy of a burn (scald) by hot ghee. [It is not the ghee which is responsible for the scald, but it is the heat inside the ghee which is responsible for this; but in usage it is generally said as "a scald by he ghee."]

सुश्रुतात्

दोषः प्रकुपितो धातून् क्षपयत्यात्मतेजसा ।
इद्धः स्वतेजसा वह्निरुखागतमिवोदकम् ॥१११॥

[सुश्रुत : सूत्र१५:३६]

According to Suśruta

The aggravated *doṣas* afflict the *dhātus* by its own *tejas* (power or *agni* or enzyme). It gets further aggravated by the association of the *agni* (enzyme) which is present in the *dhātus* to produce a disease. This is on the analogy of the water in a plate. When additional water is added to the plate full of water, then it overflows or becomes more in quantity.

पाराशरात्

द्रव्यस्यैकरसो नास्ति न रोगे[ऽ]प्येकदोषजः ।

एकः प्रकुपितो दोषस्त्वपरं दूषयेच्च सः ॥११२॥

अन्यस्थानगतं दोषं स्थानिवत्समुपाचरेत् ।

अथवा स्थानिवच्चात्र दोषं स्वस्थं प्रकल्पयेत्[103] ॥११३॥

According to Parāśara

There is no drug which has only one taste. There is no disease which is caused by the aggravation of only one *doṣa*. When one *doṣa* is aggravated it does aggravate to some extent, the other *doṣas* while producing a disease. When an aggravated *doṣa* is in the place of another *doṣa*, then the former should be treated on the lines prescribed for the latter. In other words, when a *doṣa* migrates to the place of another *doṣa*, then the former should be treated on the lines prescribed for the latter.

सुश्रुतः

विभुत्वादाशुकारित्वात् स्वातन्त्र्यादन्यकोपनात्[104] ।

सर्वत्रगमनाच्चापि[105] दोषाणां पवनो बली[106] ॥११४॥

[अष्टाङ्गहृदय : शरीर३:८४]

According to Suśruta

Among the *doṣas*, *vāyu* is the most powerful because of the following :

1. It is present all over the body;

2. It manifests its actions instantaneously;

3. It acts independent of other *doṣas*;

4. It has the power to vitiate the remaining *doṣas*; and

5. It has the ability to penetrate into all the parts of the body.

यथा महानुदकसंचयोऽतिवृद्धः सेतुमवदार्यापरेणोदकेन संमिश्रम् सर्वतोधावति, एवं

दोषाः कदाचिदेकशो द्विशः समस्ता रसादिसहिताश्चानेकधा प्रसरन्ति ॥११५॥

तत्र वायोः पित्तस्थानगतस्य पित्तवत्प्रतीकारः ॥११६॥

पित्तस्य कफस्थानगतस्य कफवत्। कफस्य वातस्थानगतस्य वातवत् ॥११७॥

[सुश्रुत : सूत्र२१:२८-३१]

For example when a lake having large quantity of water is added with more water, then because of the increase in the quantity, the dam gives way. The water from the lake then flows and gets mixed with the water of adjacent lakes and runs in all directions. Similarly, when *doṣas*—either one or two or all the three ofthem-get mixed up with *rasa* etc., then because of this, they afflict several different organs of the body. When *vāyu* migrates to the location of *pitta*, then the line of treatment prescribed for the latter should be adopted for the former. When *pitta* migrates to the place of *kapha*, then the treatment of the patient should be done on the line of treatment suggested for aggravated *kapha*. When *kapha* migrates to the place of *vāyu*, then the line of treatment suggested for *vāyu* should be adopted.

तद्यथा

107

वातोपसृष्टे हृदये वामयेत्स्निग्धमातुरम् ।

आमाशयगते वाते वमनं कारयेद्भिषक् ॥११८॥

कफस्थानत्वात् ॥११९॥

For example

If the heart is afflicted by *vāyu,* then the patient should be administered emetic therapy with unctuous drugs. If *vāyu* migrates to *āmāśaya* (the location of *kapha*) then the physician should administer ordinary emetic therapy.

अतो[ऽ]न्यथापि दृश्येत पाददाहादिषु क्रिया ।

पित्तासृक्सहितो वायुः पाददाहं करोति वै ।

कुर्यादसृक्पित्तहरां क्रियां तत्र सुखप्रदाम् ॥१२०॥

एवं बहुविधावस्था रोगाणां जायते किल ।

तेषां प्रशमनार्थाय परं यत्नं समाचरेत् ॥१२१॥

There are, however, exceptions to this general rule. For example, *pāda dāha* (burning syndrome in the sole of feet) is caused by *vāyu* along with *pitta* and *rakta.* For the treatment of this disease, therapics which alleviate *rakta* and *pitta* are administered. Many similar types of conditions appear in diseases. For the treatment of such diseases, the physician should take proper care.

स्थानबलः ॥

Thus, ends the importance or significance of the location of the *doṣas* for the treatment of diseases.

[रक्तस्य प्रकोपकालम्]

यस्माद्रक्तं विनादोषैर्न कदाचित् प्रकुप्यति ।

तस्मात्तस्य यथादोषं कालं विद्यात् प्रकोपणे ॥१२२॥

Time of Aggravation of Rakta

Rakta does not get vitiated without its association with an aggravated *doṣa.* Therefore, its time of vitiation should be determined on the basis of time of aggravation of the *doṣa* by which it is afflicted.

दोषवेदनालक्षणम्

सुश्रुतात्

तोदनभेदनताडनच्छेदनायामन-मंथन-[108]विच्छेदनचुमुचुमायन-निर्दहनाव[109]भञ्जनस्फोटन-

विदारणोत्पाटनकम्पनविविधशूलविश्लेषण-विकिरणस्तम्भनपूरणस्वप्नाकुञ्चनाङ्कु-

[110]शिकादयः संभवन्ति, अनिमित्त-विविधवेदनाप्रादुर्भावो वा मुहुर्मुहुर्यत्रागच्छन्ति

वेदनाविशेषास्तं वातिकमिति ॥१२३॥

Different Types of Pain According to Suśruta

Characteristic features of the pain caused by aggravated *vāyu* are as follows :

1. *Todana* (the pain as if pierced by a needle);
2. *Bhedana* (pain as if the skin is excised);
3. *Tāḍana* (the pain as if the organ is beaten by a staff);
4. *Chedana* (the pain as if the organ is cut by a weapon or by incision);
5. *Āyāmana* (the pain caused by the extension of a contracted organ):
6. *Manthana* (the pain as if caused by churning of the inside of an ulcer);
7. *Vicchedana* (the pain caused when something thrown out);

8. *Cumucumāyana* (the pain that is caused by application of the paste of *sarṣapa, rājikā* etc.);

9. *Nirdahana* (the pain as if caused by complete burning of the organ);

10. *Bhañjana* (breaking pain);

11. *Sphoṭana* (the pain as if caused by striking of a stone);

12. *Vidāraṇa* (the pain as if caused by incision through nail etc.)

13. *Utpāṭana* (the pain as if caused by pulling out something from the body);

14. *Kampana* (the pain associated with shivering);

15. Different types of *śūla* (colic pain as if pierced by sharp pointed weapon);

16. *Viśleṣaṇa* (pain of dislocation);

17. *Vikiraṇa* (the pain as if the surface of the ulcer is breaking at different places);

18. *Stambhana* (the pain as if caused by arrest of movement);

19. *Pūraṇa* (the pain as if something is filled up by the application of force);

20. *Svapana* (numbness);

21. *Ākuñcana* (the pain that is caused by the folding of an organ from several places);

22. *Aṅkuśikā* (the pain that is caused when a part of the organ is pierced by *aṅṅkuśa* or a sharp rounded weapon);

23. Appearance of different types of pain without any perceptible cause; and

24. Frequent appearance of the pain.

ओषचोषपरिदाहधूमायनानि यत्र गात्रमङ्गारावकीर्णमिव पच्यते । यत्रोष्माभिवृद्धिः क्षते क्षारावसिक्तवच्च वेदनाविशेषास्तं पैत्तिकमिति विद्यात् ।।१२४।।

Characteristic features of the pain caused by vitiated *pitta* are as follows :

1. *Oṣa* (burning sensation in a part of the organ);
2. *Coṣa* (the pain as if something is being sucked);
3. *Paridāha* (burning sensation all over the body);
4. *Dhūmāyana* (pain as if hot smoke is coming out of the body);
5. The pain as if the entire body is covered with hot charcoal and cooked;
6. Increase in the temperature; and
7. The painful feeling as if alkalies are spread over an ulcer.

111

कण्डूर्गुरुत्वमुपदेहोल्पवेदनत्वं स्तम्भः शैत्यं यत्र यत्र तं श्लैष्मिकमिति विद्यात् ।।१२५।।

[सुश्रुत : सूत्र२२:११]

The pain caused by the vitiation of *kapha* has the following characteristics :

1. Itching;
2. Heaviness;
3. The feeling as if something is applied externally;
4. Less of pain;

5. Rigidity; and
6. Cold in touch.

इति दोषलक्षणम् ॥१२६॥

Thus, ends the signs and symptoms of different types of *doṣas*.

[मलादीनां कार्यम्]

आत्रेयात्

शकृदुपष्टम्भकरं बलाग्नेर्धारणं परम् ।
बस्तिपूरणकृन्मूत्रं स्वेदः क्लेदयते तनुम् ॥१२७॥
अङ्गप्रसादजननमार्त्तवं गर्भकर्मकृत् ।
स्तन्यं च स्तनयोः पीनजननं जीवनं परम् ॥१२८॥

Functions of Malas (excreta)

According to Ātreya

Śakṛt (feces) causes *upaṣṭambha* (a sense of compactness of the body). It is an excellent agent for the sustenance of *bala* (strength) and *agni* (factors responsible for digestion and metabolism).

Mūtra (urine) fills up the bladder.

Sveda (sweat) gives stickiness to the body.

Ārtava (menstrual blood) promotes excellence of the organs of the body. It is also responsible for conception.

Stanya (breast milk) causes plumpness of the breasts. It is an excellent life giver.

तेषां क्षयमाह

शोधनस्यातियोगेन वेगोदीरणधारणात् ।
व्यायामाध्वमनस्तापात्तेषां संजायते क्षयः ॥१२९॥

Signs and Symptoms of the Diminution of Doṣas

Quantity of *doṣas* get diminished by the following :

1. Excessive administration of the elimination therapies;
2. Suppression of the manifested urges;
3. Improper exercise;
4. Excessive walking; and
5. Mental worry.

अप्रहर्षो[ऽ]ल्पवाङ्मोहो मूढसंज्ञाविचेष्टता ।
वातक्षये, तथा पित्तक्षये मन्दोष्मता भवेत् ॥१३०॥[112]
अग्निनाशः प्रभाहानिस्तथा श्लेष्मक्षये शृणु ।
अन्तर्दाहो रूक्षता च पक्वामाशयशून्यता ॥१३१॥
विश्लेषाश्चैव सन्धीनां कुर्यात्तत्र क्रियामिमाम् ।
स्वयोनिवर्धनद्रव्यैरन्नपानैरुपाचरेत् ॥१३२॥

The signs and symptoms of the diminution of *vāyu* are as follows :

1. Absence of excitement;
2. Less of speech;
3. Unconsciousness;
4. Absence of sensation; and
5. Irregular movement of the limbs.

The signs and symptoms of the diminution of *pitta* are as follows :

1. Less of temperature;

2. Absence of power of digestion and metabolism; and
3. Loss of lustre.

The signs and symptoms of diminished *kapha* are as follows :

1. *Antardāha* (burning sensation inside the body);
2. Ununctuousness;
3. A feeling of emptiness in *pakvāśaya* (colon) and *āmāśaya* (stomach including small intestine); and
4. Looseness of the joints.

In the above circumstances, drugs, diet and drinks which are responsible for the increase of these *doṣas* should be administered.

धातुक्षयलिङ्गमाह

सुश्रुतात्

रसक्षये तु हृत्पीडा कण्ठशोषश्च शून्यता ।
तृष्णा चातिभवेत्तत्र, शोणितस्य क्षये शृणु ।
त्वक्पारुष्यं सिरादीनां शैथिल्यं चात्र लक्षणम् ॥१३३॥

Signs and Symptoms of the Diminution of Dhātus

According to Suśruta

The following signs and symptoms are manifested by the diminution of *rasa* :

1. Pain in cardiac region;
2. Dryness of the throat;
3. Feeling of emptiness; and
4. Excessive thirst.

Signs and symptoms of the diminution of *śoṇita* (hemoglobin fraction of the blood) are as follows :

1. Roughness of the skin; and
2. Looseness of veins etc.

उरुवंक्षणकक्षासु स्फिगोष्ठोपस्थगण्डयोः ।

शुष्कता रौक्ष्यतोदौ च शैथिल्यं पिशितक्षये ॥१३४॥

The signs and symptoms of the diminution of *māṁsa* (muscle tissue) are as follows :

Dryness or emaciation, roughness, pain and looseness in thighs, hip-joint, axilla, buttock, lips, genital organ and mandibular eminence in the face.

प्लीहाभिवृद्धि सन्धेश्च शून्यता रौक्ष्यमेव च ।

मेदुरे पिशिते वाञ्छा भवेन्मेदः क्षयान्नृणाम् ॥१३५॥

The signs and symptoms produced by the diminution of *medas* (fat) are as follows :

1. Enlargements of the spleen;
2. Emptiness of the joints;
3. Roughness; and
4. Desire for taking meat of fatty animals.

113

अस्थिक्षयेऽस्थिशूलं च भङ्गः स्यान्नखदन्तयोः ।

मज्जक्षयेऽल्पशुक्रत्वं पर्वभेदोऽस्थिशून्यरुक् ॥१३६॥

The signs and symptoms of the diminution of *asthi* (bone tissue) are as follows :

1. Pain in the bones; and

2. Cracking of the nails and teeth.

The signs and symptoms of the diminution of majjā (bone marrow) are as follows :

1. Diminution of the quantity of semen;

2. Breaking pain in phalanges;

3. The feeling of emptiness in the bones; and

4. Pain in bones.

शुक्रक्षये वेदना च मेढ्रे वृषणयोस्तथा ।
अशक्तिर्मैथुने चापि चिराद्वाल्पं प्रसिच्यते ।
प्रसेके चाल्पशुक्रस्य दर्शनं शोणितस्य वा ॥१३७॥

The signs and symptoms of the diminution of *śukra* (semen) are as follows :

1. Pain in the genital organ;

2. Pain in the testicles;

3. Inability in the performance of sexual act;

4. Ejaculation of semen after a long time;

5. Ejaculation of small quantity of semen; and

6. Ejaculation of blood along with the semen which is in small quantity.

हृत्पार्श्वयोः प्रपीडा च वायोः शब्दयुतस्य च ।
भवेच्चोर्ध्वगतिः कुक्षौ विचरेत् विड्क्षये ध्रुवम् ॥१३८॥

The signs and symptoms of the diminution of *viṭ* (feces) are as follows :

1. Pain in cardiac region and the sides of the chest;

2. Ejaculation of flatus with sound; and

3. Upward movement of the wind from the lower abdomen.

मूत्रक्षये बस्तितोदस्तथा मूत्राल्पता भवेत् ।

स्तब्धता रोमकूपेषु त्वक्पारुष्यं तथैव च ॥१३९॥

The signs and symptoms of the diminution of *mūtra* (urine) are as follows :

1. Pain in the urinary bladder; and

2. Elimination of less quantity of urine.

स्नेहादिनां प्रलिप्ते च तत्क्षणं शोषता भवेत् ।

स्वेदस्य नाशः स्पर्शस्य रौक्ष्यं स्वेदक्षये भवेत् ॥१४०॥

The signs and symptoms of the diminution of *sveda* (sweat) are as follows :

1. Numbness in hair follicles;

2. Roughness of the skin;

3. If unctuous substances are applied in the form of ointment then they get dried up immediately;

4. Absence of sweating, and

5. Roughness in touch.

योनेस्तु वेदना पुष्पकालादर्शनमल्पता ।

क्षीणार्तवेषु जानीयाल्लक्षणं चात्र निश्चयम् ॥१४१॥

The signs and symptoms of the diminution of *ārtava* (menstrual blood) are as follows :

1. Pain in the female genital organ;

2. Absence of any bleeding during the period of menstruation; and

3. Less amount of bleeding during menstrual period.

स्तनयोर्म्लानता[114] स्तन्यस्याभावश्चाल्पमेव[115] च ॥१४२॥

The signs and symptoms of the diminution of *stanya* (breast milk) are as follows :

1. Looseness of the breasts;

2. Absence of lactation; and

3. Less of lactation.

[दोषधातुमलक्षयोपक्रमम्]

दोषधातुमलक्षीणो बलक्षीणोऽपि मानवः[116] ।

स्वयोनिवर्धनं भोक्तु[117]मन्नपाने प्रकाङ्क्षते ॥१४३॥

यद्यदाहारजातं तु क्षीणः प्रार्थयते नरः ।

तस्य तस्य स लाभे तु तं तं क्षयमपोहति ॥१४४॥

Line of Treatment of the Diminution of Doṣas etc.

A person, in whom *doṣas*, *dhātus*, *malas* (excreta) and *bala* (strength) are diminished, desires to take such diet and drinks which are responsible for the increase in the quantity of these elements. If the patient gets the desired diet and drinks, then this helps in overcoming the diminution of the respective elements.

यस्य धातुक्षयाद्वायुः संज्ञां कर्म च नाशयेत् ।

प्रक्षीणं च बलं यस्य नासौ शक्यः चिकित्सितुम् ॥१४५॥

[सुश्रुत : सूत्र१५:२९-३१]

If by the diminution of *dhātus*, the vitiated *vāyu* destroys the sensory and motor functions, and if the patient has become exceedingly weak, then the treatment of such persons is impossible.

[धातुषु दोषस्थानत्वम्]

[वाग्भटात्]

तत्रास्थनि स्थितो वायुः, पित्तं तु स्वेदरक्तयोः ।

श्लेष्मा शेषेषु तेनैषामाश्रयाश्रयिणां मिथः [118] ॥१४६॥

Location of Doṣas in the Dhātus

According to Vāgbhaṭa

Vāyu is located in the bones. *Pitta* is located in *sveda* (sweat) and *rakta* (hemoglobin fraction of the blood). *Śleṣman* is located in the remaining *dhātus* and *malas*. These *doṣas* and *dhātus* including *malas* are mutually dependant on each other.

यदेकस्य तदन्यस्य वर्धनं क्षपणौषधम् ।

अस्थिमारुतयोर्न्नैवं, प्रायो वृद्धिर्हि तर्पणात् ॥१४७॥

[अष्टाङ्गहृदय : सूत्र ११:२६-२७]

Factors which are responsible for the aggravation and diminution of the *doṣas* respectively increase and decrease, the quantity of *dhātus*, including *malas* in which these particular *doṣas* are located. The *asthi dhātu* and the *doṣa* which is located in it namely, *vāyu*, are however, exceptions to this rule. *Asthi dhātu* gets increased in quantity by *tarpaṇa* (nourishing therapy) which reduces the quantity of *vāyu*.

अथ डल्हणः

यवमुद्गहरेणुश्च रूक्षं च लघुभोजनम् ।

कषायकटुतिक्तं च वातक्षीणोऽभिकाङ्क्षति ॥१४८॥

[डल्हण१५:२९]

According to Dalhaṇa

A patient having diminution of *vāyu* desires to take *yava*, *mudga*, *hareṇu*, ununctuous and light food, having astringent pungent and bitter tastes.

तिलमाषकुलत्थादि पिष्टान्नविकृतिं तथा ।

मस्तुशुक्ताम्लतक्राणि पित्तक्षीणस्तथा दधि ॥१४९॥

A patient having diminution of *pitta*, desires to take *tila*, *māṣa*, *kulattha*, different types of pastry, *mastu*, *śukta*, *amla tàkra* and curd.

मांसं माहिषवाराहमाजं गुडगुरूणि च ।

श्लेष्मक्षीणोऽभिलषति क्षीरस्वप्नदधीनि च ॥१५०॥

A patient having diminution of *kapha* desires to take the meat of buffalo, pig and goat, *guḍa* (jaggery), heavy food, more of milk, sleep and curd.

इक्षुमांसरसं मन्थं मधुसर्पिगुडोदकम् ।

119

असृङ्मांसं यवागूं च रसक्षीणोऽभिकाङ्क्षति ॥१५१॥

A patient having diminution of *rasa* desires to take sugarcane juice, meat soup, *mantha*, honey, ghee, jaggery, water, blood, meat and *yavāgū* (gruel).

द्राक्षादाडिमयुक्तानि सस्नेहलवणानि च ।

रक्तसिद्धानि मांसानि रक्तक्षीणोऽभिकाङ्क्षति ॥१५२॥

A person having diminution of *rakta* desires to take food

prepared of *drākṣā* and *dāḍima* and added with fats and salts. He also desires to take meat boiled along with the blood.

अम्लानि दधिसिद्धानि तथा षाडवकानि च ।

स्थूलक्रव्यादमांसानि मांसक्षीणोऽभिकाङ्क्षति [120] ॥१५३॥

A patient having diminution of *māṁsa* desires to take food prepared by adding sour things and curd. He also desires to take different types of *ṣāḍavaka* and meat of animals having huge body and meat of meat-eating animals.

मेदःसिद्धानि मांसानि ग्राम्यानूपौदकानि च ।

सक्षाराणि विशेषेण मेदः क्षीणोऽभिकाङ्क्षति ॥१५४॥

A patient having diminution of *medas* desires to take meat boiled with fat of animals, specially those which are domesticated, which live in marshy land and which are aquatic. He specially likes to take these meats added with alkalies.

रसान्सुसिद्धान् सास्थीनि मत्स्यानीहाऽभिकाङ्क्षति [121] ।

अस्थिक्षीणस्तथा मांसं मज्जास्थिस्नेहसंयुतम् ॥१५५॥

A patient having diminution of *asthi* (bone tissue) desires to take meat soup prepared by boling along with bones and different types of fish.

स्वाद्वम्लसंयुतं द्रव्यं मज्जाक्षीणोऽभिकाङ्क्षति ।

मयूरकुक्कुटाण्डानि हंससारसयोस्तथा ।

ग्राम्यानूपोदकानां च शुक्रक्षीणोऽभिकाङ्क्षति [122] ॥१५६॥

A patient having diminution of bone-marrow desires to take meat prepared by boiling with bone-marrow and the fat of the bones. He also likes to take meat prepared along with sweet and sour things.

यवानि यवकान्नानि शाकानि विविधानि च ।

मयूरं मांसयूषांश्च वर्चः क्षीणोऽभिकाङ्क्षति ॥१५७॥

A patient having diminution of *śukra* (semen) desires to take the eggs of pea-cock, cock, swan and duck. He also desires to take eggs of other birds which are domesticated, which live in marshy land and which are aquatic.

A patient having diminution of feces, desires to take *yava*, *yavaka*, different type of vegetables and the soup of the meat of pea-cock and other types of meat.

[123]पेयामिक्षुरसं क्षीरं सगुडं बदरोदकम् ।

मूत्रक्षीणोऽभिलषति त्रपुसोर्वारुकाणि च ॥१५८॥

A patient suffering from the diminution of urine desires to take *peyā* (thin gruel), sugarcane juice, milk along with jaggery and *badarodaka*. He also likes to take *trapusa* and *ervāruka*.

अभ्यङ्गोन्मर्दनं मद्यं [124]निर्वातशयनासनम् ।

[125]गुणप्रावरणञ्चैव स्वेदक्षीणोऽभिकाङ्क्षति ॥१५९॥

A person having diminution of *sveda* desires for massage, unction, alcoholic drinks, sleep and stay in a place free from wind and thick *prāvaraṇa* (sheets for covering the body).

कट्वम्ललवणाम्लानि विदाहीनि गुरूणि च ।

[126]फलशाकानुपानानि स्त्री [127]काङ्क्षत्यार्तवक्षये ॥१६०॥

The woman having diminution of *ārtava*, desires to take food which is pungent, sour and saline in taste, sour drinks, food which cause burning sensation and which is salty. She also likes to take fruits and vegetables and similar *anupāna* (post prandial drinks).

मृगाजाविवराहाणां गर्भान् वाञ्छति संस्कृतान् ।

वसाशूल्यप्रकारादीन्[128] रक्तं गर्भपरिक्षयात्[129] ॥१६१॥

If there is diminution of foetus, then the patient desires to take preparations of the meat of foetus of deer, goat, sheep and pig. She also likes to take *vasā* (muscle fat) and different types of meat preparations like *śūlya*.

सुराशाल्यन्नमत्स्यानि[130] गोक्षीरं शर्करां तथा ।

आसवं दधि हृद्यानि क्षये स्तन्यस्य वाञ्छति ॥१६२॥

[सुश्रुत : सूत्र१५:२९-३१ डल्हणटीका]

If there is diminution of breast milk, then the patient desires to take *surā* (a type of alcoholic drink), *śāli* rice, fish, cow's milk, sugar, *āsava* (a fermented drink), curd and such other drinks which are *hṛdya* (wholesome for the heart).

[धातूनां ह्रासनम्]

पूर्वः पूर्वोऽतिवृद्धत्वाद् वर्धयेच्च परं परम् ।

तस्मादतिविवृद्धानां धातूनां ह्रासनं हितम् ॥१६३॥

Need for Reducing the Dhātus

By the excessive increase of the preceding *dhātus*, the subsequent ones also get exceedingly increased in quantity. Therefore, in a patient having excessively increase in the quantity of *dhātus*, their diminution is useful.

ओषधीर्नामरूपाभ्यां लक्षयेच्छतशो बुधः ।

जात्याकृति रसं वीर्यं गुणं संमेलनं क्रमम् ॥१६४॥

The wise physician is a acquainted with the names and characteristic features of hundreds of drugs. He is also acquainted with their species, size and shape, *rasa* (taste), *vīrya* (potency) and *guṇa* (attributes). The result of the combination of these attributes in a drug is also known to him.

पुलिन्दाश्चैव गोपाश्च ये चान्ये वनवासिनः ।
कन्दमूलफलाहारा[131] एतेभ्यो ज्ञायते बुधैः[132] ॥१६५॥

A wise physician should learn about the drugs from tribals, cow-herds and others residing in forests and living on rhizomes, roots and fruits.

यथा विषं यथा शस्त्रं यथा[ऽ]ग्निरशनिर्यथा ।
तथौषधमविज्ञातं विज्ञातममृतं यथा ॥१६६॥

[चरक : सूत्र१:१२४]

A drug which is not known is like a poison, or weapon, or fire, or thunderbolt. When properly known, it is like nectar.

[त्रिविधम् औषधम्]

अग्निवेशात्

दैवव्यपाश्रयं चैव यथा युक्तिव्यपाश्रयम् ।
सत्त्वावजयमित्येवं भेदेन त्रिविधौषधम् ॥१६७॥

Three Categories of Therapies

According to Agniveśa

Therapies are of the following three categories :

1. *Daiva vyapāśraya* or the spiritual therapy;
2. *Yukti vyapāśraya* or the therapy based on reasoning i.e., physical and chemical propriety; and
3. *Śattvāvajaya* or the psychic therapy.

मन्त्रौषध-मणि-मङ्गल[133]-बल्युपहारश्च होमनियमाश्च ।

स्वस्त्ययन-गमन-लङ्घन-प्रायश्चितं तथा च प्रणिपातः[134] ।

चरकात्रेयादिमते ज्ञेयं दैवव्यपाश्रयं नाम ॥१६८॥

Spiritual therapies are incantation of *mantras*, wearing of talisman and gems, auspicious recitations, offerings, gifts, oblations, observance of scriptural rules, chanting of auspicious hymns, going on pilgrimage, keeping of fast, atonement and paying obeisance to the gods.

आहारदिषु द्रव्याणां योजना रसकल्पना ।

भिषग्भिः क्रियते यत्र तद्धि युक्तिव्यपाश्रयम् ॥१६९॥

The prescription of the physician of proper ingredients in diet and medicine after the determination of their taste etc., constitute *yukti vyapāśraya* or the therapy based on reasoning i.e., physical and chemical propriety.

अहितेभ्यः सदार्थेभ्यो मनोनिग्रहणं तथा ।

धीर्धैर्यात्मादिविज्ञानं सत्त्वावजयमुच्यते ॥१७०॥

Withdrawal of mind from harmful objects and the practice of *dhī* (intellectual performance), *dhairya* (patience), *ātma vijñāna* (spiritual knowledge), constitute *sattvāvajaya* or the psychic therapy.

[पुनश्च त्रैविध्यम्]

अन्तः प्रमार्जनं चैव बहिः संमार्ज्जनं तथा ।

शस्त्रप्रणिधानं पुनर्ज्ञेयं त्रिविधमौषधम् ॥१७१॥

Another Classification

Therapies are again classified into three different categories as follows :

1. *Antaḥ parimārjana* or internal cleansing;
2. *Vahiḥ parimārjana* or external cleansing; and
3. *Śastra praṇidhāna* or surgical therapy.

यदौषधमथाहारं प्रविश्यान्तर्विशोधयेत् ।
135 शमयेद्वा तर्पयेद्वा तदन्तर्मार्जनं मतम् ॥१७२॥

The drugs and diet which while entering into the body cleanses it either by elimination or by nourishment is called *antaḥ parimārjana*.

अभ्यङ्गपरिषेकादि तथा लेपांजनादयः ।
वहिः संमार्ज्जनं प्रोक्तं नखादीनां च कर्तनम् ॥१७३॥

Abhyaṅga (massage), *pariṣeka* (sprinkling of medicated liquids), *lepa* (ointment) and *añjana* (collyrium) etc., and cutting of the nails etc., constitute *vahiḥ parimārjana* or external eleansing.

छेद्यभेदादिकर्माणि जलौकाद्यवचारणम् ।
136 तेषां शस्त्रप्रणिधानं नाम ज्ञेयं विशारदैः ॥१७४॥

इति भेषजपरीक्षा ॥

Incision, excision etc., and application of leeches etc., constitute *śastra praṇidhāna* or surgical therapy.

Thus, ends the examination of therapies.

[देशविभागम्]

[137] चक्षुष्येन यथा

भूमिदेहप्रभेदेन देशमाहुरिह द्विधा ।

भूमिदेशस्त्रिधानूपोजाङ्गलो मिश्रलक्षणः [138] ॥१७५॥

Classification of Deśa (land or location)

According to Cakṣuṣya

In the present context, *deśa* is of two types namely, the *bhūmi deśa* (land) and *deha deśa* (physique of the individual). *Bhūmi deśa* is again of three types, namely,

1. *ānūpa* (marshy land);
2. *jāṅgala* (arid forest); and
3. land having mixed characteristics (*sādhāraṇa*).

[आनूपदेशलक्षणम्]

नदी-पल्वल-शैलाद्य-पद्मोत्पल-मुखैर्युतः [139] ।

हंससारस-कारण्ड-बलाकाद्विजसेवितः ॥१७६॥

वराहखड्गमहिषरुरुरोहिकुलाकुलः ।

प्रभूतद्रुमपुष्पाढ्यो नानाशस्यफलोचितः ॥१७७॥

अनेकशालिकेदार-कदलीक्षुविभूषितः ।

[140] आनूपदेशो भूयिष्ठं वातश्लेष्मामयार्त्तिमान् ॥१७८॥

अल्पाग्न्यायुर्बलाः स्थूलाश्चलन्मेदस्तनोदराः ।

नराः प्रायेण तस्मात्तै[141]रन्नपानं सुखार्थिभिः ।

अनभिष्यन्दिरूक्षाम्लं देयं लघ्व[142]ग्निदीपनम् ॥१७९॥

Characteristics of Ānūpa Deśa

Ānūpa deśa or marshy land is full of rivers, lakes, mountains, lotus and lillies. Birds like *haṁsa*, *sārasa*, *kāraṇḍa* and *balākā* inhabit this land. This land is also inhabited by animals like *varāha*, *khaḍga*, *mahiṣa*, *ruru* and *rohi*. Many big trees full of flowers and many vegetations having fruit grow in this land. It has many rice fields and it is full of trees like *kadalī* and *ikṣu*. The persons inhabiting this type of land suffer from diseases caused by *vāyu* and *kapha*. They have less power of digestion, short span of life and less of strength. They are generally fatty with bulky and with mobile breasts and belly. Therefore, for their happiness, they should take such diet and drinks that are *anabhiṣyandi* (which do not obstruct the channels of circulation), ununctuous, sour, light and *agni dīpana* (which stimulate the power of digestion).

[जाङ्गलदेशलक्षणम्]

आकाशश्वभ्रसिकतास्थली विषमभूतलाः ।

शमीकरीरबिल्वार्कपीलुकर्कन्धुसंकुलाः ॥१८०॥

हारिणैण-सपृषतगोकर्ण-खर-चातकाः ।

वारुणा गोमनुष्याश्च स्थौल्यामिषपरायणाः ॥१८१॥

वरतोयाल्पसलिलो देशो जाङ्गल उच्यते ।

अत्राल्पमेदः प्रचयाः स्थिराजितपरिश्रमाः ॥१८२॥

सुसंहतवराङ्गाश्च बलिनोऽल्परुजो जनाः ।

आयुष्मन्तोऽनिलप्राया रोगास्तेषामिदं हितम् ।

बृंहणं गुरुवत् स्निग्धमन्नपानं द्रवं हितम् ॥१८३॥ 143

Characteristics of Jāṅgala Deśa

Jāṅgala deśa or arid forest land has cloudless sky, sandy zone and irregular land. It is surrounded with trees like *śamī, karīra, bilva, arka, pīlu* and *karkandhu.* The animals available in this type of land are *hariṇa, eṇa, pṛṣata, gokarṇa, khara, cātaka, vāruṇa,* cattle and *manuṣya* (?) These animals are bulky. They generally feed on meat. In this land there is less of water, but the water is healthy. The persons inhabiting this land have less of fat accumulation. They are sturdy and hard working. Their body is compact and beautiful. They are strong and they suffer from less of disease. They have a long span of life. They generally suffer from diseases caused by *vāyu.* For them, diet and drinks which are nourishing, heavy, unctuous and liquid are useful.

आनूपजाङ्गलाभ्यां तु देशाभ्यां मिश्रलक्षणः ।
साधारणः स्मृतो देशस्तथा व्याधिचिकित्सितः ॥१८४॥ 144

Sādhāraṇa Deśa

In this type of land, the characteristic features of both the *ānūpa deśa* and *jāṅgala deśa* are present. This is called *miśra deśa* (land of mixed nature) or *sādhāraṇa deśa* (land of general nature) by physicians.

सुश्रुतः

समाः साधारणे यस्माच्छीतवर्षोष्णमारुताः ।
समता तेन दोषाणां तस्मात् साधारणो वरः ॥१८५॥ 145

[सुश्रुत : सूत्र ३५:४३]

उचिते वर्त्तमानस्य नास्ति देशकृतं भयम् ।

146
आहारस्वप्नचेष्टादौ तद्देशस्य गुणे सति ॥१८६॥

[सुश्रुत : सूत्र ३५:४५]

According to Suśruta

Sādhāraṇa deśa has equal quantity of cold, rain, heat and wind. Therefore, in the persons of this land, *doṣas* are in a state of equilibrium and it is a healthy place to live. If a person resorts to diet, sleep and activities which are conducive to the characteristic features of the land, then he does not get afflicted by its evil effects.

147
अथ वृद्धवाग्भटः

यस्य देशस्य यो जन्तुस्तज्जं तस्यौषधं हितम् ।

देशादन्यत्र वसतस्तत्तुल्यगुणजन्म वा ॥१८७॥

According to Vṛddha Vāgbhaṭa

For living beings of a particular type of land, the drugs available in the locality are useful. When they are shifted to another type of land, then drugs which are of *tulya guṇa* (which have attributes similar to those growing in the earlier type of land) or which are *tulya janma* (which are grown in a land similar to the earlier one) are useful.

स्वदेशे निचिता दोषास्त्वन्यस्मिन् कोपमागताः ।

बलवन्तस्तथा न स्युर्जलजा वा स्थलाहृताः ॥१८८॥

If a *doṣa* is accumulated in a particular place and gets aggravated when the person shifts to another type of land, then these *doṣas* are not so powerful. This rule is applicable to the *doṣas* aggravated because of the water or the land in these two places.

[भूमिविभागवर्णनम्]

भूमिः पञ्चविधा तत्र कृष्णा रक्ता सिता तथा ।

पीता नीला च विज्ञेया शृणु तासां गुणागुणम् ॥१८९॥

Classification of Earth

The earth in the ground is of five types, namely, black, red, white, yellow and blue. Their attributes are being described.

श्वभ्रशर्कराश्म-विषम-वल्मीक-श्मशाना[149]घातन-देवतायतन-सिकताभिरनुपहतामनूष-

रामभङ्गुरामदूरोदकां [150]स्निग्धां प्ररोहवतीं मृद्वीं समां स्थिरां कृष्णां गौरीं लोहितां वा

भूमिमौषधग्रहणार्थं परीक्षेत। तस्यां जातमपि कृमि-विष-शस्त्रातपपवन[151]दहनतोय-

संबाधमार्गैरनुपहतमेकान्तरसपुष्टं पृथ्वागाढमूलमूदीच्यां चौषधमाददीत ॥१९०॥

[सुश्रुत : सूत्र३६:३]

Places Suitable for Collection of Herbs

Places which are free from cloud, gravel and stones, which are not irregular, which do not have ant-hills, which are not crematoria or the place of killing of animals, which are inside the compound of a temple, which are free from sound, which are not *ūṣara* (alkaline), which are not having cracks, which are not far away from water, which are unctuous, which have creepers, which are soft, fair, stable, clean, white or red, are suitable for the collection of drugs. Even if a herb is grown in this type of land, it should be ensured that the herb is not afflicted by insects, poison, weapons, excessive heat, wind, fire, water and foot path. These herbs should be saturated with *rasa* (taste) and healthy. These should be thick and they should be deep-rooted. They should be collected from the northern side of the land.

तत्राश्मवती स्थिरा गुर्वी श्यामा कृष्णा वा स्थूलवृक्षशस्यप्राया

स्वगुणभूयिष्ठा ॥१९१॥

Pañca bhautika Composition of Earth

The earth which is full of stones, which is stable, heavy, bluish-black or black and which has thick trees and vegetation is dominated by *pṛthvī mahābhūta.*

स्निग्धा शीतला[ऽऽ]सन्नोदका स्निग्धशस्यतृणकोमलवृक्षप्राया शुक्लाऽम्बुगुण-
भूयिष्ठा ॥१९२॥

The land which is unctuous and cold, which is nearer to water, which has unctuous vegetation, grass and soft trees and which is white in colour is dominated by *jala mahābhūta.*

रूक्षा भस्मरासमवर्णा [152]तनुकोटराल्परसवृक्षप्रायाऽनिलगुणभूयिष्ठा ॥१९३॥

The land which is ununctuous, which is full of ash and which has uneven colours, which has thin trees and which has in general trees with less of sap, is dominated by *vāyu mahābhūta.*

नानावर्णा [153]लघ्वश्मवती [154]प्रविरलाल्पपाण्डुवृक्षप्ररोहाऽग्निभूयिष्ठा ॥१९४॥

The land which has different types of colour, which is light, which is sandy and which has rare or small number of trees, which has yellow trees and which h?s trees with adventitious roots (*praroha*) is dominated by *agni mahābhūta.*

मृद्वी समा श्वभ्रवत्यव्यक्तरसजला सर्वतोऽसारवृक्षा महापर्वतवृक्ष-प्राया श्यामा
आकाशगुणभूयिष्ठा ॥१९५॥

[सुश्रुत : सूत्र३६:४]

The land which is soft and even, which is free from clouds, which has water of imperceptible taste, which is surrounded by emaciated trees, which has generally big mountains and trees and which is bluish-black is dominated by *ākāśa mahābhūta.*

तत्र केचिदाहुराचार्याः

155 प्रावृड्वर्षाशरद्धेमन्तवसन्तग्रीष्मेषु यथासंख्यं मूलपत्रत्वक्क्षीरपुष्प-फलान्याददीत
[इति]; तत्तु न सम्यक्, सौम्याग्नेयत्वाज्जगतः । [सौम्यान्यौषधानि
156 सौम्येष्वृतुष्वाददीत, आग्नेयान्याग्नेयेषु, एवमव्यापन्नगुणानि भवन्ति ।]
157 सौम्यान्यौषधानि सौम्येषु ऋतुषु गृहीतानि सोमगुणभूयिष्ठायां भूमौ जातान्यति-
मधुरस्निग्धशीतानि जायन्ते । एतेन शेषं व्याख्यातम् ॥१६६॥

[सुश्रुत : सूत्र३६:५]

According to Some Scholars

The root, leaf, bark, latex, flower and fruits should be collected in *prāvṛṭ* (beginning of rainy season), *varṣā* (rainy season), *śarat* (autumn), *hemanta* (winter), *vasanta* (spring) and *griṣma* (summer) seasons, respectively. This view of these scholars is not correct, because the universe has two aspects namely, *saumya* cooling element and *āgneya* (heating element). The cooling medicines should be collected during cold seasons and heating medicines should be collected during hot seasons. By doing so, the attributes of drugs do not get afflicted. If the cooling medicines are collected during cold season then these are impregnated with cooling effect of the earth and they are exceedingly sweet, unctuous and cooling in nature. In the similar way, the remaining points should be explained.

158 स्वगुणाम्बुविशिष्टायां भूमौ ग्राह्यं विरेचनम् ।
159 वाय्वग्निगुणभूयिष्ठभूमौ च वमनीयकम् ॥१६७॥

160 आकाशगुणभूयिष्ठं ग्राह्यं संशमनौषधम् ।
एवं विज्ञाय सद्वैद्यस्ततः कुर्यात्क्रियाक्रमम् ॥१६८॥

Collection of Different Types of Drugs

Purgative drugs should be collected from the earth dominated by *pṛthvi* and *jala mahābhūtas*. Emetic drugs should be collected from the earth dominated by *vāyu* and *agni mahābhūtas*. Drugs for *śamana* (alleviation of *doṣas*) should be collected from the land dominated by *ākāśa mahābhūta*. A proficient physician should ascertain this before initiating his treatment.

गन्ध-वर्ण-रसोपेता षड्विधा भूमिरुच्यते ।
तस्माद्भूमिस्वभावेन बीजिनः षड्रसैर्युता ।।१९९।।

Depending upon the smell, colour and the taste, the earth is of six types. Therefore, the herbs collected from these lands are of six different types.

161
अव्यक्तः किल तोयस्य रसो नियमनिश्चितः ।
रसः स एव चाव्यक्तो व्यक्तो भूमिरसाद्भवेत् ।।२००।।

In water the *rasa* (taste) remains in an unmanifested state. There is no exception to this rule. This unmanifested taste becomes manifested when water comes in contact with the taste of different types of earth.

सर्व-लक्षण-सम्पन्ना भूमिः साधारणा स्मृता ।
162
द्रव्याणि यातानि तत्र स्युस्तद्गुणानि विशेषतः ।।२०१।।

[सुश्रुत : सूत्र३६:१२-१४]

The earth which is endowed with all the good attributes is called *sādhāraṇa* (general). The drugs which grow in this type of land have the characteristic features specific to it.

[भेषजागारवर्णनम्]

प्लोतमृद्भाण्डफलकशङ्कुविन्यस्तभेषजम् ।

प्रशस्तायां दिशि शुचौ भेषजागारमिष्यते ॥२०२॥

[सुश्रुत : सूत्र३६:१७]

॥ इति भूमिलक्षणम् ॥

Construction of Drug Store

Drug store should be constructed in a place free from cotton, broken pieces of earthen vessels, flat stones, sharp edged stones, weapons and scattered drugs. It should be ensured that the store is constructed in an auspicious direction and in a clean place.

Thus, ends the description of characteristic features of different types of land.

अथ प्रकृतिलक्षणम्

तत्र खरनादः

शुक्रास्रगर्भिणीभोज्यचेष्टागर्भाशयर्तुषु ।

यस्याद् दोषोऽधिकस्तेन प्रकृति सप्तधोदिता ॥२०३॥

Characteristics of Different Types of Prakṛti

According to Kharanāda

Prakṛti is of seven types according to the dominating *doṣas* and as a result of the following factors:

1. *Śukra* (semen including sperm);
2. *Asra* (ovum);
3. *Garbhiṇī bhojya* (food of the mother during the period of pregnancy);
4. *Garbhiṇī ceṣṭā* (regimens followed by the mother during the period of pregnancy);
5. *Garbhāśaya* (conditions prevailing inside the uterus); and
6. *Ṛtu* (seasonal effects).

तथा च वाग्भटः

शुक्रार्तवस्थैर्जन्मादौ विषेणेव विषक्रिमेः ।

163
तैश्च प्रकृतयस्तिस्रो हीनमध्योत्तमाः पृथक् ।

समधातु समस्तासु श्रेष्ठा निन्द्या द्विदोषजाः ॥२०४॥

[अष्टाङ्गहृदय : सूत्र१:६-१०]

According to Vāgbhaṭa

Prakṛti is caused by the *doṣas* inherent in the *śukra* (semen including sperm) and *ārtava* (ovum) immediately before the conception. This is on the analogy of the production of insects in a poisonous substance. The *prakṛti* caused by *vāyu*, *pitta* and *kapha* are inferior, mediocre and superior, respectively. The *prakṛti* caused by all the three *doṣas* when they are in the state of equilibrium (*sama dhātu*) is the best among all. The *prakṛti* caused by two of the *doṣas* viz., *vāyu-pitta, pitta-kapha* and *vāyu-kapha* are the despisable ones.

आत्रेयात्

164
विषजातो यथा कीटो न विषेण मृतिं व्रजेत् ।

तद्वत्प्रकृतयो मर्त्यं शक्नुवन्ति न बाधितुम् ॥२०५॥

[सुश्रुत : शारीर४:७६]

According to Ātreya

The insect produced inside a poisonous substance does not die by the effect of the poison. Similarly, *prakṛtis* (which are manifested at the time of conception) are incapable of afflicting the individual.

[वातप्रकृतिलक्षणम्]

चक्षुष्येवेति

रूक्षापवीतशरीरः कृष्णः क्षामस्वरोऽल्पदेहबलः शीघ्रारम्भविकारो रसलोलुप मुखर [165] जागरितश्चंक्रमणोऽक्षमोदीनदीर्घनखो व्योमगः स्वप्नो स्फुटितत्वक्पाद-करश्चंचलचित्तश्चानिल प्रकृतिः ॥२०६॥

Characteristics of Vāta Prakṛti

According to Cakṣuṣya

Characteristic features of a person having *vāta prakṛti* are as follows :

1. The body is rough to touch and thin;
2. There is black complextion;
3. Poor voice;
4. Short stature and less of strength;
5. Quick in attempt and quick in giving it up;
6. Desire to have delicious food;
7. Talkative;
8. Remaining awake for a long time;
9. Inability to walk a long distance;
10. Poor disposition;
11. Long nails;
12. Having dreams of moving in the sky;
13. Having cracks in the skin, sole of feet and palm; and
14. Fickleness of mind.

[पित्तप्रकृतिलक्षणम्]

उष्णावदातसुकुमाराशिथिलगात्र प्रभूततृड्क्षुधः मृद्वल्पकपिलकेशश्मश्रु तीक्ष्णाति-तीक्ष्णाग्निः क्षिप्रवलीपलितश्च कक्षागन्धिश्च पिंगाक्षः स्निग्धोपचितशरीरो लौल्यरतो लोमवर्जितो गौरः स्तुतिप्रियस्तिक्तरसानुभोजी स्वेदी स पित्तप्रकृतिर्मनुष्यः । मध्यबलः पैत्तिकः पुरुषः । इति वा पाठः ॥२०७॥

Characteristics of Pitta Prakṛti

Characteristic features of *pitta prakṛti* are as follows :

1. The body is hot, white, tender and loose;
2. Excess of thirst and hunger;
3. The hair of the body and the hair of the face are soft, less in number and reddish in colour;
4. The *agni* (the power of digestion including metabolism) is excessively sharp;
5. Early appearance of wrinkles and greying of hair;
6. Foul smell from the axilla;
7. Coppery colour of the eyes;
8. The body is unctuous and plump;
9. Liking for different types of work and food;
10. Absence of small hair in the body;
11. White colour of the body;
12. Liking for being flattered;
13. Liking for bitter taste; and
14. Excessive sweating.

There is a variant text, according to which a person having *pitta prakṛti* has moderate type of strength.

[कफप्रकृतिलक्षणम्]

स्निग्धोपचितशरीरः प्रसन्नवर्णेन्द्रियो नरो बलवान् धृतिमान्विलंबितगतिः सुकृच्छ्रगन्धो दृढग्राही मन्दप्रलापचेष्टातृष्णास्वेददोषसंतापः देशे काले चोष्णे भवत्यरोगः कफप्रकृतिः ॥२०८॥

Characteristics of Kapha Prakṛti

Characteristic features of a person having *kapha prakṛti* are as follows :

1. Unctuous and plump body;
2. Excellence of complexion and sense organs;
3. Strength of the body;
4. Having patience;
5. Slow walk;
6. Less of foul smell and presence of good smell in the body;
7. Strong power of memory;
8. Less of talkativeness, activities, thirst, sweating, vitiation of *doṣas* and burning sensation; and
9. Absence of diseases in hot seasons and in hot countries.

[समप्रकृतिलक्षणम्]

संमिश्रवर्णाश्च सुसंहतांगो गंभीराविदीर्णरोमा रामाप्रियो भारसहोऽभिमिश्रो भोगेन युक्तः समतः प्रकृत्याः ॥२०९॥

Characteristics of Sama Prakṛti

Characteristic features of a person having *sama prakṛti* caused by the *doṣas* in a state of equilibrium, are as follows :

1. Mixed colouration of the body;
2. Compact limbs;
3. The small hairs of his body are deep-rooted and there are no cracks in the hair;
4. He is loved by ladies;
5. Capable of carrying heavy weight; and
6. He is endowed with luxurious life.

[पञ्चभूतात्मिकाप्रकृतिवर्णनम्]

अपरापि पञ्चभूतात्मिका सुश्रुतेनोक्ता

प्रकृतिमिह नराणां भौतिकीं केचिदाहुः
पवनदहनतोयैः कीर्तितास्तास्तु तिस्रः ।
स्थिरविपुलशरीरः पार्थिवश्च क्षमावान्
शुचिरथ चिरंजीवी नाभसः खैर्महद्भिः ॥२१०॥

[सुश्रुत : शारीर ४:८०]

Prakṛti caused by Five Mahābhūtas

Suśruta has described five types of *prakṛtis* on the basis of the predominance of the five *mahābhūtas*. According to him, "Some scholars divide the *prakṛtis* of human beings on the basis of the predominance of the *mahābhūtas*. Out of them, the *prakṛtis* caused by predominance of *vāyu mahābhūta*, *agni mahābhūta* and *jala mahābhūta* are similar to *vāyu prakṛti*, *pitta prakṛti* and *kapha prakṛti*, respectively. A person having *prakṛti* with the predominance of *pṛthvī mahābhūta* has a stable and large-size body. He is capable of tolerating heavy odds. The person having *prakṛti* caused by the predominance of *ākāśa mahābhūta* likes cleanliness and he has a long span of life. The openings in his body are bigger in size."

[षोडशविधप्रकृतिवर्णनम्]

तथा च त्रिगुणात्मिका षोडशविधप्रकृतिरुद्दिष्टा ।

[166]शुद्धा सप्तविधा ज्ञेया षड्विधा राजसस्य हि ।
तामसस्य त्रिधा ज्ञेया तासां लक्षणमुच्यते ।।२११।।
शौचमास्तिक्यमभ्यासो देवता[167]गुरुपूजनम् ।
प्रियातिथित्व[168]मिज्या च ब्रह्मकायस्य लक्षणम् ।।२१२।।
माहात्म्यं शौर्यमाज्ञा च सततं शास्त्रबुद्धिता ।
भृत्यानां भरणं चापि माहेन्द्रं कायलक्षणम् ।।२१३।।
शीतसेवा सहिष्णुत्वं पैङ्गल्यं हरिकेशता ।
प्रियवादित्वमित्येतद्वारुणं कायलक्षणम् ।।२१४।।
मध्यस्थता सहिष्णुत्वमर्थस्यागमसंचयौ ।
महाप्रसव[169]शक्तिश्च कौबेरं कायलक्षणम् ।।२१५।।
गन्धमाल्यप्रियत्वं च नृत्यवादित्र[170]कामिता ।
विहारशीलता चैव गान्धर्वं कायलक्षणम् ।।२१६।।
प्राप्तकारी दृढोत्थानो [171]निर्भयः स्मृतिमान् शुचिः ।
राग[172]मोहभयद्वेषैर्वर्जितो [173]यमसत्त्ववान् ।।२१७।।
जपव्रतब्रह्मचर्यहोमाध्ययनसेविनम् ।
ज्ञानविज्ञानसंपन्न[174]मृषिकायस्य लक्षणम् ।।२१८।।
सप्तैते सात्त्विकाः कायाः,

Sixteen Types of Prakṛtis

Prakṛti is also divided into sixteen types, depending upon the three *guṇas*, namely, *sattva*, *rajas* and *tamas*. *Sāttvika* type is of seven varieties, *rājasa* is of six varieties and *tāmasa* is of three varieties. Their characteristic features are described below :

Types of Prakṛti (1)	*Characteristic features of the Individual* (2)
A. *Sāttvika type of prakṛti*	
1. *Brāhma* (sharing the traits of Brāhma)	1. Purity and love for truth;
	2. Sincerity in effort;
	3. Offering prayers to the gods and preceptors;
	4. Respect for guests; and
	5. Endeavour for acquiring knowledge.
2. *Māhendra* (sharing the traits of Mahendra).	1. Having great fame and courage;
	2. Obedience;
	3. Constant devotion to scriptural study; and
	4. Proper maintenance of servants.
3. *Vāruṇa* (sharing traits of *Varuṇa*).	1. Liking for cold things;
	2. Tolerability;

(1)	(2)
	3. Coppery colour;
	4. Greenish colour of the hair; and
	5. Pleasing talks.
4. *Kaubera* (sharing the traits of Kubera).	1. Disposition to work as a moderator;
	2. Tolerability;
	3. Acquiring and accumulation of wealth; and
	4. Great power to deliver goods.
5. *Gāndharva* (sharing the traits of Gandharva)	1. Liking for scents and garlands;
	2. Desire for dance and music; and
	3. Desire to move about.
6. *Yāma* (sharing the traits of Yama).	1. Observance of the propriety of actions;
	2. Initiation of strong action;
	3. Fearlessness;
	4. Memory and purity; and
	5. Freedom from attachment, illusion, fear and envy.
7. *Ārsa* (sharing the traits of *ṛṣi*)	1. Devotion to penance and sacred rituals;
	2. Celibacy, oblation to fire and study; and
	3. Material and spiritual knowledge.

राजसांस्तु निबोध मे ।[175]

ऐश्वर्यवन्तं रौद्रं च शूरं चण्डमसूयकम् ॥२१९॥

एकाशिनं चौदरिकमासुरं सत्त्वमीदृशम् ।

तीक्ष्णं[176] मायाविनं भीरुं चण्डं[177] मेधाविनं तथा ॥२२०॥

विहाराहार[178]चपलं सर्पसत्त्वं विदुर्नरम् ।

प्रवृद्धकामसेवी चाप्यजस्राहार एव च ॥२२१॥

अमर्षणोऽनवस्थायी शाकुनं कायलक्षणम् ।

एकान्तग्राहिता रौक्ष्य[179]मसूया धर्मबाह्यता ॥२२२॥

भृश[180]मात्मरति[181]श्चापि राक्षसं कायलक्षणम् ।

उच्छिष्टाहारता तैक्ष्ण्यं साहसप्रियता तथा ॥२२३॥

स्त्रीलोलुपत्वं नैर्लज्ज्यं पैशाचं कायलक्षणम् ।

असंविभागमलसं दुःखशीलमसूयकम् ॥२२४॥

लोलुपं चाल्प[182]दातारं प्रेतसत्त्वं विदुर्नरम् ।

षडेते राजसाः कायाः,

Types of Prakṛti	*Characteristic features of the Individual*
(1)	(2)
B. *Rājasika type of prakṛti*	
1. *Āsura* (sharing the traits of *Asura*)	1. He is endowed with wealth; 2. He is terrifying, brave, cruel and envious; 3. Liking for enjoyment alone; and 4. Desire for satisfying the belly.

(1)	(2)
2. *Sārpa* (sharing the traits of a a *sarpa* or snake)	1. Sharpness, deceptiveness, cowardice, cruelty and intelligence; and 2. Fickleness in movement and eating food.
3. *Śākuna* (sharing the traits of a *śakuni* or a bird)	1. Excessive indulgence in sex; 2. Intake of food very frequently; and 3. Anger and unstability.
4. *Rākṣasa* (sharing the traits of *rākṣasa*)	1. Onesided thinking; 2. Anger and envy; 3. Absence of religious mind; and 4. Indulgence in self-praise.
5. *Paiśāca* (sharing the traits of *piśāca*)	1. Liking for taking left-out food; 2. Sharpness; 3. Liking for bravery; 4. Fondness for women; and 5. Shamelessness.
6. *Praita* (sharing the traits of *pretas*)	1. Desire for not sharing the enjoyments; 2. Laziness; 3. Miserable disposition; 4. Jealousy; 5. Greediness; and 6. Less liking for charity.

तामसांस्तु निबोधमे ॥२२५॥

दुर्मेधस्त्वं मन्दता च स्वप्ने मैथुनमेव[183] च ।
निराकरिष्णुता चैव विज्ञेयाः पाशवो[184] गुणाः ॥२२६॥

अनवस्थितता मौर्ख्यं भीरुत्वं सलिलार्थिता ।
परस्पराभिमर्दश्च मत्स्यसत्त्वस्य लक्षणम् ॥२२७॥

एकस्थानरतिर्नित्यमाहारे केवले रतिः[185] ।
वानस्पत्यो नरः सत्त्वधर्मकामार्थवर्जितः ॥२२८॥

इत्येतास्त्रिविधाः[186] कायाः प्रोक्ता वै तामसस्तथा ।
कायानां प्रकृतिं[187] ज्ञात्वा[188] अनुरूपं क्रियां चरेत्[189] ॥२२९॥

[सुश्रुत : शारीर४:८१-९८]

Types of Prakṛti (1)	*Characteristics features of the Individual* (2)
C. *Tāmasika Type of prakṛti*	
1. *Pāśava* (sharing the traits of *paśu* or animal)	1. Lack of intelligence; 2. Sluggishness; 3. Indulgence in sex during dreams; and 4. Disobedience.

(1)	(2)
2. *Mātsya* (sharing the traits of *matsya* or a fish)	1. Instability;
	2. Lack of wisdom;
	3. Cowardice;
	4. Desire for water; and
	5. Mutual destruction of each other.
3. *Vānaspatya* (sharing the traits of *vanaspati* or vegetation)	1. Liking to stay in only one place;
	2. Liking only for taking food; and
	3. Absence of *sattva* (mental faculty), *dharma* (religion), *kāma* (desire) and *artha* (wealth).

The physician should first of all ascertain the *prakṛti*, of the individual, as mentioned above, and thereafter, initiate treatment conducive to him.

बाल्यं वृद्धिः छविर्मेधात्वक्दृष्टिः शुक्रविक्रमौ ।
190
बुद्धिः कर्मेन्द्रियं चैव जीवितं दशधादिशेत् ॥२३०॥

वासुदेव ॥

According to Vāsudeva

The process of living (life) has the following ten different aspects :

1. Tenderness of age;
2. Growth;
3. Aura;
4. Intellect;
5. Characteristic features of the skin;
6. Characteristic features of the eye sight;

7. Semen;

8. Forceful attempt;

9. Wisdom; and

10. Functioning of the motor organs.

191

इति श्रीमहाराजाधिराज टोडरमल्लविरचिते टोडरानन्दे आयुर्वेदसौख्ये दोषत्रयपंचात्मकदोषस्थान-कर्म-अविकृतदोषलक्षण-विकृतदोषोपचयगति-हेतु-प्रकोपलक्षणोपशमनं दोषावस्था.दोषवेदना-दोषधातुक्षयलक्षण-भेषजपरीक्षादेश-लक्षण-भूमिलक्षण-नानाप्रकृतिलक्षण-कथनं नाम द्वितीयो हर्षः ।।२३१।।

Thus, ends second Chapter of *Āyurveda saukhyaṁ* in *Ṭoḍarānanda* composed by the great king *Ṭoḍara malla*, which deals with the following topics :

1. Three *doṣas*;

2. Five types of each of the *doṣas*;

3. Location and functions of the *doṣas*;

4. Signs and symptoms of normal *doṣas*;

5. Vitiation of *doṣas* along with the causes of accumulation, causes of spread, signs and symptoms of vitiation and their alleviation;

6. Different states of *doṣas*;

7. Characteristic features of the pain caused by different types of *doṣas*;

8. Signs and symptoms of the diminution of the *doṣas* and *dhātus*;

9. Examination of the drugs;

10. Characteristic features of different types of *deśa* including different types of land; and

11. Description of different types of *prakṛti*.

NOTES AND REFERENCES

1. नहि मति इति पञ्चमपुस्तके पाठः ।
2. प्रयायाद् इति द्वितीयपुस्तके पाठः ।
3. भूपवर्यः इति द्वितीयषष्ठपुस्तकयोः पाठः ।
4. स्त्यानस्य इति आदर्शपुस्तकेषु पाठः ।
5. अत्र पञ्चमपुस्तके 'प्रथम गतिः' इति अधिकः पाठः ।
6. द्रष्टव्यम्—सुश्रुत : सूत्र ३१:३१ इति गद्यांशोपरि डल्हणः । किंचित् परिवर्तितम् ।
7. ०साम्यविभेदतः इतिप्रथमपुस्तके पाठः ।
8. श्लोकार्धोऽयं प्रथमषष्ठपुस्तकयोरेवास्ति नान्यत्र ।
9. द्रष्टव्यम्—अष्टाङ्गहृदयः सूत्र १:३-७ ।
10. ०संश्रया इति आकरे धृतः पाठः ।
11. प्रकम्पतः इति द्वितीयपुस्तके, प्रकोपणः इति पञ्चमपुस्तके च पाठः ।
12. रामं इति द्वितीयपुस्तकपाठः ।
13. साधकश्चेति इति आदर्शपुस्तिकासु पाठः तत्तु सम्यक् न प्रतिभाति ।
14. ०भूपम् इति षष्ठपुस्तके पाठः ।
15. ०भियानर्दि इति द्वितीयपुस्तके पाठः ।
16. ०स्वरुप० इति प्रथमपुस्तके पाठः ।
17. च बलेन इति द्वितीयपुस्तके पाठः ।
18. करोत्यचलं बलम् इति द्वितीयपुस्तके पाठः ।
19. क्लेदकृत् इति षष्ठपुस्तके पाठः ।
20. सद्यस्तु इति द्वितीयपुस्तके पाठः ।
21. श्लोकोऽयं द्वितीयषष्ठपुस्तकयोर्नोपलभ्यते ।
22. स्तम्भो इति द्वितीयषष्ठपुस्तकयोः पाठः ।

23. श्लक्ष्णस्तु इति षष्ठपुस्तके पाठः ।

24. पिच्छल इति षष्ठपुस्तके पाठः ।

25. शुक्तः इति षष्ठपुस्तके पाठः ।

26. स्वभावजः इति षष्ठपुस्तके पाठः ।

27. विसर्गानन्द० इति षष्ठपुस्तके पाठः ।

28. ०परिचारणात् इति द्वितीयपुस्तके पाठः ।

29. कालेऽपि वा न तु इति अष्टाङ्गहृदयसंमतः पाठः, स तु साधीयान् ।

30. द्रष्टव्यम्—सुश्रुत : सूत्र २१:१८ ।

31. अत्र यद्यपि 'विवर्ततेऽपि' इति सर्वपुस्तकपाठः तथाऽपि सोऽर्थसङ्गतिरहित इति अष्टाङ्गहृदयतट्टीकासंमतः पाठ एवाङ्गीकृतः ।

32. श्लोकोऽयं यद्यपि कस्यामपि आदर्शपुस्तिकायां नोपलभ्यते तथापि तदभावेऽर्थ-संङ्तिविरहादयम् अष्टाङ्गहृदयादुद्ध्रियते ।

33. छायामत्येति नात्मीयां यथा वा कृत्स्नमप्यदः इत्याकरे पाठः :

34. ०कृच्छ्र० इति पञ्चमं विहाय सर्वेषु आदर्शपुस्तकेषु पाठः । तत्तु न सम्यक् प्रतिभाति ।

35. द्रष्टव्यम्—चरक : सूत्र १७:११२ ।

36. द्रष्टव्यम्—अष्टाङ्गहृदय : सूत्र १३:२१ ।

37. कोष्ठप्रयत्नांश्च इति द्वितीयपुस्तके पाठः ।

38. पथ्यं स्बन्तं इति आदर्शपुस्तिकासु पाठः तत्तु सम्यक् न प्रतिभाति । 'यथा-सन्नं' तु आकरे पाठः ।

39. द्रष्टव्यम्—चरक : सूत्र १७:११३ ।

40. ये तत् इति पञ्चमपुस्तके पाठः ।

41. अन्तः श्रितामया इति द्वितीयपुस्तके पाठः ।

42. स्मृताः षष्ठपुस्तके पाठः ।

43. मर्म इति द्वितीयषष्ठपुस्तकयोः पाठः ।

44. दोषवृद्धिर्हि इति द्वितीयपुस्तके पाठः ।

45. वयं इति प्रथमपञ्चमषष्ठपुस्तकेषु पाठः ।

46. भुवि इति आदर्शपुस्तिकासु पाठः तत्तु सम्यक् न प्रतिभाति ।
47. मूर्द्धार्द्धे इति सर्वादर्शपुस्तकेषु पाठः ।
48. प्रशान्ता भवति इति सर्वादर्शपुस्तकेषु पाठः ।
49. श्लोकार्धोऽयं द्वितीयपुस्तके नास्ति ।
50. तनुँ इति प्रथमपुस्तके पाठः ।
51. तृडतिशिशिरेच्छा इति प्रथमद्वितीयपुस्तकयोः पाठः ।
52. मोहनिद्रा इति षष्ठपुस्तके पाठः ।
53. च इति द्वितीयपुस्तके पाठः ।
54. श्लोकार्धोऽयं षष्ठपुस्तके नास्ति ।
55. तथैव च इति आकरे पाठः ।
56. नहि इति प्रथमद्वितीयषष्ठपुस्तकेषु पाठः ।
57. परिज्ञातं इति द्वितीयपुस्तके पाठः ।
58. सूक्ष्मं इति द्वितीयषष्ठपुस्तकयोः पाठः ।
59. द्रष्टव्यम्—चरक : विमान १:१३-१५ ।
60. भेषजान्नाति इति द्वितीयपुस्तके पाठः ।
61. दीपनैः पाचनैर्द्रव्यैः सिद्धाः स्नेहास्त्वनेकधा । इति द्वितीयपुस्तके पाठः ।
62. श्लोकोऽयं प्रथमद्वितीयषष्ठपुस्तकेषु नोपलभ्यते ।
63. अयमेव अष्टाङ्गहृदयसंमतः पाठः, अन्यत्र सर्वत्र तु 'अयन्त्रणमुखं' इत्युपलभ्यमानः पाठोऽसङ्गतेः परिहृतः ।
64. इत आरभ्य 'दीर्घिका' इत्यन्तः पाठः षष्ठपुस्तके नोपलभ्यते ।
65. सैकतम् इति द्वितीयपुस्तके पाठः ।
66. द्रष्टव्यम्—अष्टाङ्गहृदयः सूत्र १३:५-८
67. श्लोकोऽयं केवलं पञ्चमपुस्तकएवोपलभ्यते ।
68. पाठोऽयं चिकित्साकलिकायाम् नोपलभ्यते ।
69. ०निरूहनस्य० इति योगशतकधृतपाठः ।
70. जीवनं योगशतकधृतपाठः ।

71. दुष्ट इति द्वितीयषष्ठपुस्तकयोः पाठः ।
72. श्लोकपादोऽयं षष्ठपुस्तके नास्ति ।
73. ०नियुक्त० इति षष्ठपुस्तके पाठः ।
०ध्वतियुद्ध० इति द्वितीयपुस्तके पाठः ।
74. धूमः ताप० इति योगशतकधृतः पाठः ।
75. स्वेदोपनाहादिकं इति योगशतकधृतः पाठः ।
76. श्लोकोऽयं प्रथमपञ्चमपुस्तकयोः नोपलभ्यते ।
77. संश्लिष्ट० इति प्रथमपुस्तके पाठः ।
78. विरेचनवस्ती इति प्रथमपञ्चमपुस्तकयोः पाठः ।
79. सर्वाण्यमूनि इति प्रथमपुस्तके पाठः ।
80. द्रष्टव्यम्—अष्टाङ्गहृदय : सूत्र १३:२४ ।
81. ०भ्यश्चाति० इति प्रथमपञ्चमपुस्तकयोः पाठः ।
82. ०गौरवातिर्य० इति षष्ठपुस्तके पाठः ।
०गौरवानिल० इति अष्टाङ्गहृदयधृतः पाठः ।
83. दन्तत्वक्चक्षुषां इति अष्टांगहृदयधृतपाठः ।
84. तमः इति सर्वादर्शपुस्तकेषु पाठः ।
85. पाठोऽयं आकरे उपलभ्यते न तु आदर्शपुस्तिकासु ।
86. पाठोऽयं आकरे उपलभ्यते न तु आदर्शपुस्तकेषु ।
87. 'बहु' इति पञ्चमपुस्तके क्वचित् संशोधितः पाठः ।
88. मूत्रभावैः इति योगशतकधृतपाठः ।
89. इत आरभ्य ०मूत्रता इत्यन्तः पाठः द्वितीयषष्ठपुस्तकयोः नास्ति ।
90. ०स्तम्भ० इत्यष्टाङ्गहृदये पाठः ।
91. सूर्यमेद्योदये इति अष्टाङ्गहृदयधृतपाठः ।
92. प्रचक्षते इति षष्ठपुस्तके अधिकः पाठः ।
93. ०ऽवतिष्ठते इत्याष्टाङ्गहृदये सूत्र १३:२७ उर्ध्वम् पाठः ।
94. दुर्गन्धि क्षुदुद्गारविघातकृत् इत्याष्टाङ्गहृदये सूत्र १३:२७ ऊर्ध्वम् पाठः ।

95. स एव विज्ञेयश्छेदवान् वक्त्रशुद्धिदः अष्टांगहृदयः सूत्र १३:२७ ऊर्ध्वम् पाठः।
96. वमनैश्चविरेकैश्च इति पञ्चमेतरपुस्तकेषु पाठः ।
97. हि इति आकरे पाठः ।
98. स्व० इति षष्ठपुस्तके पाठः ।
99. व्याधिस्तत्रोपजायते इति आकरे पाठः ।
100. वाऽपि इति सुश्रुत संमतः पाठः ।
101. सर्वाङ्गे इति आदर्शपुस्तकेषु पाठः ।
102. स्वलिङ्गै इत्यपि पाठः ।
103. क. दोषाणां पवनो बली इति द्वितीयपुस्तकपाठो न सङ्गच्छते ।
ख. प्रथमपञ्चमपुस्तकयोः श्लोकोऽयं नोपलभ्यते ।
104. अत्र 'स्वातं आदन्य' इति पाठस्तु लिपिकरप्रमादविजृम्भित एव ०बलित्वादन्य० इति पञ्चमपुस्तके तथा अष्टांगहृदयधृत पाठः ।
105. अथवा स्थानिवच्चापि इति द्वितीयपुस्तकपाठः ।
106. स्वान्तत्र्याद् बहूरोगत्वाद् दोषाणां प्रबलोऽनिलः इति पञ्चमपुस्तकेऽधिकः पाठः ।
107. कारयेदिति इति षष्ठपुस्तके पाठः ।
108. विक्षेपण० इति सुश्रुतधृतपाठः ।
109. अवसंजन इति द्वितीयषष्ठपुस्तकयोः पाठः ।
110. ०कुन्थिकादयः इति षष्ठपुस्तके पाठः ।
111. वेदना इति द्वितीयषष्ठपुस्तकयोः अधिकः पाठः ।
112. श्लोकार्धोऽयं द्वितीयपञ्चमपुस्तकयोर्नोपलभ्यते ।
113. रौक्ष्यं इति पञ्चमपुस्तके पाठः ।
114. स्तन्याद्यभावे इति द्वितीयपुस्तके पाठः ।
115. द्रष्टव्यम्—अष्टांगहृदय : सूत्र ११:१५-२३ तथा सुश्रुत : सूत्र १५:६ ।
116. वा नरः इति सुश्रुत्रधृतः पाठः ।
117. यत्तदन्नपानं प्रकाङ्क्षति इति सुश्रुतधृतपाठः ।
118. ०श्रयेषु तेनैषामाश्रयाश्रयितां इति द्वितीयपुस्तके पाठः ।

119. रसासृङ्मांसं यूषं च इति आदर्शपुस्तके पाठः :

120. श्लोकद्वयं षष्ठपुस्तके नास्ति ।

121. मांसानि इति डल्हणे पाठः ।

122. श्लोकद्वयं द्वितीयषष्ठपुस्तकयोर्नोपलभ्यते ।

123. पेयानिक्षुरसं इति आदर्शपुस्तिकासु पाठः ।

124. निवात० इति पञ्चमपुस्तके पाठः ।

125. गुप्त० इति प्रथमद्वितीयपुस्तकयोः पाठ ।

126. फलशाकान्नपानानि इति षष्ठपुस्तके पाठः ।

127. वाञ्छत्यार्तंवक्षये इति डल्हणे धृतः पाठः ।

128. भोक्तुम् इति डल्हणे पाठः ।

129. ०परिक्षये इति डल्हणे पाठः ।

130. मांसानि इति पञ्चमपुस्तके डल्हणे च पाठः ।

131. ये तेभ्यः इति प्रथमपुस्तके पाठः ।

132. द्रष्टव्यम्—चरक : सूत्र १:१२० ।
सुश्रुत : सूत्र ३६:१० ।

133. मङ्गल्य इति द्वितीयषष्ठपुस्तकयोः पाठः ।

134. विनिपातः इति प्रथमद्वितीयषष्ठपुस्तकेषु पाठः ।

135. तदन्तर्मार्जनं इति प्रथमपुस्तके पाठः ।

136. द्रष्टव्यम्—चरक : सूत्र ११:५५ ।

137. क. चक्षुष्येतो इति प्रथमपुस्तके पाठः ।
ख. चक्षुष्योतो इति द्वितीयपुस्तके पाठः ।

138. द्रष्टव्यम्—चरक : विमान ८:९२-९३ ।
अष्टाङ्गहृदय : सूत्र १:२३ ।

139. कुलैः इति पञ्चमपुस्तके पाठः ।

140. आनूपदेशो इति प्रथमपञ्चमपुस्तकयोः पाठः ।

141. तान् इति समीचीनः पाठः ।

142. सद्यो इति षष्ठपुस्तके पाठः ।

143. श्लोकार्धोऽयं षष्ठपुस्तके नास्ति ।

144. द्रष्टव्यम्—चरक : कल्प १:८ ।
हारीतसंहिता ४:२-७ ।
सुश्रुत : सूत्र ३५:४२ ।
अष्टाङ्गहृदय : सूत्र १:२३-२४ ।

145. मतः इत्याकरे पाठः ।

146. कृते इति आदर्शपुस्तिकासु पाठः ।

147. ०वाहडः इति प्रथमपञ्चमपुस्तकयोः पाठः ।

148. द्रष्टव्यम्—सुश्रुत : सूत्र ३५:४४ ।

149. ०नायतन इति द्वितीयषष्ठपुस्तकयोः पाठः ।

150. प्ररोहन्ती प्रथमपुस्तकपाठः ।

151. परीक्षयेत् इति आदर्शपुस्तकेषु पाठः ।

152. तनुवृक्षाल्परसकोटरवृक्ष० इत्याकरे पाठः ।

153. स्निग्धाश्मवती द्वितीयषष्ठपुस्तकयोः पाठः ।

154. षण्ड इति सर्वपुस्तकपाठोऽर्थसंगतिविरहित इति आकरस्थपाठोऽङ्गीकृतः ।

155. ०सार इति सुश्रुते ।

156. एतावान् पाठो यद्यपि कुत्रचिदपि पुस्तके नावलोक्यते तथापि प्रसंगप्राप्तत्वाद् आकराद् गृहीतः ।

157. सौम्य इति षष्ठपुस्तके पाठः ।

158. या धरा इति षष्ठपुस्तकपाठः ।

159. 'अग्न्याकाशमारुतगुणभूयिष्ठायां वमनद्रव्याणि, उभयगुणभूयिष्ठायामुभयतोभागानि' इत्याकरस्थः सन्दर्भोऽवलोकनीयः ।

160. 'आकाशगुणभूयिष्ठायां इति प्रथमपञ्चमपुस्तकयोः पाठः समीचीनतरः, किन्तु स छन्दोदोषदुष्टः ।

द्रष्टव्यम्—सुश्रुत : सूत्र ३६:६ ।

161. निश्चयनिश्चितः इत्याकरे पाठः।

162. यत्र तत्रैव तद्गुणानि इत्याकरे पाठः।

163. तिस्त्रः प्रकृतयः इत्याकरे पाठः।

164. विपद्यते इति सुश्रुते।

165. प्रथमपुस्तके अधिकपाठः।

166. सत्त्वा इति पञ्चमपुस्तकपाठः।

167. वेदेषु इत्याकरधृतः पाठस्तु साधीयान्।

168. इच्छा इति द्वितीयपुस्तकपाठो न समीचीनः।

169. ०त्वं इत्याकरे पाठः।

170. ०वादिप्रकामिता इति सुश्रुते।

171. निर्दयः इति प्रथमद्वितीयषष्ठपुस्तकेषु पाठः:

172. ०मद इति सुश्रुते।

173. याम्य० इति सुश्रुते।

174. सत्त्वं नरं विदुः इति सुश्रुते।

175. श्लोकोऽयं द्वितीयषष्ठपुस्तकयोः नोपलभ्यते:

176. तीक्ष्णमायासिनं इति सुश्रुते।

177. मायान्वितं इत्याकरे पाठः।

178. ०चार० इत्याकरे पाठः।

179. रौद्र० इति सुश्रुते।

180. भृशमात्रं इति सुश्रुते।

181. तम० इति सुश्रुते।

182. चाप्य० इति सुश्रुते।

183. ०नित्यता इति सुश्रुते।

184. पाशवा इति सुश्रुते।

185. रतः इति सुश्रुते।

186. इत्येते त्रिविधाः इति सुश्रुते ।

187. प्रकृतीर्ज्ञात्वा इति सुश्रुते ।

188. त्व० इति सुश्रुते ।

189. द्रष्टव्यम्—चरक : शारीर ४:३६-४० ।

190. श्लोकोऽयं केवलं षष्ठपुस्तके उपलभ्यते । तत् तु प्रक्षिप्तं प्रतिभाति ।

191. दोषपश्चात्मक इति आदर्शपुस्तकेषु पाठः ।

CHAPTER 3

गोपालसूनुर्भुवि वल्लवीनां[1] निदेशकृद्वेदशिरोऽभितरवम् ।
संस्तूयमाभो[2] दिवि[3] देवसंघैस्तनोतु शं[4] टोडरमल्लभूपे[5] ॥१॥

Invocation

Śri Kṛṣṇa the son of *gopāla* (cow-herd), who is loved by everybody in this universe, who is the embodiment of all knowledge and who is offered prayers by the gods in the heaven, may bestow peace on the king *Ṭoḍara malla*.

[द्रव्यमहत्त्वम्]

द्रव्यं पुरस्कृत्य यतश्चिकित्सा संप्रवर्त्तते ।
व्यक्ताव्यक्तविभेदेन लिख्यतेऽथ समासतः ॥२॥

पञ्चीकृतं भवेद् व्यक्तमव्यक्तं तदभावतः ।
चिकित्सा भवति व्यक्ते ह्यतो व्यक्तं च कथ्यते ॥३॥

Importance of Dravya or Matter

A physician initiates his treatment by keeping the *dravya* or the matter inculding the drug in his view. Therefore, this matter is being described here in brief. It is of two types namely, *vyakta* or manifested and *avyakta* or unmanifested. The matter becomes manifested after the process of *pañci karaṇa* (combination of five subtle *tanmātrās*). In the absence of this *pañci karaṇa*, the matter remains unmanifested. It is the manifested matter on the basis of which treatment is initiated. Therefore, in this text, only the manifested matter will be described.

[द्रव्यभेदवर्णनम्]

काय-बाल-ग्रहोर्ध्वाङ्ग-शल्य-दंष्ट्रा-जरा विषे ।
अष्टाङ्गमण्डपे या तु सरसा सौषधी द्विधा ॥४॥
लता-वृक्षविभेदेन तथा स्थावरजङ्गमात् ।
कन्दमूलविभेदेन फलपुष्पविशेषतः ।
बन्ध्यावन्ध्याविभेदेन ग्रामारण्यविभागतः ॥५॥

Āyurveda has the following eight branches, namely; (1) *kāya cikitsā* (internal medicine); (2) *bāla cikitsā* (paediatrics), (3) *graha cikitsā* (treatment of afflictions by unfavourably positioned planets and evil spirits); (4) *ūrdhvāṅga cikitsā* (treatment of diseases of the head and neck); (5) *śalya cikitsā* (surgery); (6) *danṣṭrā cikitsā* (treatment of afflictions by poisonous animals); (7) *jarā cikitsā* (treatment of old age); and (8) *viṣa cikitsā* (treatment of poisoning).

[This classification is slightly different from the one accepted generally in *āyurveda*—vide Chapter 1:13-40.]

In this arena of āyurveda, drugs play the role of sweet music and they are differently classified into two types, as follows : (1) as creeper and tree; (2) as *sthāvara* (which do not move namely, metals, minerals and vegetable kingdom) and *jāṅgama* (animals),

(3) as *kanda* (rhizome) and *mūla* (root); (4) as fruit and flower; (5) as *bandhyā* (sterile) and *abandhyā* (fertile; and (6) as *grāmya* (domesticated) and *āraṇya* (wild).

अग्निवेशात्

पञ्चभूता[त्मिका]योनिर्भूतानां[सा]चतुर्वि[धा] ।
जरायुजान्यण्डजानि स्वेदजान्यौद्भिदानि[7] च ।
अतश्चतुर्विधं द्रव्यं मतं स्थावरजङ्गमम्[8] ॥६॥

According to Agniveśa

Living creatures which are composed of five *mahābhūtas* have four types of *yoni* (sources of origin). They are (1) *jarāyuja* (living creatures which are covered by amniotic membrane in the womb of the mother), (2) *aṇḍaja* (living creatures which take birth from eggs), (3) *svedaja* (living creatures which come out of sweat or moist heat), and (4) *audbhidja* (living creatures including vegetables which come out by perforating the earth). Thus, *sthāvara* and *jaṅgama dravyas* are divided into the above four categories.

पञ्चीकृतेषु यस्यांशोऽप्यधिकः स्यात् तदाह्वयः ।
आग्नेयं चैव सौम्यं च पुनर्द्विविधमुच्यते[9] ॥७॥

Mahābhūtas are created by the *pañcī karaṇa* of subtle *tanmātrās*. Depending upon the predominance of the one or the other of these *tanmātrās* in the *mahābhūta* it is called either *pārthiva* or *āpya* or *āgneya* or *vāyavīya* or *ākāśiya mahābhūta*. Drugs having these *mahābhutas* are also called *pārthiva āpya*, *taijasa*, *vāyavīya* and *ākāśiya* respectively.

Drugs are also broadly classified into two categories, namely *āgneya* (having heating effect) and *saumya* (having cooling effect).

शोधनं शमनं चैव समासात् तत् द्विधा पुनः ।
पार्थिवं [चौद्भिदं][10] चैव स्थिरं द्विविधमौषधम् ॥८॥

Depending upon their therapeutic effects, drugs are also of two categories namely, *śodhana* (which cure by elimination of *doṣas*) and *śamana* (which cure by alleviation of *doṣas*).

Drugs which are stable in nature are also of two types namely (1) *pārthiva* (which are available on or inside the earth); and (2) *audbhida* (which come out by penetrating the earth).

[भेषजनामानि[11]]

चिकित्सितं व्याधिहरं पथ्यं साधनमौषधम्[12] ।
प्रायश्चित्तं प्रशमनं प्रकृतिस्थापनं हितम्[13] ।
विद्याद् भेषजनामानि भेषजं द्विविधं च तत् ॥६॥

[चरक : चिकित्सा १:१:३-४]

Synonyms of Therapy

The term therapy which is of two types, has the following synonyms viz., *cikitsita*, *vyādhi hara*, *pathya*, *sādhana*, *auṣadha*, *prāyaścitta*, *praśamana*, *prakṛti sthāpana* and *hita*.

[पार्थिवद्रव्यवर्णनम्[14]]

मृत्सुधा शर्कराऽश्मानो लवणं कूटशर्करा ।
अञ्जनं गैरिकं लोहं विमला काञ्चनादिकम् ॥१०॥
रसाश्चोपरसाश्चैव विविधा मणयस्तथा ।
कपालाद्यास्तथाऽन्ये[15] च भेषजं पार्थिवं विदुः ॥११॥

Pārthiva dravya

The following drugs, among others, come under *pārthiva* category :

1. *Mṛt* (mud);

2. *Sudhā* (lime);
3. *Śarkarā* (sand);
4. *Aśman* (stone);
5. *Lavaṇa* (salt);
6. *Kūṭa śarkarā* (alkaline substances collected from caves);
7. *Añjana* (collyrium);
8. *Gairika* (red ochre);
9. *Loha* (metals like iron);
10. *Vimalā* (a type of pyrite);
11. *Kāñcana* (gold);
12. *Rasa* (mercury etc.);
13. *Uparasa*;
14. Different types of gems and jewels; and
15. *Kapāla* (broken pieces of earthen pot).

[16]
[औद्भिदद्रव्यवर्णनम्]

वनस्पत्यौषधीवीरुद्वानस्पत्यस्तथा पुनः ।
मूलं पत्रं फलं पुष्पं त्वक् सारः स्वरसः पयः ।
[17]
क्षीरं तैलानि निर्यासनालकन्दानि चौद्भिदम् ॥१२॥

Audbhida dravya

The following drugs, among others, come under *audbhida* category :

1. *Vanaspati* (trees having fruits without flowers);
2. *Auṣadhi* (plants which die out when their fruits mature);

3. *Vīrut* (creepers);
4. *Vānaspatya* (trees having both flowers and fruits); and
5. Roots, leaves, fruits, flowers, barks, *sāra* (aqueous extract or heart-wood), juice, latex, milk (of plants), oil, gum, stalks and rhizomes.

[18] [जाङ्गमद्रव्यवर्णनम्]

त्वग्रक्तमांसमेदोऽस्थिमज्जाशुक्राणि गोरसः ।
पित्तं मधु मधूच्छिष्टं विण्मूत्रं रोचनादिकम् ॥१३॥
केशलोमनखस्नायुशृङ्गाणि दशनाः खुराः ।
कोष्ठमण्डानि[19] वर्हाणि[20] चौषधं जङ्गमात् स्मृतम् ॥१४॥

Jāṅgama dravya

The following drugs, among others, come under the *jāṅgama* category:

1. Skin, blood, meat, fat, bone, bone marrow and semen;
2. Milk and bile;
3. Honey, bee's wax, stool and urine;
4. *Gorocana* (solidified ox-bile);
5. Hair, small hair, nail, ligament, horn, tooth and hoof;
6. *Koṣṭha* (abdominal and thorasic viscera); and
7. Testicles and feather.

[पंचभूतात्मकद्रव्यलक्षणम्]

[पार्थिवद्रव्यम्]

तत्र द्रव्यं गुरुस्थूलं स्थिरं गन्धगुणोल्वणम् ।
पार्थिवं गौरवस्थैर्यसंघातोपचयावहम् ॥१५॥

Mahābhautika Characteristics of Drugs

Pārthiva dravya

Drugs which are heavy, gross, stable and having more of smell, are dominated by *pṛthvī mahābhūta*. Such drugs cause heaviness, stability, compactness and plumpness of the body.

[आप्यद्रव्यम्]

द्रवशीतगुरुस्निग्धमन्दसान्द्ररसोल्वणम् ।
आप्यं स्नेहमभिष्यन्दिक्लेदप्रह्लादबन्धकृत् ॥१६॥ [21]

Āpya dravya

Drugs which are liquid, cold, heavy, unctuous, sluggish, dense and having more of taste are dominated by *jala mahābhūta*. Such drugs cause unctuousness, obstruction to the channels of circulation (*abhiṣyandi*), stickiness (*kleda*), happiness (*prahlāda*) and cohesiveness (*bandha*).

[आग्नेयद्रव्यम्]

रूक्षतीक्ष्णोष्ण-विशद-सूक्ष्म-रूप-गुणोल्वणम् ।
आग्नेयं दाह-भावर्णप्रकाशं,

Taijasa dravya

Drugs which are ununctuous, sharp, hot, non-slimy, subtle and having more of colour are dominated by *agni mahābhūta*. Such drugs cause burning sensation, aura (*bhā*) and complexion of the body.

[वायव्यद्रव्यम्]

पवनात्मकम् ॥१७॥
व्यवायि रूक्ष विशदं लघुस्पर्शगुणोल्वणम् ।
खरं सूक्ष्मं [22] शीतलं च [23] विचारग्लानिकारकम् ॥१८॥

Vāyavya dravya

Drugs which are *vyavāyi* (which pervade the body before getting digested), ununctuous, non-slimy, light and which have more of tactual attributes are dominated by *vāyu mahābhūta.* Such drugs cause roughness, subtlity, cooling, movement and *glāni* (feeling of exhaustion without effort).

[नाभसद्रव्यम्]

नाभसं सूक्ष्म-विशद-लघु-शब्दगुणोल्वणम् ।
सौषिर्यलाघवकरं तथा व्यक्तरसं भवेत् ॥१९॥

Nābhasa dravya

Drugs which are subtle, non-slimy, light and having more of sound are dominated by *ākāśa mahābhūta.* Such drugs cause porosity and lightness. These drugs have unmanifested tastes.

व्यामिश्रगुणभूयिष्ठं द्रव्यं व्यामिश्रमुच्यते ।

Drugs having mixed attributes are dominated by a mixture of *mahābhūtas.*

[वमनद्रव्यम्]

वाय्वग्निगुणभूयिष्ठं स्वभावादूर्ध्वमार्गगं ॥२०॥

24

वमनीयं भवेत्तद्धि विषपुष्पफलादिकम् ।

Vamana dravya

Emetic drugs like the fruit of *viṣa puṣpa,* are dominated by *vāyu* and *agni mahābhūtas,* and by nature, they have a tendency to move upwards.

[विरेचनद्रव्यम्]

अधोगामि च यद् द्रव्यं तद्भूजलगुणाधिकम् ॥२१॥

विरेचनं भवेत्[25] तच्च[26] कार्णिकादि फलं यथा ।

Virecana dravya

Purgative drugs like the fruit of *karṇika* are dominated by *pṛthvī* and *jala mahābhūtas*, and by nature, they have a tendency to move downwards.

[संग्राहीद्रव्यम्]

संग्राहकं भवेद्द्रव्यं प्रभञ्जनगुणाधिकम् ॥२२॥

Saṁgrāhī dravya

Astringent (bowel binding) drugs are dominated by *vāyu mahābhūta*.

[बृंहणशमनद्रव्यम्]

बृंहणं च जलाधिक्यादाकाशात् शमनं मतम् ।

Bṛṁhaṇa and Śamana dravyas

Bṛṁhaṇa or nourishing drugs are dominated by the *jala mahābhūta*.

Śamana (which alleviate *doṣas*) drugs are dominated by *ākāśa mahābhūta*.

[दीपनं द्रव्यम्]

अग्न्याधिक्यात् दीपनं च किञ्चिद्वारिगुणैर्युतम् ॥२३॥

Dīpana dravya

Dīpana drugs which stimulate digestion are dominated by *agni mahābhūta*. They are slightly associated with the attributes of *jala mahābhūta*.

[बल्यद्रव्यम्]

बहूर्वीसत्त्वसहितं द्रव्यं बलकरं मतम् ।

एतेषां लक्षणं चाथ संक्षेपेण च लिख्यते ॥२४॥

Balya dravya

Drugs dominated by *pṛthvi mahābhūta* in excess are the promoters of strength. Their characteristic features will now be described in brief.

[दीपनद्रव्यम्]

पक्त्वामं पावकं कुर्यात् तत् तु दीपनमुच्यते ।

Dipana dravya

The drug which stimulates the digestive power by causing *pāka* (digestion) of *āma* (undigested food material or matabolic biproduct) is called *dipana.*

[पाचनद्रव्यम्]

कुर्यान्न वह्निमामं यत्पचेत्तत्पाचनं मतम् ॥२५॥

Pācana dravya

A drug which does not stimulate the digestive fire but helps in the *pāka* (digestion) of *āma* (undigested food material or metabolic biproduct) is called *pācana.*

[दीपनपाचनभेदवर्णनम्]

अथ जिज्ञासा ॥ पाचनदीपनयोः को भेदः ॥२६॥

Distinctive features between Dipana and Pācana Drugs

The query that may arise as to what is the difference between the *dipana* and *pācana* drugs?

तत्रोच्यते

आग्नेयगुणभूयिष्ठमामादीस्तद् विपाचयेत् ।

तदुक्तं[27] पाचनं द्रव्यं यथा[28] स्यात् कासमर्दकः ॥२७॥

कासमर्दः कथं नाम, पाचनो नास्ति दीपनः ।
वाय्वग्निगुणभूयिष्ठं द्रव्यं पाचनमुच्यते ॥२८॥
औष्ण्यात् कटुविपाकित्वात् पाचनोऽयमुदाहृतः ।
माधुर्याच्छितिभावाच्च न पुनर्दीपनो मतः ॥२९॥

It is stated in this connection that the *pācana* drug is dominated by *agni mahābhūta* and it causes digestion and metabolic transformation of *āma* e.g. *kāsa mardaka*. Why *kāsa mardaka* is only a *pācana* drug and not a *dipana* drug? *Pācana* drugs are dominated by *vāyu* and *agni mahābhūtas*. *Kāsa marda* is categorised as a *pācana dravya* because of its *uṣṇa* (hot) property and *kaṭu vipāka* (which becomes pungent in taste after digestion). It is not a *dipana* drug because of its sweet taste and cooling property.

कृष्णात्रेयात्

यदग्निकृत् पचेन्नामं दीपनं तद्यथा घृतम् ।
पाचनं विपरीतं स्याद्यथा वक्ष्यामि लङ्घनम् ॥३०॥

[29] लङ्घनं पाचने सत्यपि न दीपनं ॥३१॥

तद्यथा

संशोधनास्रविस्रावस्नेहयोजनलङ्घनैः ।
यात्यग्निर्म्मंदतां तस्मात्क्रमं पेयादिमाचरेत् ॥३२॥
स्रोतसां कफदुष्टानां[30] निर्मलीकरणं परम् ।
पाचनं तत्समाख्यातं धातोः पाचक ईष्यते ॥३३॥

According to Kṛṣṇātreya

The drug, which stimulates the digestive fire but does not help in the digestion of *āma*, is called *dipana* e.g. ghee. The drug acting otherwise is called *pācana*. *Laṅghana* or fasting is *pācana* but not *dipana*. But, by *saṁśodhana* (elimination therapies), *asra visrāva* (blood-letting), *snehana* (oleation therapy) and *laṅghana* (fasting), the *agni* or the digestive fire gets diminished. Therefore, *peyā* (thin gruel) etc., should be administered as diet to such patients. *Pācana* drugs cleanse the channels of circulation vitiated by *kapha*. These drugs also help in the *pāka* (metabolic transformation) of *dhātus* (tissue elements).

अथ गोपुरः

जिज्ञासा वर्त्तते चात्र पाचने वदतां वर ।
दोषान्पचति आमं वा सप्तधातूनथाऽपि वा ॥३४॥
'दोषान्पचति धातूंश्च पाचनो दृश्यते यदि[31] ।'
दोषपाकाद्धातुपाकान्मरणं दृश्यते तदा ।
इति सर्वत्र कथितं पाचनो दोषपाचनः ॥३५॥

According to Gopura

O ! Preceptor, "We desire to know the mode of action of *pācana* drugs. Do they cause *pāka* (metabolic transformation) of *doṣas* or *āma* or the seven categories of *dhātus*? If they cause *pāka* of *doṣas* and *dhātus*, then this should result in the death of the patient. Generally, people believe the drugs to cause *pāka* of *doṣas*."

अस्योत्तरम्

स्वहेतूपच्चितान् दोषान् सामान् रसपथगानुगान्[32] ।
रसमामं पाचयित्वा कुर्याद्दोषं पृथक्ततः ।
स एव पाचनो[33] ज्ञेयो न च दोषान् विपाचयेत् ॥३६॥

The preceptor replied, "*Doṣas* accumulated as a result of their respective causative factors get associated with *āma* and enter into the channels of circulation of *rasa*. As a result of this, the *rasa* becomes associated with *āma*. The drug, which causes *pāka* (metabolic transformation) of this *āma* as a result of which *doṣas* become free from it, is called *pācana*. Such drugs do not cause *pāka* of *doṣas*.

अत्राह

दोषस्य पाको दृश्येत ऊर्द्ध्वाधोगमनं तथा ।
अतिप्रवृद्धवातस्य पित्तस्य श्लेष्मणस्तथा ॥३७॥
पाचनीयेन द्रव्येण दृश्यते पाचनं तथा ।
वमनीयेन द्रव्येण दृश्यते वमनाद्यपि ॥३८॥

Thus it is said

The *pāka* of *doṣas* can be associated by the upward and downward movement of even exceedingly vitiated *vāyu, pitta* and *kapha*. Similarly, the effect of *pācana* drugs can be ascertained by the process of *pāka* (metabolic transformation) as the effects of *vamana* (emetic) drugs can be ascertained by emesis.

अत्रोच्यते

स्वयोनिवर्द्धनद्रव्यैः सुरातक्रजलासवैः ।
34
घृतादिभिः प्रवृद्धास्ते प्रकृत्या वृद्धिमाप्नुयुः ॥३९॥
यथा क्षीरे जलं क्षिप्तं क्षीरवद्दृश्यते बहु ।
35
सुस्वादुगुणनिर्मुक्तं भस्माग्नितपनात्पुनः ॥४०॥
जले दग्धे भवेत्क्षीरं तत्स्वादुस्वगुणैर्युतम् ।
36
तथाप्यधातुसंश्लिष्टाः सामाः स्वहेतुदूषिताः ॥४१॥
लंघनात्पाचनोल्लेखात्स्वप्रमाणं भजन्त्यपि ।
पच्यन्ते नैव दोषास्तु पचन्त्यामरसादयः ॥४२॥

It is also said

By the factors which aggravate their various attributes, the *doṣas* naturally get aggravated by drugs like *surā*, *takra*, *jala*, *āsava* and ghee. This is on the analogy of increasing the quantity of milk by adding water to it. This milk, no doubt, appears to be more in quantity, but it will not have the taste of the original milk. If this diluted milk is again boiled and the water is evaporated, then it regains its original taste. On the same analogy, *doṣas* which are vitiated by the respective causative factors, which are associated with *āma* and which are not associated with any other *doṣa*, return to their own state of equilibrium (normal quantity) by *laṅghana* (fasting), *pācana*, *ullekhana* (emetic therapy) etc. It is not the *doṣas* themselves but the *āma rasa* associated with them which undergoes the process of *pāka*.

कुर्यान्न वह्निमामं यत् पचेत् तत् पाचनं मतम् ।

The drug, which does not stimulate the *agni* (digestive fire) but causes *pāka* (metabolic transformation) of *āma* (immature digestive and metabolic products), is called *pācana*.

[शमनद्रव्यम्]

न शोधयति यद्दोषान् समान्न[37] दूषयत्यपि ।
'शमनं तद्विजानीयात्, कोभेदः स्वस्थरक्षणात्[38] ॥४३॥'

Śamana drugs

The drug, which does not eliminate the *doṣas* and which does not vitiate the normal *doṣas* but alleviates the vitiated ones, is called *śamana*.

How these *śamana* drugs (which alleviate *doṣas*) are different from *svastha rakṣaṇa* drugs (which help in the maintenance of positive health) ?

अत्राहात्रिः

क्षयस्थाने विवृद्ध्यर्थं दोषाणां यत्प्रयुज्यते ।

39

विना संशोधनद्रव्यैस्तत्संशमनमुच्यते ॥४४॥

According to Atri

Drugs, which are employed for increasing the quantity of the diminished *doṣas* and which do not remove *doṣas* by the process of *saṁśodhana* or elimination, are called *saṁśamana* or *śamana.*

[अनुलोमनद्रव्यम्]

तच्चानुलोमनं द्रव्यं यद्वातमनुलोमयेत् ।

Anulomana dravya

The drug, which causes the downward movement of *vāyu,* is called *anulomana.*

[स्रंसन भेदनद्रव्यम्]

यद्बन्धभेदनं कृत्वा मलान् पक्वान् नयत्यधः ॥४५॥

स्रंसनं तद्विजानीयद्भेदनं प्रोच्यते ह्यतः ।

अधो नयति यद्बद्धमबद्धं भेदनं मतम् ॥४६॥

Sraṁsana and Bhedana dravyas

The drug, which eliminates the excreta that are *pakva* (digested) after disintegrating the solid state, is called *sraṁsana.*

The drug, which eliminates both the solid and disintegrated excreta through the downward tract, is called *bhedana.*

[विरेचनवमनद्रव्यम्]

40

मलं पक्वमपक्वं वा यद्यद् विद्रावयत्यधः ।

41 42

श्लेष्मपित्ताद्यपक्वं यदूद्‌र्ध्वं नयति वमनम् ॥४७॥

Virecana and Vamana dravyas

The drug, which eliminates both the *pakva* (digested) and *apakva* (undigested) excreta by dissolving through downward tract is called *virecana.*

The drug, which eliminates the *apakva* (undigested) *kapha, pitta* etc., through the upward tract, is called *vamana.*

[छेदनद्रव्यम्]

दोषानुन्मूलयति यत्[43] श्लिष्टान् तत् छेदनं बलात् ।

Chedana dravya

The drug, which by force uproots the adhered *doṣas,* is called *chedana.*

[ग्राहिद्रव्यम्]

उष्णत्वाद् दीपनं यच्च पाचनं ग्राहि तद्भवेत् ॥४८॥

Grāhi dravya

A drug, which as a result of its heating nature, works as *dīpana* (digestive stimulant) and *pācana* (carminative) and which causes constipation, is called *grāhi.*

[स्तम्भनद्रव्यम्]

लघुपाकात् कषायत्वाद्भवेद्यत्स्तम्भनं मतम्[44] ।

Stambhana dravya

A drug, which is light for digestion and which because of its astringent taste causes constipation, is called *stambhana.*

[रसायनद्रव्यम्]

रसायनं तदुद्देश्यं जराव्याधिविनाशि यत् ॥४९॥

Rasāyana dravya

The drug, which destroys the process of ageing as well as diseases, is called *rasāyana.*

[वाजीकरद्रव्यम्]

द्रव्येण येन हर्षः स्यात्स्त्रीषु वाजीकरं हि तत् ।

[शुक्रलद्रव्यम्]

यस्माच्छुक्रस्य वृद्धिस्याच्छुक्रलं हि तदुच्यते ॥५०॥
यथाऽश्वगंधा मुशली शर्करा च शतावरी ।
प्रवर्त्तकानि कथ्यन्ते जनकानि च[45] रेतसः ॥५१॥
शुक्रप्रवर्तिनी योषा[46] क्षुद्रा शुक्रस्य रेचनी ।
तत्स्तम्भकृज्जातिफलं कालिङ्गं तत्क्षयप्रदम् ॥५२॥

Vājikara and Śukrala dravya

The drug, which causes excitement and passionate desire for woman, is called *vājikara.*

The drug, which increases the quantity of semen, is called *śukrala*, for example, *aśvagandhā*, *muśalī*, *śarkarā* and *śatāvarī*.

Some of these drugs stimulate the ejaculation of semen and some others help in the production of more of semen.

A beautiful woman induces the ejaculation of semen. *Kṣudrā* causes the actual ejaculation. *Jāti phala* increases the power of retention of semen. The seeds of *kaliṅga* reduce the quantity of semen.

[सूक्ष्मद्रव्यम्]

तनुच्छिद्रेषु सूक्ष्मेषु विशेत्तत्सूक्ष्ममुच्यते[47] ।

Sūkṣma dravya

The drug, which has the ability to enter through the thin and subtle channels, is called *sūkṣma*.

[व्यवायिद्रव्यम्]

तद् व्यवायि तनुं व्याप्य पूर्वं यत् पाकतां व्रजेत् ॥५३॥

Vyavāyi dravya

The drug, which pervades the entire body before being digested, is called *vyavāyi*.

[विकाशिद्रव्यम्]

विकाशि तद्यत् करोति बन्धान् सन्धिस्थितान् शुभान्[48] ।

हस्तपादान् शिथिलयेद् भवेद् विश्लेषितं[49] मतम् ॥५४॥

Vikāśi dravya

The drug, which loosens the ligaments of the joints, which causes slackness of the hands and legs and which separates them, is called *vikāśi*.

[मदकारिद्रव्यम्]

यद्बुद्धिनाशने दक्षं मदकारि तदुच्यते ।

Madakāri dravya

The drug, which is effective in destroying the wisdom is called *madakāri*.

[प्रमाथिद्रव्यम्]

वीर्येण दोषान् स्रोतोस्थान्[50] निरस्यति प्रमाथि तत् ॥५५॥

Pramāthi dravya

The drug, which by its own potency, eliminates the *doṣas* located in the channels of circulation, is called *pramāthi*.

[अभिष्यन्दिद्रव्यम्]

रुणद्धि गौरवाद् द्रव्यं स्नैग्ध्याद्रसवहाः सिराः ।
कलेवरे गुरुत्वं च धत्तेऽभिष्यन्दि तन्मतम् ॥५६॥

Abhiṣyandi dravya

The drug, which because of its heaviness and unctuousness, obstructs the channels of circulation carrying *rasa* (plasma) and which produces heaviness in the body, is called *abhiṣyandi*.

[उदाहरणम्]

उदाहरणमेतेषां क्रमाद् द्रव्येण वक्ष्यते ।
दीपनश्चित्रको ज्ञेयः पाचनं नागकेशरम् ॥५७॥
गुडूची शमनी ज्ञेया हरीतक्यनुलोमिनी ।
स्रंसनं कृतमालः स्याद्भेदिनी कटुरोहिणी ॥५८॥
रेचनी त्रिवृता [51]ज्ञेया वामकं मदनं फलं ।
[52]'छेदनं सलिलं क्षौद्रं ग्राहि स्याज्जीरकं च यत्' ॥५९॥
स्तम्भनो वत्सको ज्ञेयो गुग्गुलुः स्याद्रसायनम् ।
वाजीकरं पयो [53]माषास्तालमूली शतावरी ॥६०॥
सैंधवं मधु सूक्ष्मं स्यादहिफेनो व्यवायी च ।
विश्लेषि क्रमुकं ज्ञेयं मदकारि सुरादिकं ॥६१॥

योगवाहि विषं ज्ञेयं प्रमाथि मरिचं स्मृतम् ।

दध्यभिष्यन्दि विज्ञेयं शिराणां सन्निरोधनात् ॥६२॥

Examples

The examples of different categories of drugs described above are given below, seriatim :

1.	*Dīpana*	*Citraka*
2.	*Pācana*	*Nāga keśara*
3.	*Śamana*	*Guḍūcī*
4.	*Anulomana*	*Harītakī*
5.	*Sraṁsana*	*Kṛtamāla*
6.	*Bhedana*	*Kaṭu rohiṇī*
7.	*Recana*	*Trivṛtā*
8.	*Vāmana*	*Madana phala*
9.	*Chedana*	Water and honey
10.	*Grāhi*	*Jīraka*
11.	*Staṁbhana*	*Vatsaka*
12.	*Rasāyana*	*Guggulu*
13.	*Vājīkara*	Milk, *māṣa, tālamūlī* and *śatāvarī*
14.	*Sūkṣma*	*Saindhava* and honey
15.	*Vyavāyī*	*Ahiphena*
16.	*Vikāśī (Viśleṣī)*	*Kramuka*
17.	*Madakārī*	*Surā etc.*
18.	*Yogavāhī*	*Viṣa*

19.	*Pramāthi*	*Marica*
20.	*Abhiṣyandi*	*Dadhi* (because it obstructs the channels of circulation).

[रस]

रसादीनां च विज्ञानमभ्यासाज्जायते न वा ।
तस्मात्तत्र परं यत्नं कारयेत् मतिमान्[54] द्विजः[55] ॥६३॥
आश्रयाणामसंख्यानां[56] तथैव गुणकर्मणाम् ।
असंख्येया इति रसाः केचिदाहुर्महर्षयः ।
तत्त्वाह तत्र आत्रेयः षडेवेह रसा मताः ॥६४॥

तद्यथा

रसाः स्वाद्वम्ललवणतिक्तोषणकषायकाः ।
षड्द्रव्यमाश्रितास्ते[57] च यथापूर्वं बलावहाः ॥६५॥

[अष्टाङ्गहृदय : सूत्र१:१४-१५]

Rasa (*tastes*)

The knowledge of *rasa* (taste) etc., is acquired by constant practice. Some times, in spite of it, one fails to get this knowledge. Therefore, a wise physician should strive hard to acquire this knowledge. The sources of *rasa* (tastes) as well as *guṇa* (attributes) and *karma* are innumerable. Therefore, according to some great sages, *rasas* are innumerable. However, according to *Ātreya*, there are only six types of *rasas*. They are sweet, sour, saline, bitter, pungent and astringent. They are located in six categories of matter. In the reverse order, they are more and more powerful in nature.

अग्निवेशात्

स्वादुर्भूम्यम्बुभूयस्त्वाद् भूमिदाहात् तु तैजसः ।
अम्लो रसोऽथ लवणः सलिलाग्न्यतिरेकजः[58] ॥६६॥

वाय्वग्न्योः कटुकस्तिक्तो वाय्वाकाशातिरेकजः ।
भूमारुतगुणाधिक्यात् कषायो जायते रसः ॥६७॥

According to Agniveśa

Predominance of *pṛthvī* and *jala mahābhūtas* gives rise to sweet taste. The sour taste which is *taijasa* in nature is produced as a result of the predominance of *pṛthvī* and *agni mahābhūtas*. By the predominance of *jala* and *agni mahābhūtas* saline taste is manifested. Predominance of *vāyu* and *agni mahābhūtas* gives rise to pungent taste. The bitter taste is manifested as a result of the predominance of *vāyu* and *ākāśa mahābhūtas*. Predominance of *pṛthvī* and *vāyu mahābhūtas* causes the manifestation of astringent taste.

स्पर्शनार्थे यथा स्पर्शो रसनार्थे तथा रसः ।

As the tactile sensation is perceived through the skin, similarly, the taste of a substance is perceived by the tongue.

स्नेहनप्रीणनैः तृप्तिह्लादमार्दवलेपनैः ॥६८॥
जिह्वास्यतालुकण्ठानां मुखस्थं मधुरं वदेत् ।

Sweet taste is ascertained by unctuousness, deliciousness, sense of satisfaction, delightfulness, softness and production of stickiness in the tongue, mouth, palate and throat while the substance is in the mouth.

अम्लं रुचिमुखास्रावदन्तहर्षास्यबोधनैः ॥६९॥

Sour taste is ascertained by the relish, salivation, *danta harṣa* (setting of teeth on edge) and clarity of mouth.

लवणं रेचनं क्लेदि दाहाश्लिष्यंदिलाघवैः ।

Saline taste is ascertained by purgation, stickiness, burning sensation, moistness and lightness.

59

कटुको मुखनासाक्षितोददाहार्त्तिसंस्रवैः ॥७०॥

Pungent taste is ascertained by the production of *toda* (pinching pain), *dāha* (burning sensation), *arti* (cutting pain), and *saṁsrava* (exudation of watery fluid) of mouth, nose and eyes.

60

तिक्तो रसनविश्लेषवैशद्याह्लादशोषणैः ।

Drugs and diet, having bitter taste, weaken the taste perception and cause non-sliminess, delightfulness and dryness.

कषायं तु विकाशित्वशैत्यस्तम्भत्वमार्दवैः ॥७१॥

Drugs and diet, having astringent taste, are *vikāśi* (which cause looseness of joints) and they produce *śita* (cooling), *stambha* (rigidity) and *mārdava* (softness).

षण्णां रसानामित्युक्तं मुखस्थानां स्वलक्षणम् ।

Thus, the signs and symptoms that are manifested by these six tastes, when they are in the mouth, are described

स्वाद्वम्ललवणाः सौम्याः स्नेहप्रक्लेदभावतः ॥७२॥

कषायतिक्तकटुकास्त्वाग्नेयास्तद्विपर्ययात् ।

Sweet, sour and saline tastes are *saumya* (cooling), because they produce unctuousness and stickiness. On the other hand, astringent, bitter and pungent tastes are *āgneya* (heating), because they work in the opposite manner.

61

समीरणे तु नादेयाः कटुतिक्तकषायकाः ।

पित्ते कट्वम्ललवणाः स्वाद्वम्ललवणाः कफे ॥७३॥

When *vāyu* is aggravated, then pungent, bitter and astringent tastes are contra-indicated. In aggravated *pitta*, pungent, sour and saline tastes are contra-indicated. When *kapha* is aggravated, then sweet, sour and saline tastes are contra-indicated.

वाग्भटः

'मधुरं श्लेष्मलं प्रायो जीर्णाच्छालियवादृते ।
मुद्गाद्गोधूमतः क्षौद्रात्सितायाः जाङ्गलामिषात् ॥७४॥

According to Vāgbhaṭa

Sweet taste generally aggravates *kapha*. But old *śāli* rice, old barley, *mudga*, *godhūma*, honey, sugar and meat of animals inhabiting dry land forests are exceptions to this rule.

प्रायोऽम्लं पित्तजननं दाडिमामलकादृते ।

Sour taste generally aggravates *pitta*. But *dāḍima* and *āmalaka* are exceptions to this rule.

62

अपथ्यं लवणं प्रायश्चक्षुषोऽन्यत्र सैन्धवात् ॥७५॥

Salts are generally unwholesome for eye sight. But *saiṅdhava* (rock salt) is an exception to this rule.

तिक्तं कटु [च] भूयिष्ठमवृष्यं वातकोपनम् ।
ऋतेऽमृतापटोलीभ्यां शुण्ठीकृष्णारसोनतः ।

Bitter and pungent tastes are exceedingly non-aphrodisiac and they cause aggravation of *vāyu*. But *amṛtā*, *paṭolī*, *śuṇṭhī*, *kṛṣṇā* and *rasona* are exceptions to this rule.

63

कषायं प्रायशः शीतं स्तम्भनं चाऽभयां विना ॥७६॥'

[अष्टाङ्गहृदय : सूत्र १०:३३-३६]

Astringent taste is generally cooling and bowel-binding. But *abhayā* is an exception to this rule.

'रसाः कट्वम्ललवणा वीर्येणोष्णा यथोत्तरम् ।
तिक्तः कषायो मधुरस्तद्वदेव च शीतलाः ॥७७॥'

[अष्टाङ्गहृदय : सूत्र१०:३६-३७]

Pungent, sour and saline tastes are progressively more and more *uṣṇa* (hot) in potency. Similarly, bitter, astringent and sweet tastes are progressively more and more *śītala* (cold) in potency.

कटोः[64] कषायस्तस्माच्च मधुरः परमो[65] गुरुः ।
लघुरम्लः कटुस्तस्मात्तस्मादपि च तिक्तकः ॥७८॥

Astringent taste is heavier than saline taste and sweet taste is heavier than astringent taste. Sour taste is light for digestion and pungent taste is lighter than that. The bitter taste is the lightest of all.

आत्रेयात्

समाः षडभ्यवहृता यान्त्यम्लस्य वशं रसाः ।
कटुकस्याम्लवर्ज्यास्तु तौ विना लवणस्य तु ॥७९॥
विना कट्वम्ललवणैर्द्वौ स्वादुवशगौ रसौ ।
तिक्तानुगः कषायस्तु विषमेषु च योऽधिकः ॥८०॥

According to Ātreya

If all the tastes are taken in equal quantity, then the final product becomes sour in taste. If sour taste is excluded, then the final taste becomes pungent. If pungent taste is excluded, then the final product becomes saline in taste. If pungent, sour and saline tastes are excluded, then the final taste becomes sweet. If only bitter and astringent tastes are taken in equal quantity, then the final product becomes bitter.

If however, diet having different tastes are consumed in inequal quantity, then the taste of the final product will be according to the predominating taste in the compound.

अथ वीर्यलक्षणम्

शमनं दीपनं चैव ऊर्ध्वाधः शोधनं च वै ।
संग्राहकाग्निजननं लेखनं चावपीडनम् ॥८१॥
रसायनं बृंहणं च तथा वाजीकरं हि यत् ।
श्लेष्मलं शोफशमनं दारणं भेदनं तथा ॥८२॥
मंथनं प्राणघातं च विषप्रशमनानि च ।
भवन्ति वीर्यप्राधान्यात्तद्वीर्यं द्विविधं मतम् ॥८३॥

Characteristic Features of Vīrya (potency)

The drugs or the diet, because of their predominating *vīrya* (potency), produce various therapeutic effects, like *śamana* (alleviation of *doṣas*) *dīpana* (stimulation of digestive fire), *ūrdhvādhaḥ śodhana* (elimination of *doṣas* through upward and downward tracts), *saṁgrāhaka* (constipation), *agni janana* (production of digestive fire), *lekhana* (depletion), *avapīḍana* (extraction by application of pressure), *rasāyana* (rejuvenation), *bṛṁhaṇa* (nourishment), *vājīkaraṇa* (manifestation of aphrodisiac effect), *śleṣmala* (aggravation of *kapha*), *śopha śamana* (alleviation of oedema), *dāraṇa* (excision), *bhedana* (penetration), *manthana* (churning), *prāṇaghāta* (killing) and *viṣa praśamana* (anti-toxic effect).

उष्णं शीतं जगद्यस्मादुष्णं शीतं भवेत्ततः ।
केचिदष्टविधं वीर्यं वदन्ति शृणु तत्त्वतः ॥८४॥

This *vīrya* (potency) is of two types. In view of the *uṣṇatā* (heating property) and *śaitya* (cooling property) of the universe, the two types of *vīrya* or potency are *uṣṇa* (hot) and *śīta* (cold) respectively.

'मृदु-रूक्ष-गुरु-स्निग्ध-तीक्ष्णोष्ण-लघु-शीतलम् ।

बलमष्टविधं त्वेतद् द्रव्याणां वीर्यमुच्यते[66] ॥८५॥

According to some scholars, *vīrya* or potency, is of eight types as follows :

1. *Mṛdu* (soft) ;
2. *Rūkṣa* (ununctuous);
3. *Guru* (heavy);
4. *Snigdha* (unctuous);
5. *Tīkṣṇa* (sharp);
6. *Uṣṇa* (hot);
7. *Laghu* (light); and
8. *Śītala* (cold).

The above mentioned eight specific powers of the matter are called *vīrya* or potency.

ते गुणाः विंशतिविधा श्रृणु चात्रेयकीर्तिताः ।
शीतोष्णस्निग्धरूक्षाख्यो मंदस्तीक्ष्णो लघुर्गुरुः ॥८६॥
पिच्छिलो विशदः श्लक्ष्णः परुषः कठिनो मृदुः ।
द्रवः सान्द्रः स्थिरसरः स्थूलसूक्ष्मश्च विंशतिः ॥८७॥

Characteristic Features of Guṇa

According to *Ātreya*, *guṇas* or attributes are twenty in number. These are as follows :

1. *Śīta* (cold)
2. *Uṣṇa* (hot)
3. *Snigdha* (unctuous)
4. *Rukṣa* (ununctuous)
5. *Manda* (sluggish)
6. *Tīkṣṇa* (sharp)
7. *Laghu* (light)
8. *Guru* (heavy)

9. *Picchila* (slime)
10. *Viśada* (non-slime)
11. *Ślakṣṇa* (smooth)
12. *Paruṣa* (rough)
13. *Kaṭhina* (hard)
14. *Mṛdu* (soft)
15. *Drava* (liquid)
16. *Sāndra* (dense)
17. *Sthira* (stable)
18. *Sara* (mobile)
19. *Sthūla* (gross)
20. *Sūkṣma* (subtle).

[67] अत्र “इन्द्रियार्था व्यवायी च विकाशी चापरे गुणाः” इति न लिखितम् । यतो

[68] व्यवायीसरगुणस्यैव प्रकर्षः, विकाशी तीक्ष्णस्यैव ॥८८॥

In this context, two other attributes which are perceptible by senses viz., *vyavāyi* and *vikāśi* are not described because *vyavāyi* is the excellent state of *sara* (mobile) attribute and *vikāśi* is the excellent state of *tikṣṇa* (sharp).

तथोक्तं वाग्भट्टेन

सरस्तीक्ष्णप्रकर्षौ तु कैश्चित्तौ परिकल्पितौ ॥८९॥

[अष्टाङ्गसंग्रह : सूत्र१:४१]

According to Vāgbhaṭa

According to some, *vyavāyi* and *vikāśi* are the excellent states of *sara* and *tikṣṇa* attributes respectively.

‘ये रसा वातशमना भवन्ति यदि तेषु वै ।

रौक्ष्यलाघवशैत्यानि न ते हन्युः समीरणम् ॥९०॥

Rasas and Doṣas

Rasas (tastes) which should normally alleviate *vāyu*, do not do so if there is predominance of attributes like ununctuousness, lightness and coldness in the drug.

ये रसाः पित्तशमना भवन्ति यदि तेषु वै ।

तीक्ष्णोष्णलघुता[69] चैव न ते तत्कर्मकारिणः ॥६१॥

Rasas (tastes) which should normally alleviate *pitta* do not do so if there is predominance of sharpness, heat and lightness in the drug.

"ये रसाः श्लेष्मशमनाः[70] भवन्ति यदि तेषु वै ।

स्नेहगौरवशैत्यानि न ते तत्कर्मकारिणः"[71] ॥६२॥'

[सुश्रुत : सूत्र४०:६-८]

Rasas (tastes) which should normally alleviate *kapha*, do not do so if there is predominance of unctuousness, heaviness and coldness in the drug.

अथ पाकः

त्रिधा विपाको द्रव्यस्य स्वाद्वम्लकटुकात्मकः ।

अन्ये प्रतिरसं पाकं प्रवदन्ति मुनीश्वराः ॥६३॥

Vipāka

Vipāka (the taste that emerges after digestion) is of three types viz., *svādu* (sweet), *amla* (sour) and *kaṭu* (pungent). According to some sages, each *rasa* (taste) has its own *pāka*.

तत्राह वाग्भटः

'स्वादुः पटुश्च मधुरमम्लोऽम्लं पच्यते रसः ।

तिक्तोषणकषायाणां विपाकः प्रायशः कटुः ॥६४॥'

[अष्टाङ्गहृदय : सूत्र९:२१]

According to Vāgbhaṭa

The *vipāka* of sweet and saline tastes is sweet. The *vipāka* of sour taste is sour. The *vipāka* of pungent, bitter and astringent tastes is generally pungent.

चरकात्

> घृतक्षीरादि मधुरमम्लं दधिसुरादि च ।
>
> कटुचित्रकचव्यादिरसतः पाकमादिशेत् ॥६५॥

According to Caraka

Ghee, milk etc., have sweet taste. *Dadhi* (curd), *surā* (alcohol) etc., are sour in taste. *Citraka*, *cavya* etc., are pungent in taste. The *vipāka* of these substances are similar to their *rasa* or taste.

सुश्रुतमते अम्लपाको नास्ति ॥६६॥

तद्यथा

> पित्तं विदग्धमेति यत्[72] तदम्लत्वं भजत्यपि ।
>
> आग्नेयत्वाच्छृणुष्वान्यां[73] गतिं श्लेष्मविपाकजाम् ॥६७॥
>
> यद्येवं लवणः पाको[74] भविष्यति हि चापरः ।
>
> विदग्धोऽपि[75] कफः पाके लवणत्वमवाप्नुयात्[76] ॥६८॥

Suśruta does not recognise sour as a type of *vipāka*. According to him, *pitta* becomes *vidagdha* (a state of imperfect digestion) as a result of which it becomes sour in taste because, it is dominated by *agni mahābhūta*. If *amla* (sour) is accepted as a type of *vipāka*, then *lavaṇa* (saline) should also be treated as another type of *vipāka*, because the taste of *kapha* becomes saline when it becomes *vidagdha* (a state of imperfect digestion).

यद्येवं तर्हि सुश्रुतेनाप्येवं कथमुक्तम्? ॥६९॥

If the above quoted view of *Suśruta* is correct, then why did he describe as below :

मधुरश्चाम्लपाकश्च व्रीहिः पित्तकरो गुरुः ।

77

उष्णाः कुलत्थाः पाकेऽम्लकफशुक्रानिलापहाः ॥१००॥

"*Vrihi* is sweet in taste and *amla* (sour) in *pāka*. It aggravates *pitta* and it is heavy. *Kulttha* is hot and *amla* (sour) in *pāka*. It reduces *kapha*, *śukra* (semen) and *vāyu*."

78

तत्राम्लकारित्वसामर्थ्यादम्लपाकावुक्तौ; नार्थोऽम्लपाकेनैति चन्द्रटः ॥१०१॥

Candraṭa has solved this problem of contradiction by saying, that the sour taste referred to in the above verses from *Suśruta* does not pertain to sour *vipāka*. It only explains that, they have the ability to produce sourness.

यदि प्रतिरसं पाकः कथमेवं प्रदिश्यते ।

79

अभया क्षीणरूढा ये शालयो जाङ्गलास्तथा ॥१०२॥

धात्री निम्बपटोलौ च सामुद्रं लवणं तथा ।

कषायस्वादुकट्वम्लतिक्तादेश्चान्यपाकता ॥१०३॥

If the *vipāka* of a substance is determined by its taste, then why astringent, sweet, pungent, sour and bitter substances like *abhayā*, dwarf variety of *śāli* rice, meat of animals living in arid land forests, *dhātrī*, *niṁba*, *paṭola* and sea salt should have *pāka* not in conformity with their tastes ?

सुश्रुते द्विविधः पाकः प्रोक्तो भगवता पुरा ।

80

मधुरः कटुकश्चैव तयोर्मिष्टो गुरुर्भवेत् ।

कटुकाख्यो लघुः प्रोक्तः पृथिव्यादेः स्वभावतः ॥१०४॥

The sage has stated in *Suśruta saṁhitā* that, there are two types of *pāka* viz., sweet and pungent. The drugs or diet with sweet *vipāka* are heavy and those having pungent *vipāka* are light.

This happens because, of the nature of the *mahābhūtas* like *pṛthvi* etc., which enter into the composition of such drugs and diet.

'द्रव्येषु पच्यमानेषु येष्वम्बुपृथिवीगुणाः ।
निर्वर्तन्तेऽधिकास्तत्र पाको मधुर उच्यते ॥१०५॥'

[सुश्रुत : सूत्र४०:११]

'तेजोऽनिलाकाशगुणाः पच्यमानेषु येषु तु ।
निर्वर्तन्तेऽधिकास्तत्र पाकः कटुक उच्यते ॥१०६॥'

[सुश्रुत : सूत्र४०:१२]

If, during the process of the digestion of a substance, the attributes of *jala* and *pṛthvi mahābhūtas* are excessively manifested then the *vipāka* becomes sweet. If during this process, attributes of *agni*, *vāyu* and *ākāśa mahābhūtas* are manifested in excess, then the *vipāka* becomes pungent.

विपाकमधुरा स्निग्धा कफघ्ना पिप्पली कथम् ।
कफस्थानमतिक्रम्य माधुर्यमुपयाति सा ॥१०७॥

The question that might arise now as to why *pippali* which is sweet in *vipāka* and unctuous in quality alleviates *kapha* ? This is because, the drug becomes sweet (in *vipāka*) only after it has crossed the location of *kapha*.

जठराग्नेस्तु संयोगाद्यदुदेति रसान्तरम् ।
रसानां परिणामान्ते स विपाक इति स्मृतः ॥१०८॥

81

Definition of Vipāka

The taste, that emerges in the drug or articles of food by their interaction with the *jaṭharāgni* (digestive enzymes) at the end of the process of digestion, is called *vipāka*.

अथ प्रभावः कथ्यते

कर्त्तुं येन प्रसरति हितं वा यदि वाऽहितम् ।

हिताहितप्रभूतत्वात् स प्रभाव इति स्मृतः ॥१०९॥

Prabhāva

The factor, which is responsible for the manifestation of useful or harmful effects of a drug, which is exceedingly useful or harmful, is called *prabhāva* or specific action.

[82] 'रसादिसाम्ये यत्कर्म विशिष्टं तत् प्रभावजम् ।'

[अष्टाङ्गहृदय : सूत्र९:२६]

हिताहितात्स द्विविधः प्रभावः परिकीर्तितः ॥११०॥

The specific action, which is manifested in a drug in spite of its similarity with others in *rasa* (taste) etc., is called *prabhāva*.

[83] क्षीरमूलकशुण्ठ्यादितक्रादीनां हितं तथा ।

सर्षपादिषु शाकेषु अहितं चाथमूलकम्[84] ॥१११॥

This *prabhāva* is of two types viz., wholesome effect and unwholesome effect. Milk, (tender) *mūlaka, śuṇṭhī,* butter milk etc., are generally wholesome. The leaf of the *sarṣapa,* when used as a vegetable, and over-matured *mūlaka* are unwholesome.

ज्वरं हंति शिरोबद्धा सहदेवीजटा बलात् ।

तस्करः स्नायुजं मूलं तथा निद्रां प्रवर्त्तयेत् ॥११२॥

The root of *sahadevi,* when tied to the head of a patient suffering from fever, cures the disease. In the same manner, the roots of *taskara* and *snāyu* induce sleep.

लघूष्णकटुकादन्तीप्रभावात्तु विरेचनी ।

Dantī, which is light, hot and pungent, produces purgative effect by its specific action.

विषं विषहरं प्रोक्तं त्रिदोषं स्वगुणैर्विषम् ॥११३॥

जयेच्च कासमर्दो हि वृश्चिकोत्थं महाविषम् ।

कर्णफूत्कारयोगेन प्रभावस्तत्र कारणम् ॥११४॥

The cure of poisoning by the administration of a poison, cure of poisoning and alleviation of all the three *doṣas* by *kāsa marda*, and cure of the serious type of scorpion poisoning by the blowing of air (impregnated with a *mantra*) into the ear of the patient, are the examples of *prabhāva* or specific action.

'मण्यौषधीनां मंत्राणां धर्म्मादीनां तथैव च ।

दृश्यते यन्महत्कर्म्मप्रभावस्तत्रकारणम्'[85] ॥११५॥

॥इति रसवीर्यादिलक्षणम्॥

Similarly, the magnificient effects of jewel, talishman, *mantras* and religious rituals, are manifested because of their *prabhāva*.

Thus, ends the topic dealing with the description of *rasa* (taste), *vīrya* (potency) etc.

अथ कालपरीक्षा

आत्रेयात्

कालः कलयते लोकं[86] कालः कलयते जगत् ।

कालः कलयते विश्वं तेन कालोऽभिधीयते ॥११६॥

Examination of Kāla (time)

According to Ātreya

Kāla or time, regulates (*kalayate*) the phenomena in the world, *kāla* regulates (*kalayate*) the phenomena in the moving universe and *kāla* regulates (*kalayate*) all types of phenomena. Therefore, it is called *kāla*.

सुश्रुतात्

संवत्सर शरीरस्य ऋत्वंगिनः कालस्य ग्रहणम् तस्योपयोगित्वात्

चिकित्सायां ॥११७॥

तद्यथा

'तस्य संवत्सरात्मनो भगवानादित्यो गतिविशेषेण निमेषकाष्ठाकलामुहूर्त्ताहोरात्र-

87

पक्षमासर्त्वयनसम्वत्सरयुगप्रविभागं करोति ॥११८॥'

[सुश्रुत : सूत्र६:४]

According to Suśruta

Kāla or the time, has its body or unit quantity in the form of year. Its limbs or parts are the various seasons. This has been accepted, because of its relevance in the treatment of diseases. For example, depending upon the movement of the almighty sun, this unit of year is divided and subdivided into *nimeṣa*, *kāṣṭhā*, *kāla*, *muhūrta*, *ahorātra* (day and night), *pakṣa* (unit of 15 days depending upon the appearance and disappearance of the moon), *māsa* (month), *ṛtu* (season), *ayana* (solstice), *saṁvatsara* (year) and *yuga* (unit of 12 years).

सूर्योपलक्षणं कृत्वा तेन चन्द्रोऽपि गृह्यते ।

निशाकरादि हेतुत्वादथवा भगवान् रविः ॥११९॥

In the above description, the term *āditya* (lit. sun) includes both the sun and moon. Even if the literal meaning i.e. the sun alone is accepted, there is no error because, the moon is dependant upon the sun.

स्वरश्मिभिः स्वमाहत्म्यात्कुर्याच्छीतोष्णवर्षणम् ।
तथा कालविभागं च करोति स्वबलेन च ॥१२०॥
शिशिरश्च वसन्तश्च ग्रीष्मवर्षाशरद्हिमाः ।
ऋतवः षट्क्रमादेते कालसम्वत्सरः[88] स्मृतः[89] ॥१२१॥

By its rays, the sun creates disturbance in the atmosphere (*kha*=lit. sky) and thereby produces cold, heat and rain. Accordingly, it causes seasonal variations. *Śiśira* (late winter), *vasanta* (spring), *grīṣma* (summer), *varṣā* (rainy season), *śarat* (autumn) and *hemanta* (early winter)—these are the six consecutive seasons which constitute the unit of time i.e. year.

आत्रेयः

[90]वर्षंद्विधा त्रिधा षट्धा प्रोक्तं द्वादशधापि च ।
द्विधा त्वयनभेदेन वर्षाशीतोष्णतस्त्रिधा ।
षट्धा चैवर्त्तुभेदेन मासैर्द्वादशधा पुनः ॥१२२॥
संचयादि सुबोधार्थं शोथनार्थं तथैव च ।
दोषाणां ऋतुभिर्वर्षः[91] षड्भि श्रेष्ठतमो[92] मतः ॥१२३॥

According to Ātreya

The year is divided into two, three, six and twelve divisions. Depending upon the *ayana* (solstice), it is divided into two. Depending upon the rain, cold and heat, it has three divisions. On the basis of seasons, it is divided into six. On the basis of months, it has twelve divisions.

To facilitate the comprehension of *sañcaya* (accumulation of *doṣas*) etc., and administration of *śodhana* (elimination) therapies, the six divisions of the year, on the basis of seasons, is the best.

वाग्भटात्

'शिशिराद्यैस्त्रिभिस्तैस्तु विद्यादयनमुत्तरम् ।

[93]आदानं हि तदादत्ते नृणां प्रतिदिनं बलम् ॥१२४॥

[94]तस्मिन्नत्यर्थतीक्ष्णोष्णरूक्षा मार्गस्वभावतः ।

आदित्यपवनाः सौम्यान् क्षपयन्ति गुणान् भुवः ॥१२५॥

तिक्तः कषायः कटुको बलिनोऽत्र रसाः क्रमात् ।

तस्मादादानमाग्नेयम्

According to Vāgbhaṭa

Śiśira (late winter), *vasanta* (spring) and *griṣma* (summer)—these three seasons constitute the *uttarāyaṇa* (northern solstice). During this period, the strength of the human being is taken away day by day. Because of the characteristic features of *mārga* (northern solstice), the sun and the wind become exceedingly sharp, hot and ununctuous during this period. They take away the *saumya* (cooling) attributes from the earth. During these seasons, bitter, astringent and pungent tastes become more prominent gradually. Therefore, the *ādāna kāla* (northern solstice or the period of absorption) is *āgneya* (heating) by nature.

ऋतवो दक्षिणायनं ॥१२६॥

वर्षादयो विसर्गश्च यद्बलं विसृजत्ययम् ।

सौम्यत्वादत्र सोमो हि बलवान् हीयते रविः ॥१२७॥

मेघवृष्ट्यनिलैः [95]शीतैः शान्ततापे महीतले ।

स्निग्धाश्चेहाम्ललवणमधुरा बलिनो रसाः ।'

[अष्टाङ्गहृदय : सूत्र३:२-६]

96

जीवानामतुलं तेजः गोजातीनां पयोद्भवः ॥१२८॥

Varṣā (rainy season), *śarat* (autumn) and *hemanta* (early winter)—these three seasons constitute *dakṣiṇāyana* (southern solstice). This is the period of elimination. It impregnates the human beings with strength. Because of the *saumya* (cooling) nature, *soma* (moon) is more powerful during this period and the power of the sun is reduced. The cloud, the rain and the wind have cooling effects. They reduce the temperature of the earth. There is more unctuousness in the drugs and food articles. Sour, saline and sweet are the more powerful tastes during this period. The living beings acquire considerable energy and cows etc., produce more of milk.

सुश्रुतात्

97

'शीतांशुः क्लेदयत्युर्वीं विवस्वान् शोषयत्यपि ।

तावुभावपि संश्रित्य वायुः पालयति प्रजा ॥१२९॥'

[सुश्रुत : सूत्र६:८]

According to Suśruta

The moon with its cooling rays produces moistness and the sun absorbs it. On the basis of these two, the *vāyu* regulates the activities of the living beings.

अग्निवेशः

98

हेमन्ते शिशिरे चाग्र्यं ग्रीष्मवर्षासु चावरम् ।

99

शरद्वसन्तयोर्मध्यं बलं स्यात्प्राणिनां ध्रुवम् ॥१३०॥

According to Agniveśa

The strength in *hemanta* and *śiśira* is in a superior state and in *grīṣma* and *varṣā*, it is in an inferior state. During *śarat* and *vasanta*, the strength of the living beings is certainly in mediocre state.

‘चयप्रकोपोपशमा[100] वायोर्ग्रीष्मादिषु त्रिषु ।
वर्षादिषु[101] तु पित्तस्य, श्लेष्मणः शिशिरादिषु ॥१३१॥’

[अष्टाङ्गहृदय : सूत्र१२:२४-२५]

In *grīṣma*, *vāyu* gets accumulated, in *varṣā* it gets aggravated and in *śarat* it gets alleviated. *Pitta* gets accumulated in *varṣā* season, it gets aggravated in *śarat* and it is alleviated in *hemanta*. *Kapha* gets accumulated in *śiśira*, aggravated in *vasanta* and alleviated in *grīṣma*.

[हेमन्तर्तुचर्या]

‘धूमधूम्रा रजोमन्दास्तुषाराविलमण्डलाः ।
दिगादित्या मरुच्छैत्यात् दन्तरोमप्रहर्षणः ॥१३२॥
लोध्रप्रियङ्गुपुन्नागलवल्यः कुसुमोज्ज्वलाः ।
हृष्टा गजाजमहिषवाजिवायसशूकराः[102] ॥१३३॥’

[अष्टाङ्गसंग्रह : सूत्र४:९-१०]

विस्तीर्णं शालिकेदारानीलधान्योज्ज्वला[103] मही ।
स्वादुपाको रसानां च वायुः श्लेष्मात्रचीयते ॥१३४॥
हेमन्ते हि चितः श्लेष्मा शिशिरेऽपि न कुप्यति ।
आहारैश्च गुरुस्निग्धैः भृशमेवोपचीयते ॥१३५॥

वसंते रविसंतापाद्विलीनश्चाशु कुप्यति ।
ग्रीष्मे ऋतुस्वभावेन स श्लेष्माऽऽशु प्रणश्यति ॥१३६॥
[104]
'बलिनः शीतसंरोधाद्धेमन्ते प्रबलोऽनलः ।
भवत्यल्पेन्धनो धातून् स पचेद्वायुनेरितः ॥१३७॥
अतो हिमेऽस्मिन्सेवेत स्वाद्वम्ललवणान् रसान् ।
दैर्घ्यान्निशानामेतर्हि प्रातरेव बुभुक्षितः ॥१३८॥
[105]
अवश्यकार्यं संभाव्य यथोक्तं शीलयेदनु ।
वातघ्नतैलैरभ्यङ्गं मूर्ध्नि तैलं विमर्दनम् ।
नियुद्धं कुशलैः सार्धं पादाघातं युक्तितः ॥१३९॥'

[अष्टाङ्गहृदय : सूत्र३:७-१०]

Regimens for Hemanta

The following are the characteristic features and regimens for *hemanta* (early winter) :

1. The sky becomes smoky by smoke;

2. There is less of dust in the atmosphere;

3. The atmosphere is foggy;

4. The sun ray is less hot and as a result of cold wind, there is tingling sensation in teeth and horripilation;

5. The earth is surrounded with the beautiful flowers of *lodhra, priyaṅgu, punnāga, lavalī* etc.;

6. There is more of energy among the elephants, goats, buffalos, horses, crows and pigs;

7. The earth looks beautiful with the blue coloured grains and wide-spread paddy fields;

8. All the *rasas* become sweet in *vipāka*;

9. *Vāyu* and *kapha* get accumulated in this season. This *kapha* does not get aggravated even in *śiśira* (late winter) but gets further accumulated by heavy and unctuous food articles. It gets immediately aggravated only in *vasanta*, because it gets liquified as a result of the hot rays of the sun. Because of the characteristic features of *grīṣma* (summer season), it immediately gets alleviated;

10 In persons having a strong physique, the *anala* (digestive enzymes) becomes more powerful as from outside it gets covered by cold. If sufficient fuel (food) is not provided, then these digestive enzymes, being stimulated by *vāyu*, consume the *dhātus* (tissue elements). Therefore, in this season, a person should take more of sweet, sour and saline food articles;

11. The nights become longer in duration because of which the person feels hungry in the morning. Therefore, he should take some snacks before performing the other routines of the day;

12. The person should have a massage of the body with oil which alleviates *vāyu*. He should also have oil massage in the head; and

13. The person should practice wrestling with experts and his body should be kneaded with feet appropriately.

अभ्यङ्गानन्तरं मूर्ध्नि तैलविमर्दनमित्ययुक्तम् । उत्तमाङ्गस्य प्रथमत्वात् ॥१४०॥

अत्रोच्यते

प्रयोगपारिजातः

मस्तकाभ्यङ्ग[106] शेषेण[107] कचिन्नोद्वर्त्तयेत्तनुम् ।

पुण्यहानिरलक्ष्मीः स्यात्तस्मात्तत्परिवर्जयेदिति ॥१४१॥

कषायोपहितस्नेहस्ततस्नातो यथा विधिः ।

Application of oil in the head has been described after the massage of the body. This may not appear to be appropriate, because the head has a position superior to that of the body. In this connection, it is stated in *Pryogapārijāta* that the residual oil which is left out after the massage of the head should not be used for the massage of the body. By doing so, one loses the *puṇya* (virtues) and gets inauspiciousness. Therefore, it should be avoided. The oil etc., which are used for massage, should be prepared by boiling with decoctions of medicinal plants. Thereafter, he should take bath according to the prescribed procedure.

पादाघातस्तैलयुक्तो दीपनो देहपुष्टिकृत् ॥१४२॥

शुक्रौजस्तेजसां वृद्धिकरः श्रोत्रविशोधनः[108] ।

Kneading the body with legs after smearing it with oil is *dīpana* (stimulant of digestion and metabolism) and nourishing. It also promotes semen, *ojas* and energy, and it cleanses the ears.

पौष्टिकोद्वर्षणं[109] वर्ण्यं कण्डूकोष्ठमलापहम् ॥१४३॥

व्यायामादौ तदन्ते च कल्कं वा मुद्गमाषजम् ।

Unction of the body by the nourishing drugs promotes complexion and cures *kaṇḍū* (itching) and *kuṣṭha* (obstinate skin diseases) and removes *mala* (excreta). Therefore, in the beginning and at the end of exercise, one should use the paste of either *mudga* or *māṣa* for this purpose.

सेवेतादित्यकिरणान्निर्धूमं च हुताशनम् ॥१४४॥

पृष्ठतोऽर्कं निषेवेत जठरेण हुताशनम् ।

One should bake himself in sun's rays and sit before the fire which is free from smoke. Sun's ray should be enjoyed from the back side and heat of the fire from the front side.

स्वामिनं [110] सत्यभेदेन परलोकममायया ॥१४५॥

One should serve his master by being truthful and without any deception for benefit in the next world (life).

[111] गुरुष्णमन्नं संसेव्यं चन्दनागुरुधूपितम् ।

ग्राम्यानूपौदकं मांसं स्नेहो गोधूमशालयः ॥१४६॥

[112] स्नेहो गोधूमविकृतिस्तीक्ष्णं मद्यं [113] च शीलयेत् ।

'पीवरोरुस्तनश्रोण्यः समदाः प्रमदाः प्रियाः ।

हरन्ति शीतमुष्णाङ्ग्यो [114] धूपकुङ्कुमयौवनैः ॥१४७॥'

[अष्टाङ्गहृदय : सूत्र३:१५]

One should take heavy and hot food, and get himself fumigated with *candana* and *aguru*. One should take the meat of domesticated, marshy and aquatic animals, fat, wheat, different types of *śali* rico, preparation of wheat fried with ghee and habitually take strong alcohol. Women who have bulky thighs, breasts and buttocks, who have strong sexual passion, who are pleasing, who are youthful, who are fumigated with insence and saffron and who have warm physique, take away the cold.

[115] वाग्भटात्

'अङ्गारतापसंतप्तगर्भभूवेश्मचारिणः [116] ।

शीतपारुष्यजनितो न दोषो जातु जायते ॥१४८॥'

[अष्टाङ्गहृदय : सूत्र३:१६]

According to Vāgbhaṭa

If a person resides in a house heated with charcoal, in an

underground cellar or in a house constructed of earth, then he does not get afflicted with ailments caused by the roughness of the cold weather.

कामतः सुरतं कुर्यात्तृप्तो वाजीकरैर्हिमे ।

'प्रावाराजिनकौशेयप्रवेणीकुथकास्तृतम् ।

उष्णस्वभावैर्लघुभिः[117] प्रावृतः शयनं भजेत् ॥१४६॥'

[अष्टाङ्गहृदय : सूत्र३:१३-१४]

In winter, one should take aphrodisiac drugs and indulge in sex as much as he likes. During winter season, he should sleep on a bed covered with *prāvāra* (blankets), *ajina* (leather), *kauśeya* (silken), *praveṇi* and *kuthaka* types of bed covers. While sleeping, he should cover himself with quilt which is hot and light in nature.

चरकात्

'प्रवातं प्रमिताहारमुदमन्थं हिमागमे ।'

[चरक : सूत्र६:१८]

कषायकटुतिक्तानि रूक्षाणि च लघूनि च ।

[चरक : सूत्र६:२१]

'वर्ज्जयेच्छीतसंस्पर्शान् शीतान्युपवनानि च[118] ॥१५०॥'

॥इति हेमन्तर्तुः॥

According to Caraka

One should reside in a house which is not windy and take adequate quantity of food and *udamantha* (liquid preparations of corn flour during *hemanta* (early winter). He should also take food which is astringent, pungent and bitter in taste and which is ununctuous.

He should avoid the touch of cooling things, and he should not move in cooling parks.

Thus, ends the regimens for *hemanta* (early winter) season.

[शिशिरर्तुचर्या]

अयमेव विधिः कार्यः शिशिरेऽपि[119] विशेषतः ।

तथाहि शीतमधिकं रौक्षं चादानकालजम् ॥१५१॥

Regimens for Śiśira

During *śiśira* (late winter) season, one should adopt more particularly, the regimens prescribed for *hemanta*. During *śiśira*, there is more of cold and there is ununctuousness as a consequence of *ādāna kāla* (time of absorption).

आत्रेयः

बहुलशिशिरवातात्[120] किञ्चिदुद्भूतशस्या, भवति वसुमतीयं पक्वशस्यैस्तु[121] पीता ।

कथमपि तुहिनस्याल्लिङ्गं वैशेषिकं स्यात्, पवनकफविकारो जायते शैशिरे च ॥१५२॥

तत्रापि तैलं लशुनं कोलवघ्नप्रलेहितान्[122] ।

कृशरां चातिदुग्धान्नां[123] भुञ्जानः सुखमाप्नुयात् ॥१५३॥

According to Ātreya

Because of excessive cold wind very few tender plants start growing in *śiśira*, Therefore, with the ripe plants of corn and grains the earth becomes yellow in colour. During this season more of characteristic features of winter season are manifested and diseases of *vāyu* and *kapha* afflict human beings, for which oil, garlic and the linctus of *kola* are useful. Intake of *kṛśarā* prepared with liberal quantity of milk is also useful.

क्षेमेन्द्रात्

सार्द्रकार्द्रा सुसंधाना[124] सबाह्लीका ससैन्धवाः[125] ।

सस्नेहा कामिनीचेयं कृशरा शिशिरे हिता ॥१५४॥

॥इति शिशिरर्तुः॥

According to Kṣemendra

Alcoholic drinks well fermented and added with *ārdraka, bāhlika* and *saindhava* along with pleasing women and *kṛśarā* are useful in *śiśira.*

Thus, ends the description of regimens for *śiśira* (late winter) season.

[वसन्तर्तुचर्या]

कदलीदलनीलकोकिलाभिः कृतकोलाहलकाहलप्रपञ्चः ।

मलयानिलमत्तवारणस्थो मदनश्चात्र चकार जैत्रयात्राम् ॥१५५॥

Characteristics and Regimens for Vasanta

The *vasanta* (spring) is characterised by the blue leaves of *kadalī* and the koojing sound of *koel* birds. During this season, the wind coming from *malaya* hills excites passion even of elephants. The god of sex has an overwhelming effect during this season.

आत्रेयः

मुदितकोकिलकूजितकाननं मदनशोभितं किंशुकशोभितम् ।

कुसुमसौरभरञ्जितभूधरं क्वणितमत्तमधुव्रतलालसम् ॥१५६॥

मकरकेतनवाससमाकुलं मुदितमेवसमस्तमिदं जगत् ।

मलयमारुत[126]तुर्यगुणान्वितं कफकरो हि वसंतऋतुर्भवेत् ॥१५७॥

According to Ātreya

During spring season, the forest resounds with the koojing sound of excited *koel* birds and it is full of the flowers of *madana* and *kiṁśuka*. The atmosphere is full of the fragrance of flowers and the earth is gracefully covered with the coloured flowers. The intoxicated black bees roam round the flowers in search of honey. The atmosphere is surrounded with the fragrance of the flower of *makara ketana* (mango) etc. The entire earth appears as if in a jubilant mood. This is multiplied by the effect of the wind coming from the *malaya* mountains. *Kapha* is aggravated during this season.

वाग्भटः

नवप्रवालत्वक्पत्राः पादपाः ककुभो[127]ऽमलाः ।

किंशुकाशोकचूतादिवनराजिविराजिताः ॥१५८॥

[अष्टाङ्गसंग्रह : सूत्र४:२२]

According to Vāgbhaṭa

During the spring season, beautiful trees like *kakubha, kiṁśuka, aśoka* etc., get fresh buds, bark and leaves. With these, the forest looks beautiful.

वसन्ते कुपितः श्लेष्मा हृल्लासाग्निवधादिकान् ।

रोगान्करोति त्वरया ग्रीष्मे शान्तिमुपैति च ॥१५९॥

गुरुशीतदिवास्वप्नस्निग्धाम्लमधुरं त्यजेत् ।

तीक्ष्णैर्वमननस्याद्यै[128]र्लघुरूक्षैश्च भोजनैः ॥१६०॥

व्यायामोद्वर्तनाघातैर्जित्वा श्लेष्माणमुल्बणम् ।

129

पुराणयवगोधूमक्षौद्रजाङ्गलशल्यभुक् ॥१६१॥

Kapha gets aggravated during spring season and produces diseases like *hṛllāsa* (nausea) and *agni vadha* (suppression of the power of digestion). This *kapha* gets alleviated immediately after the onset of the summer season. During spring season, heavy and cold things, sleep during day time and unctuous, sour as well as sweet things should be avoided. To overcome the aggravated *kapha*, one should resort to the following :

1. Emesis with drugs which are sharp in quality;
2. Strong inhalation therapy;
3. Intake of food which is light and ununctuous; and
4. Exercise, unction and kneading.

During spring season, one should take old barley and wheat, honey, the meat of animals dwelling in arid forests and *śalya* type of meat preparation.

स्नातोऽनुलिप्तः कर्पूरचन्दनागुरुकुंकुमैः ।

सहकाररसोन्मिश्रानास्वाद्य प्रिययार्पितान् ॥१६२॥

प्रियास्यसंगसुरभीन् प्रियानेत्रोत्पलाङ्कितान् ।

सौमनस्यकृतो हृद्यान्वयस्यैः सहितः पिबेत् ॥१६३॥

निर्गदानासवारिष्टसीधुमार्द्वीकमाधवान् ।

शृङ्गवेराम्बु साराम्बु मध्वम्बु जलदाम्बु च ॥१६४॥

[अष्टाङ्गहृदय : सूत्र३:१९-२३]

After taking bath, the body should be smeared with the paste of *karpūra*, *candana*, *aguru* and *kuṁkuma*. He should take the drink prepraed of the juice of mango, served by passionately attached women. Alcoholic drinks shared by the beloved ladies and offered by these ladies having eyes like lotus should be taken along with friends. This drink taken in such circumstances, provides mental well being and it works as cardiac tonic. *Āsava*, *ariṣṭa sīdhu*, *mārdvika* and *mādhava* types of alcoholic drinks which are well fermented should be taken during this season. Water boiled with ginger, *sārāmbu*, water mixed with honey and water collected from rain, are useful in spring.

विचित्रपुष्पवृक्षेषु काननेषु सुगन्धिषु ।

गोष्ठीकथाभिश्चित्राभिर्मध्याह्नं[130] गमयेत्सुखी ॥१६५॥

[अष्टाङ्गहृदय : सूत्र३:२५]

॥इति वसन्तवर्णनम्॥

One should spend happily mid-day in gardens with variegated flowers and trees emitting fragrance while hearing interesting stories along with friends.

Thus, ends description of characteristics and regimens for the spring season.

[ग्रीष्मर्तुचर्या]

निर्वर्त्तते रसो ग्रीष्मे कटुको न तथेतरः ।

आपश्च कटुपच्यन्ते रौक्ष्यात्तैक्ष्ण्यात्तथा रवेः ॥१६६॥

तस्मात् श्लेष्मा शमं याति मारुतश्चोपचीयते ।

समेघवाताभिहतो वायुर्वर्षासु कुप्यति ॥१६७॥

शरत्कालेऽर्कसंतापात्स च वायुः प्रशाम्यति ।

Characteristics and Regimens for Grīṣma

During *grīṣma* or summer season, the pungent taste is manifested much more than the others. The water undergoes *kaṭu pāka* because of the ununctuousness and sharpness of the rays of this sun. Therefore, *kapha* gets alleviated and *vāyu* gets accumulated during the season. This *vāyu* gets aggravated during rainy season by the impact of the clouds and the wind, and gets alleviated during autumn season because of the hot rays of the sun.

भवेत्तीक्ष्णांशुरादित्यो मारुतो नैर्ऋतो[131] सुखः ॥१६८॥

भूस्तप्ता सरितस्तन्व्यः पांशुवृष्ट्याऽऽकुला दिशः ।

[132]भ्रान्तचक्राह्वयुगलाः पयःपानाकुला मृगाः ॥१६९॥

ध्वस्तवीरुत्तृणलता विपर्णाङ्कितपादपाः ।

[सुश्रुत : सूत्र६:२९-३०]

वहवो मारुतोन्वाताः[133] पत्रांवरविभूषिताः[134] ॥१७०॥

वसन्तस्य वियोगेन तापसा इव शोभिताः ।

त्यज्येत्तु पटुकट्वम्लव्यायामार्ककरानपि ।

भजेन्मधुरमेवान्नं लघु स्निग्धं हिमं द्रवम् ॥१७१॥

[अष्टाङ्गहृदय : सूत्र३:२८]

During summer season, the sun becomes very sharp and the wind which blows from *nairṛta* direction (south-west) is pleasing. The earth gets heated up and the ponds become thin with water. All the directions become hazy by dust and rain. The couple of *cakra vāka* becomes worried and animals become anxious to drink water. Trees, grass and creepers get destroyed and big trees get denuded of leaves. Wind blows from different directions and it carries along with it dried leaves of trees. Because of the disappearance of spring season, the trees appear like hermits. During summer season, one should avoid saline, pungent and sour things, exercise and exposure to sun rays. During this season, one should take excessively sweet food which is light, unctuous, cold and liquid.

उदमंथः सिता सर्पिः जाङ्गलाः शालय पयः ।

स्निग्ध गोधूमिका भक्ष्यास्तथा मुद्गाढकीयवाः[135] ॥१७२॥

सेव्याः खर्जूरमृद्वीका[136]रागषाडवसैन्धवाः[137] ।

न च मद्यं पिवेद्ग्रीष्मे पिवेद्वाल्पं जलोत्तरम्[138] ॥१७३॥

पाटलावासितं चाम्भः सकर्पूरं सुशीतलम् ।

पिबेद्रसं नातिघनं पंचसारकपानकम् ॥१७४॥

'ससितं माहिषं क्षीरं चन्द्रनक्षत्रशीतलम् ।

अभ्रङ्कषमहाशालतालरुद्धोष्णरश्मिषु ॥१७५॥

वनेषु माधवीश्लिष्टद्राक्षास्तबकशालिषु ।

सुगन्धिहिमपानीयसिच्यमानपटान्तिके[139] ॥१७६॥

कायमाने चिते चूतप्रवालफललुम्बिभिः ।

कदलीदलकह्लारमृणालकमलोत्पलैः ॥१७७॥

कोमलः कल्पिते तल्पे हसत्कुसुमपल्लवे ।'

[अष्टाङ्गहृदय : सूत्र ३:३२-३६]

One should take *udamantha* (diluted corn-flour), sugar, ghee meat of forest dwelling animals, *śāli* rice, milk, pastries which are unctuous and prepared of wheat, *mudga*, *āḍhakī*, *yava*, *kharjūra*, *mṛdvikā*, *rāga*, *ṣāḍava* and *saindhava*. One should not take alcohol during summer season. Even if one is required to take it, it should be diluted very well with water. Water which is made fragrant by soaking the flower of *pāṭalā* and which is made cold by adding camphor, should be used. One should use the drink called "*pañca sāraka*" which is very thick in consistency. Buffalo milk added with sugar and made cold by exposure to moon and stars should be taken. One should walk in forests which have very thick trees of *śāla* and *tāla*. The hot rays of the sun get obstructed by the leaves of these trees from coming down. In these forests, creepers of *mādhavī* and bunches of *drākṣā* around the trees are very useful. In the houses, one should have curtains sprinkled with fragrant cold water. All around, the fruits of mango and *pravāla* should be hanged. The bed should be spread with the tender leaves of *kadalī*, *kalhāra*, *mṛṇāla*, *kamala* and *utpala*, which should be surrounded by beautiful flowers and leaves.

'मध्यन्दिनेऽर्कतापार्तः स्वप्याद्धारागृहेऽथवा ।
निशाकरकराकीर्णे सौधपृष्ठे निशासु च ॥१७८॥'

[अष्टाङ्गहृदय : सूत्र३:३६,३७]

During mid-day, because of the painful rays of the sun, one should sleep in a *dhārā gṛha* (the house which has fountains or streams of water inside it). At night, one should sleep on the roof of the building which is exposed to the rays of the moon.

कृष्णात्रेयात्

ग्रीष्मे चूतफलं चाद्याच्छुष्कशाकानि वर्जयेत् ।
सेव्याढकी[140] तथा मुद्गाः सिता गोधूमशालयः ॥१७९॥
सौवीरं घोलतक्रं च क्षीरं च ससितं[141] जलम् ।
सेव्यानि श्वेतवस्त्राणि नालिकेरोदकानि[142] च ॥१८०॥

॥इति ग्रीष्मर्तुः॥

According to Kṛṣṇātreya

During summer season, one should eat mango and avoid dry vegetables including leafy vegetables. One should take *āḍhakī*, *mudga*, sugar, wheat, *śāli* rice, *sauvīra*, butter-milk, milk and water added with sugar. During this season, one should use white cloth. The water of coconut may be used as a drink during this season.

Thus, ends the description of the characteristics of and regimens for the summer season.

[वर्षार्तुचर्या]

सघनवारिदवारिसमाकुला [143] विमलसत्प्रवरोदकपूजिताः ।
समदवातकरा हि [144] दिशोदशप्रमुदिताः कृमिकीटभृता मही ॥१८१॥

नीलशष्पहरितोज्ज्वलामही [145] कुल्यकासलिलसप्लुता मही ।
इन्द्रगोप[146]क[147]विराजिराजिता पञ्चभूषणविभूषिता [148] बभौ ॥१८२॥

उन्मत्तभूतांकुरभूधरस्याद्रेजेवनं [149] वा मधुरं विकूजत् ।
मृगा मयूरा जलदस्य घोषात्सर्वेऽपि जीवा जलमाप्नुवन्ति ॥१८३॥

केकी कूजति कानने च सरसि [150] म्लानाम्बुपूर्णा तथा ।
हंसा मानसमाव्रजन्ति कमलान्याम्लानतां यान्ति च ॥१८४॥

Characteristics and Regimens for Varṣā

The following are the characteristic features of *varṣā* or rainy season :

1. The sky remains covered with clouds and rain;
2. All around the earth, there will be clear water in large quantity;

3. All the ten directions become filled with intoxicating wind;

4. The earth becomes filled with worms and insects, and it looks beautifully green by tender and blue plants;

5. The earth gets flooded with water and canals ;

6. It looks beautiful with *indra gopa, kavirāji* and five groups of natural ornaments;

7. The earth becomes full of germinated plants and koojing sound of different types of birds;

8. The deer and peacocks become happy by the sound of the cloud and all animals get water;

9. In the forests, *kekī* produces beautiful sounds and the ponds become full of pure water;

10. The swans go back to *māna sarovara*;

11. The lotus flower gets withered; and

12. There is a resonance from the caves and crevices of mountains which are greenish blue in colour because of the abundance of vegetation.

151
गर्जन्महीध्रकन्दरदरी शस्यातता श्यामला ।

भात्येवं पवनस्य कोपनकरी वर्षाऋतुः श्रेयसी ॥१८५॥

किञ्चिद्गर्भोद्भवानि स्युः शस्यातिदृढतां शनैः

शिलिन्द्रछत्रसंयुक्ता भूरव्यक्तजलस्थलाः ॥१८६॥

कदम्बनीपकुटजसर्जकेतकिभूषिता ।

वाप्यः प्रोत्फुल्लकुमुदनीलोत्पलविराजिताः ।

एवं गुणसमायुक्ता नातिवर्षाऋतुः शुभा ॥१८७॥

The rainy season is very beautiful because of its above-mentioned features, and during this season, *vāyu* gets aggravated. Some of the plants start yielding seeds and they become gradually sturdy. The earth becomes full of different types of mushrooms. It becomes very difficult to recognise the uplands and ditches because all of them are full of water. During this season, the earth becomes decorated with the flowers of *kadamba*, *nīpa*, *kuṭaja*, *sarja* and *ketakī*. The ponds look beautiful because of the flowers of *kumuda* and blue variety of *utpala*. With the above characteristics, the rainy season is very auspicious if there is no excess of rain.

सुश्रुतः

भूमौ जलोपक्लिन्नायां क्लिन्नो[152] देहश्च जायते[153] ।
तरुण्यश्चाल्पवीर्यास्तु[154] औषध्योऽपि भवन्ति हि ॥१८८॥

According to Suśruta

Since the earth becomes moist, it increases the moisture inside the body. The *taruṇis* (fresh or new *yava*, *godhūma*, *śāli* etc.) and herbs become reduced in potency.

ननु वर्षासु यवादयः पुरातना एव भवन्ति; कथमभिनवा इत्युच्यन्ते? नैषदोषः । गोधूमयवशाल्यादयः सूक्ष्मजललवानुप्रवेशात्प्रोच्छूनतामुपगताः किञ्चित् तिरस्कृतशक्तयः प्ररोहधर्म्मिण्यः अनवा अपि तरुण्य इत्युच्यन्ते[155] ॥१८९॥

During rainy season, barley etc., are usually old. Why are they described as *taruṇi* or new in the above verse? It is not a mistake. The wheat, barley, rice etc., get impregnated with small particles of water and become swollen. Therefore, they are deprived of their potency. They have a tendency to germinate. Therefore, even the old ones are called *taruṇi* or new.

भूबाष्पेणाम्लपाकेन मलिनेन च वारिणा ।
वह्निनैव च मन्देन तेषु तेऽन्योऽन्यदूषिषु ॥१९०॥

[अष्टाङ्गहृदय : सूत्र३:४३-४४]

Because of the heat that comes out of the earth and because of the sour *vipāka* of the water which has become muddy, there is suppression of the power of digestion. Each one of them affects the other.

भजेत्साधारणं तत्र तस्मादाहारचेष्टितम् ।
स्वेदनं मर्दनं पथ्यं निर्वातशयनं तथा ॥१६१॥
गौरीरामारतं शस्तं व्यायामस्य क्रमं त्यजेत् ।
कट्वम्लक्षारस्वरसाः सेव्या वातकफापहाः ॥१६३॥
पुराणयवगोधूमशाल्यन्नं [156] जाङ्गलामिषम् ।
[157] माषान्नवटकांश्चापि लशुनांश्च प्रलेहयेत् ।
जीर्णमद्यासवारिष्टं दधि सेवेत युक्तितः ॥१६३॥

Therefore, during this season, one should use diet and regimens which are of moderate nature. One should resort to fomentation, massage and sleep in a place free from wind which are wholesome. One should indulge in sex with *gaurī rāmā* (a white-coloured and pleasing woman). One should gradually give up exercise. One should use things having pungent, sour and alkaline tastes for the alleviation of *vāyu* and *kapha*. Old barley, wheat, *śāli* rice, meat of animals dwelling in forest land, food prepared of *māṣa*, *vaṭaka*, linctus of *laśuna*, old alcoholic drinks, *āsava* and *ariṣṭa* types of wine and curd should be taken in appropriate quantity during this season.

वीरभद्रः

दिव्य-त्र्यूषसूरणसैन्धवकरकाक्षदीप्यकोपेतम् ।
माधवभीमशिवाभिश्चूर्णं दधिमंडसंयुतम् पीतं ॥१६४॥

प्रावृड्काले सुखावहमिदमौषधमग्निदोषहरम् ।
दिव्यं लवंगं, करकं दाडिमी, माधवं जीरकं, भीमं पूकं[158], अक्षं सौवर्चलम् ॥१६५॥

According to Vīra bhadra

During *prāvṛṭ* (beginning of rainy season), *dadhi maṇḍa* (the scum of curd or butter-milk) mixed with *divya*, *tryūṣaṇa*, *sūraṇa*, *saindhava*, *karaka*, *akṣa*, *dīpyaka*, *mādhava*, *bhīma* and *śivā* in powder form should be taken which is useful in correcting *agni doṣa* (defects in the digestive power).

Divya is *lavaṅga*. *Karaka* is *dāḍima*. *Mādhava* is *jīraka*. *Bhīma* is *yūka* (?). *Akṣa* means *sauvarcala*.

अग्निवेशात्

[159]सोपदंश निषेवेत् मैरेयारिष्टमाधवम् ।
पिबेत्प्रावृषि धीरोऽल्पं रात्रौ तदपि वर्जयेत् ॥१६६॥
मस्तुसौवर्चलाढ्यं वा पञ्चकोलावचूर्णितम् ।
भौमं कौपं सारसं वा[160] शृतं शीतं जलं पिबेत् ॥१६७॥
अतिदुर्दिनकालेन, सुदिनेत्वशृतं हितम् ।
अथ त्यजेद्दिवास्वप्नं जलतृप्ति गुरूणि च ।
नदीतोयं व्यवायं च वर्जयेन्मंथमातपम् ॥१६८॥

॥इति वर्षाऋतुः॥

According to Agniveśa

In the rainy season one should take *maireya*, *ariṣṭa* and *mādhava* types of wine along with snacks. These should, however, be taken in small quantity and should be avoided at night. *Mastu* (thin butter-milk) mixed with liberal quantity of *sauvarcala* and added with the powder of *pañca kola* should be used. The water of *bhauma* type (which comes out from the earth), well and pond should first be boiled and then cooled, before using it for drinking, during the days when it rains in excess. When there is no excess of rain, unboiled water is useful. One should avoid sleep during day time. One should not take water to the full of his satisfaction. One shouid avoid heavy things, water from river, sexual intercourse, *mantha* (roasted corn flour) and exposure to sun.

TLus, ends the description of the characteristic features of and regimens for the rainy season.

[शरदृतुचर्या]

मेघाः सूर्यशिलासमानरुचयो ह्यम्लप्रधानाः[161] रसाः,

हंसालीजलजालिमण्डितजलं पद्माकरं शोभनम् ॥१९९॥

तीव्रस्निग्धमयूखइन्दुविमला सानंदिनीकौमुदी,

चित्राघर्मविपक्वतोयसरसी स्यान्निर्मलं पुष्करम् ॥२००॥

'पङ्कशुष्कद्रुमाकीर्णा निम्नोन्नतसमेषु[162] भूः ।

[163]बाणसप्ताह्वबन्धूककाशासनविराजिता' ॥२०१॥

[सुश्रुत : सूत्र६:३६]

भूर्निम्नोन्नतसमेषु[164] यथा संख्यं पंकादिभिः कीर्णा भवति। द्रुमा वल्मीककारिण्यः सूक्ष्मा पिपीलिका कपिलारित्यर्थः[165] ॥२०२॥

Characteristics and Regimens for Śarat

During *śarat* (autumn), clouds are beautiful like sun-stone, and the sour taste predominates over others. The ponds become beautiful with groups of *haṁsa* and lotus over its water. The rays of the moon become strong, unctuous, clean and exceedingly pleasing. The water of ponds and lakes becomes pure because it becomes impregnated with the rays of the *citrā* (?). The lower parts of earth are full of mud, the upper parts are dried up and even parts of the earth are full of trees. During this season, trees like *bāṇa*, *saptāhva*, *bandhūka*, *kāśa* and *asana* grow luxuriously.

[Note : The second sentence of the passage No. 203 is also available in the *Dalhaṇa* commentary on *Suśruta saṁhitā* in a slightly modified form. But the relevant text is missing both in the *Suśruta saṁhitā* and the present work].

दर्शयन्ति शरन्नद्यपुलिनानि शनैः शनैः ।
नवसंगम सव्रीड[166] जघनानीव योषितः ॥२०३॥

During autumn the watei in the rivers gets reduced slowly and it appears as if a blashful lady is reluctantly exposing her thighs during her first intercourse.

'वर्षाशीतोचिताङ्गानां सहसैवार्करश्मिभिः ।
तप्तानामाचितं[167] पित्तं[168] प्रायः शरदि कुप्यति' ॥२०४॥

[चरक : सूत्र६:४१]

The parts of the body adopted for rains and cold are suddenly exposed to the heat of the sun with the beginning of autumn. Therefore, the *pitta* accumulated during the rains generally gets vitiated in the autumn.

तत्क्षयाय[169] घृतं तिक्तं विरेको रक्तमोक्षणं ।
तिक्तं स्वादुकषायं च[170] क्षुधितोन्नं[171] भजेल्लघु ॥२०५॥
शालिमुद्गासिताधात्रीपटोलमधुजाङ्गलम्[172] ।
शृतक्षीरं सितायुक्तं चंद्रिकासेवनं निशि ॥२०६॥

श्यामारामारतं शस्तं सेव्या क्षौद्र हरीतकी ।

173
स्नानपानावगाहेषु हितमंशूदकं सदा ॥२०७॥

तप्तं तप्तांशुकिरणै शीतं शीतांशुरश्मिभिः ।

174
समंतादप्यहोरात्रमगस्त्योदयनिर्विषम् ॥२०८॥

175
शीताच्छं दोषरहितं सर्वं कौप्य विवर्जितम् ।

For alleviation of aggravated *pitta*, one should use ghee, bitter things, purgation therapy and blood-letting therapy. When hungry, he should take food which is bitter, sweet, astringent and light. *Śāli*, *mudga*, sugar, *dhātri*, *paṭola*, honey, meat of animals dwelling in arid land forests and boiled milk mixed with sugar are useful. At night, exposure to the rays of the moon is useful. One should have sexual intercourse with *śyāma* type of woman. *Haritaki* mixed with honey should be regularly used. For bath, drink and washing, *aṁśūdaka* is always useful. The water which is exposed to the heat of the sun during day time and to the cooling rays of the moon during night time and which is detoxicated by the effect of the star Canopus (*agastya*) is called *aṁśūdaka*. It is cooling, clean and free from all defects. But the water of well, exposed in the same way, does not fall under this category.

तुषारक्षारसौहित्यदधितैलवसातपान् ।

176
तीक्ष्णमद्यदिवास्वप्नपुरोवातान्विवर्जयेत् ॥२०९॥

॥इति शरदृतुः॥

One should avoid exposure to dew, habitually intake of alkalies, curd, oil, *vasā* (muscle fact), exposure to sun, strong alcohol, sleep during day time and wind coming from the eastern direction.

Thus, ends the description of characteristic features of and regimens for the autumn season.

ज्येष्ठाषाढेषु यत्सुप्तं यद्भुक्तं पौषमाघयोः ।
शरत्काले जलं पीतं तेन जीवन्ति जन्तवः ।

The amount of sleep one enjoys during the months of *jyeṣṭha* and *āṣāḍha*, the quantity of food one takes during the months of *pauṣa* and *māgha* and the quantity of water one drinks during the autumn season, determine the life (well being) of living beings.

नित्यं सर्वरसाभ्यासः स्वस्वाधिक्यमृतावृतौ ॥२१०॥

One should consume daily all the tastes habitually. However, depending upon the nature of the season, certain *rasas* (tastes) should be taken in excess.

ऋतुसंधि]

ऋत्वोरंत्यादिसप्ताहावृतुसन्धिरिति स्मृतः ।
तत्र पूर्वविधिस्त्याज्यः सेवनीयोऽपरः क्रमात् ॥२११॥

असात्म्यजा हि रोगाः स्युः सहसा त्यागशीलनात् ।
मासराशिस्वरूपाख्यमृतोर्यल्लक्षणत्रयम् ॥२१२॥

177
यथोत्तरं भजेच्चर्यां तत्र तस्य बलादिति ।

Ṛtu sandhi

The last week of a season and the first week of the consecutive season, constitute *ṛtu sandhi* (transitional phase of the season). During this period, one should gradually give up the prescriptions of the previous season and resort to the measures prescribed for the consecutive season. If the regimens of the season which is coming to an end, are abruptly given up or if the regimens prescribed for the incoming season are suddenly resorted to then they give rise to diseases because of *asātmya* (unwholesomeness). Depending upon the characteristic features of the three seasons constituted of months or *rāśis*, one should follow the regimens according to his strength.

पुष्टधातुः समाग्निश्च निश्चिन्तो नीरुजः सुखी ॥२१३॥

भजेदृतौ[178] वै युवतीं यथा शास्त्रं तथोपरि ।

त्र्यहाद्वसन्तशरदोः पक्षाद्वृष्टिनिदाघयोः ॥२१४॥

प्रकामं तु निषेवेत मैथुनं शिशिरागमे ।

A person who has nourished tissue elements, who has the equilibrium of *agni* (the power of digestion and metabolism), who is free from worry and diseases and who is happy, should desire in *ṛtu kāla* (appropriate time), young woman and should have intercourse with her according to the prescriptions in scriptures. During spring and autumn, sexual intercourse should be performed on third days; during rainy and summer seasons, it should be done fortnightly and during the onset of winter, one should have sexual intercourse as much as he desires.

शीते रात्रौ दिवा ग्रीष्मे प्रावृडासारगर्जिते[179] ॥२१५॥

वसन्ते च दिवारात्रौ शरत्सु सरसः स्मरः ।

During winter season, intercourse should be done at night; during summer in day time; during rainy season, at the time of the roaring of the cloud, during spring season, it is permitted both in day and night time; and during autumn, when the person is excited.

शरीरे जायते नित्यं वाञ्च्छा[180] चैव चतुर्विधा ॥२१६॥

आहाराम्बु च निद्रा च कामश्चेति चतुर्विधः[181] ।

अन्नहीनं दहेद्धातुं शोणितं चाम्बुहीनतः[182] ॥२१७॥

कामहीनं दहेच्चक्षुरनिद्रारोगकारिणी ।

सम्यक्प्रकारं सेवेत यथारोग्यं प्रजायते ॥२१८॥

In the living beings, there are four types of invariable desires viz., desire for food, desire for drinking water, desire for sleep and desire for sex. Without food, the tissue elemeuts are burnt, without water the blood is reduced, without sex eyesight is afflicted and sleeplessness is caused which give rise to many diseases. Therefore, these desires are to be satisfied appropriately for the maintenance of health.

[183] तत्रान्नपानमूलं हि स्वास्थ्यं इति[184] विनिश्चितम् ।

तत्र शीतोष्णवर्षाणां हीनमिथ्याधिकेन च ॥२१९॥

जलानामौषधादीनां विपरीतो गुणो भवेत् ।

तस्योपरोधाद्विविधरोगाणां चाशुसंभवः[185] ॥२२०॥

तस्माद्वैद्यैर्बुद्धिमद्भिः सम्यगृतुषु संग्रहम् ।

भगां बाह्यौषधीनां च कारयेच्च प्रयोजयेत्[186] ॥२२१॥

Certainly, the health of an individual is dependant upon the food and the drink he consumes. Because of the diminution, perversion or excess of cold, heat and rain, the properties of different types of water and drugs including corns and cereals become of opposite nature. By the impact of this phenomenon different types of diseases abruptly appear. Therefore, a wise physician should collect different types of water and drugs in appropriate seasons and administer them.

अनुत्पत्तौ यतन्ते ये ते वैद्यास्ते च मंत्रिणः ।

विपाकं को विजानाति गदानां विपदामपि ॥२२२॥

Who can predict the result of a disease or a danger to the country ? Therefore, those who take preventive measures before such diseases or dangers appear, they are the true physicians and efficient ministers.

शीतोद्भवं दोषचयं वसंते विशोधयेद्ग्रीष्मजमभ्रकाले ।

घनात्यये वार्षिकमाशु सम्यक्प्राप्नोति रोगान्न रुजां कदाचित् ॥२२३॥

Doṣas accumulated during the winter season should be eliminated in the spring; those accumulated in the summer should be eliminated in rainy season and those accumulated during rainy season should be eliminated after the rains are over. By doing so, one can overcome the diseases and pains.

सुश्रुतात्

अतिपातिषु रोगेषु नेच्छेद्विधिमिमं भिषक् ।

प्रदीप्तागारवच्छीघ्रं तत्र कुर्यात् प्रतिक्रियाम् ॥२२४॥

[सुश्रुत : सूत्र५:४०]

According to Suśruta

The description of elimination of *doṣas* during different seasons, given above, is meant for a healthy person. When a disease has already afflicted the patient, then without waiting for the appropriate season, the requisite therapies should be administered as one would like to extinguish the fire if it has already started burning.

अग्निवेशात्

अव्यापन्नेषु ऋतुषु कदाचिदपि जायते ।

विविधा व्याधिपीडा च मरणोत्पातदारुणः ॥२२५॥

According to Agniveśa

Sometimes, diseases occur even if there is no perversion in the seasonal effects. The patient gets afflicted with the different types of pains, and the disease may even become serious resulting in the death of the patient.

नानाजातिप्रकृत्यन्नविहाराणां शरीरिणाम् ।
कथं जनपदोध्वंसः सामान्यस्याधिमान्मवेत् ॥२२६॥
हेतुलिङ्गौषधं चात्र यत्तदृतुषु नो गुरो! ।[187]
आत्रेयश्चोदितं स्त्वेवं हृष्टात्मा शिष्यमब्रवीत् ॥२२७॥
कालो देशो जलो वायुश्चैते दुष्टाः विलक्षणैः ।[188]
कुर्युर्जनपदोद्ध्वंसमेकरूपेण यक्ष्मणा ॥२२८॥

Oh ! Preceptor, please tell us the reasons for which persons who are of different castes, natures and whose diet and regimens are different, but all of them get afflicted by epidemics ? What are the causative factors, signs, symptoms and treatment of such epidemics in different seasons ? Having heard this from the disciple, *Ātreya*, who was in a happy mood, told, "Because of perversion, *kāla* (time), *deśa* (land), *jala* (water) and *vāyu* (air) get vitiated resulting in the manifestation of epidemics in the form of one type of disease.

एकरूपेणयक्ष्मणा कोऽर्थः? सर्वेषां शीतज्वरादीनां रूपेणेत्यर्थः ॥२२६॥

What is the meaning of the term *"eka rūpeṇa yakṣmaṇā"*? This term means "affliction of all people by one of the diseases like *śita jvara* (epidemic flue) etc."

राजा धर्मं परित्यज्य यदाऽधर्मे प्रवर्तते ।[189]
अधर्ममनुवर्तन्ते तद्देशपुरवासिनः ॥२३०॥

उत्क्रान्तधर्ममर्यादा प्रजा वा यद्युपेक्ष्यते ।

सराजं तं जनपदं संत्यजन्तीह देवताः ॥२३१॥

तयोरधर्मात्सम्प्राप्ते काले व्यापद्यते ध्रुवम् ।

उत्क्रान्तधर्ममर्यादा तं प्रजास्त्यक्तजीवितम्[190] ॥२३२॥

When the king gives up his duties and indulges in sinful acts, the citizens of that kingdom also get involved in sinful acts. When the king exceeds the limit of his royal duties, or neglects his subjects, then the gods abandon that king as well as that kingdom. By the sinful acts, the king and his citizens themselves get certainly afflicted, and when the limits of the duties are exceeded, the subjects become as if devoid of life.

[कालव्यापत्तिलक्षणम्]

विध्वंसयन्ति विकृताः कालदेशास्तु[191] मारुताः ।

ग्रह[192]नक्षत्रसंस्थानप्रधान[193]जनवैकृतैः ॥२३३॥

तयोरधर्मात्सम्प्राप्ते कालो व्यापद्यते ध्रुवम् ।

Characteristic Features of the Vitiated Kāla (*Time*)

As a result of the improper position of the planets and the stars, by the perversion of the leaders, *kāla* (time), *deśa* (land) and *maruta* (air) get vitiated resulting in the destruction of the people. Because of the sinful acts of the king and his subjects, the *kāla* (time) certainly gets afflicted.

कालः सम्वत्सरः शीतः घर्मवर्ष[194]श्च लक्षणम् ॥२३४॥

स हीनातिविपर्यस्त स्वलिङ्गो दुष्ट उच्यते ।

शीतेऽतिवातता शीतमथवाऽस्य विपर्ययः ।

तथा चोष्णे च वर्षे च कालव्यापत्तिलक्षणम् ॥२३५॥

Kāla (time) is the same as *saṁvatsara* (year), and it is characterised by winter, summer and rainy seasons. When there is diminution, excess or perversion of the characteristic features of these seasons, they are called vitiated. If during winter season, there is excess of wind or excess of cold or there are opposite features, then this is called vitiation of *kāla*. Similarly, may be explained the vitiation of summer and rainy seasons.

[प्रदुष्टदेशलक्षणम्]

प्रकृत्या विकृतस्पर्शगन्धवर्णरसाश्रयः ।

[195]तृणोपललतागुल्मजालव्रततिसंकुलः ॥२३६॥

मक्षिकादंशमशककृमिकीटाद्युपद्रुतः ।

शुकाखुशलभोल्लुकश्मशानिकमृगद्विजैः ॥२३७॥

पीडितो वातनिर्वातकंपोल्काशनिवृष्टिभिः ।

निःश्रीकपुष्पो गबनो नष्टशस्यौषधीफलः ॥२३८॥

संशुष्को [199]दीर्घसंक्षु[ब्ध]घोरस्वनजलाशयः ।

नीलिकादिभिराच्छन्नो वाप्यादीनां जलोद्गमः ॥२३९॥

घोरनादकृमिर्वायुर्मेघाच्छन्ननभस्तलः ।

अकालपुष्पफलवान्गर्भाद्यद्भुतदर्शनः ॥२४०॥

निस्तन्य [197]इव निःश्रीकः तप्तोद्भ्रान्तमृगद्विजः ।

अजस्रं संभ्रमोद्भ्रान्त उत्क्रुष्टाश्वगणो भृशम् ॥२४१॥

भैरवाद्भुतं संत्रासो रुदितानिष्टनिःस्वनः ।

द्वीपादीनां[198] वरोत्पत्तिरश्वादीनां[199] द्विधालकाः ॥२४२॥

प्रासादानां[200] प्रपातश्च अकस्माच्चैव जायते ।

त्रासश्च गोवृषादीनां अश्वानां च पलायनम् ॥२४३॥

भवेद्धर्मार्जवादीनां नाशः सत्यौजसां तथा ।

उत्पातैस्तद्विधैश्चान्यैः प्रदुष्टो देश उच्यते ॥२४४॥

Characteristic Features of Vitiation of Deśa (land)

The following characteristic features are manifested when the land gets vitiated :

1. There will be change in the natural touch, smell, colour and taste;

2. The grass, herb, creeper and bush get surrounded with net-like substances;

3. There will be more of flies, insects, mosquitos, worms and germs;

4. There will be more of parrots, rats, locusts, *ullūka* (owl bird) and animals as well as birds inhabiting crematorium;

5. There will be more of strong winds, tornado, earthquake, fall of meteor, thunder storm and rain;

6. The flowers and wind will lose their beauty and tenderness respectively, and there will be no fruits or grains in the plants and trees ;

7. The lakes will either be dry or get increased in size with turbulance and big roaring sound;

8. Ponds etc., will be covered with *nilikā* (blue moss) and there will be abrupt rise in water level;

9. The sky will be full of roaring sound, germs, strong wind and cloud;

10. Fruits and flowers will appear untimely (unseasonal);

11. There will be birth of monsters and disfigured foetus;

12. The deer and birds will have no lactation and they will lose their graceful appearance. They would be in an irritable mood running here and there;

13. Even the best of the horses will commit several mistakes and will go wild very often. They will look fierceful, make surprising gestures, be fearful, cry and make inauspicious sounds;

14. Elephants and horses will produce unusual sounds;

15. Sudden fall of buildings;

16. Cows and bulls become fearful and horses run away; and

17. There will be destruction of religion, purity, truth and energy.

If the above mentioned and other similar afflictions are manifested, the *deśa* (land or country) should be considered as polluted.

[दुष्टाम्बुलक्षणम्]

स्वभावविरसस्पर्शगन्धवर्णरसोदितम् ।
आगन्तुभिः [201] कृमिक्लेदपैच्छिल्यैश्चाप्युपद्रुतम् ॥२४५॥

परित्यक्तं जलचरैरकस्माद्वापि सेवितम् ।
पातस्तटद्रुमाणां च क्षीयमाणं जलाशयम् ॥२४६॥

[202] अनारोग्यकरं चाम्बु प्राणिनां दुष्टमुच्यते ।
[203] विवर्षितः कुण्डलितश्चण्डघोरजवस्वनः ॥२४७॥

Characteristics of Polluted Udaka (water)

The following are the characteristic features of polluted water :

1. The water loses its natural taste, touch, smell and colour and there will be foul smell in it;
2. Affliction of water by extraneous germs, stickiness and sliminess;
3. Sudden disappearance or appearance of aquatic animals and birds;
4. Fall of trees in the bank of water reservoirs and their drying up;
5. The water becomes hostile for good health of animals; and
6. Sudden rise in water level, appearance of whirlpools, and ferocious as well as loud sound inside the reservoir.

The water having the above-mentioned characteristic features should be deemed as polluted.

[प्रदुष्टवायुलक्षणम्]

अतिशीतोष्णरूक्षातिपरुषोऽतिबलः खरः ।
असात्म्यगन्धसिकतापांशुधूमरजोवहः ॥२४८॥
यथर्तुविपरीतश्च प्रदुष्टोवायुरुच्यते ।

Characteristics of Polluted Vāyu (air)

The following are the characteristic features of polluted air :

1. Excessive coldness, heat, ununctuousness, roughness, strength and dryness of the wind;

2. Association of unpleasant smell, sand, ash and smoke in the air; and

3. Manifestation of features opposite to the seasonal characteristics.

The air having the above mentioned characteristic features should be deemed as polluted.

ऋतुकालप्रदेशेन वायुर्मुह्यति वायुना ॥२४९॥

सलिलं सलिलेनोर्वी तैः सर्वैश्चौद्भिदोगणः[204] ।

कालदेशाम्बुमरुतां दुष्टानां धर्मसंक्षये ।

एषां दुष्परिहार्यत्वात्पूर्वपूर्वो[205] भवेद्बली ॥२५०॥

The *ṛtu kāla* (time in the form of seasons) gets polluted by the pollution of *deśa* (land).

The polluted air and water further pollute the remaining air and water respectively. By the pollution of *deśa*, *kāla*, *udaka* and *vāyu* as a result of the diminution of *dharma* (religious virtues), the plants get polluted. Because of their unavoidability the earlier ones are more powerful than the later ones.

[जनपदोध्वंसे चिकित्सा]

अकालमृत्युतस्तस्मात्संरक्षेज्जीवितं बुधः ।

रसवीर्यविहीनानामौषधीनां च वर्जनम् ॥२५१॥

[206] सम्यगर्तुप्रभूतानां गृहीतानां च सेवनम् ।

जलानामौषधीनां च व्रतचर्य्याञ्च कारयेत् ॥२५२॥

देवगोविप्रसिद्धानां गुरूणां चार्चनं तपः ।

बलयः शान्तिकर्माणि होमस्वस्त्ययनानि च ॥२५३॥

जपोपवासाध्ययननियमध्यानमार्जवम् ।

हितं जनपदोद्ध्वंसे इन्द्रियाणां च निग्रहः ॥२५४॥

Management of Epidemics

The wise physician should save the life of patients who are destined to succumb to untimely death as a result of the epidemics. For this purpose, the following measures should be adopted :

1. One should avoid use of such drugs as are devoid of *rasa* (taste) and *vīrya* (potency);

2. One should use only such of the drugs and water as are grown and collected in appropriate seasons;

3. One should perform religious rites and offer prayer to the gods, cows, *brāhmaṇas*, *siddhas* and preceptors;

4. One should perform penance, sacrifice (*bali*), rituals for peace, oblation to fire, auspicious invocation, incantation, fasting, study of religious scriptures, observance of scriptural rules, meditation and purification; and

5. Abstinence of the sense organs from their objects.

वह्वम्बुनगमत्स्यास्तु सक्षारमधुरोदकाः ।

हिमवत्सागरानूपसंसृता येषु चापगाः ॥२५५॥

[207] विषवृक्षाल्पहारिण्यो याश्चाप्यचलनिम्नगाः ।

[208] बहुरोगा नरस्तेषु देशेष्वल्पायुषस्तथा ॥२५६॥

Person inhabiting the land having the following characteristic features suffer from many diseases and have a short span of life;

1. A place having a lot of water, crocodiles and fish and where water is alkaline or sweet in taste; and

2. A place which has many rivers (or streams), which flow from the *Himālayas*, sea or marshy areas, which carry water through poisonous trees, which carry less quantity of water and which are just descending from a mountain.

विषौषधियुते[209] देशे विषपुष्पादिभिर्युते ।
तत्राक्रम्य यदा वायुः शुभे[210] देशे प्रवर्तते[211] ॥२५७॥
तदा शिरसि पीडा च कासश्वासवमिज्वराः ।
भवन्ति मरको[212] वापि तस्मात्तास्तु परित्यजेत् ॥२५८॥

Headache, bronchitis, asthma, emesis and fever, including *maraka* (a serious type of epidemic disease) occur even in an unpolluted land, if the air which blows over it has come after passing through a place having poisonous trees, poisonous flowers etc. Therefore, such places should be avoided.

गृहदाराञ्जनपदान् शयनासनसेवकान् ।
परीक्षेत गुणैर्दोषैः रत्नानि च मणीनपि ॥२५९॥
स्थानत्यागो पुरस्त्यागो कुर्याद्धोमं जपस्तथा ।
अन्यथा दोषयुक्तानां ग्रहणाद्विघ्नसंभवः ॥२६०॥

A wise person should examine both the good and bad qualities before taking a decision on the construction of a house, marriage, living in a particular country, bed, seat, servants, jewels and gems. If any of these items having bad qualities is accepted then this will lead to dangerous situations. Therefore, in such events, one should give up that place or that country and perform *homa* (oblation to fire) and *japa* (incantation of *mantras*).

213

कालार्थकर्मणां योगो हीनमिथ्यातिमात्रकः ।

सम्यग्योगश्च विज्ञेयो रोगारोग्यैककारणम् ॥२६१॥

[अष्टाङ्गहृदय : सूत्र१:१६]

॥इति कालपरीक्षा॥

Less utilisation, wrong utilisation and excessive utilisation of the time (season) and objects of senses and activities, are the exclusive causes of ill health. Their proper utilisation is known to maintain good health.

Thus, ends the examination of the characteristic features of *kāla* (time).

अथ दिनचर्या

[शौचविधिः]

प्रातःकाले समुत्तिष्ठेत्स्वस्थो रक्षार्थमायुषः ।

शरीरशुद्धिं निर्वर्त्य कृतशौचविधिर्न्नरः ॥२६२॥

Regimens for the Day

Purification of the Body

A healthy person should get up in *prātaḥ kāla* (early morning) for the preservation of his life. Thereafter, he should attend the toilet which should be followed by the cleaning of the body.

[प्रसाधनविधि]

214

केशपाशे प्रकुर्वीत प्रसाधन्या विशोधनम् ।

Hair dressing

Thereafter, he should dress his hair with the help of the comb.

[दन्तनिर्लेखनविधिः]

ततो हि दन्तनिर्लेखं प्रकुर्याद्विधिना स्मृतम् ॥२६३॥

क्षीरतिक्तकषायाणां[215] द्वादशाङ्गुलमायतम् ।

कनिष्ठिकासम[216] स्थौल्यं ख्यातवृक्षस्य[217] शोभनम् ॥२६४॥

Tooth brushing

Thereafter, the person should brush his teeth according to the procedure prescribed for the purpose. The tooth cleaning stick should be twelve *aṅgulas* (about six inches) in length and it should have the thickness of his little finger. It should be collected from the well known trees having latex and bitter as well as astringent tastes.

वनस्पतिस्तुतिः

आयुर्बलं यशोवर्चः प्रजापशूवसूनि च ।

ब्रह्मप्रज्ञां च मेधां च त्वं नो देहि वनस्पते! ॥२६५॥

इत्यादिस्तुतिवाक्येन ये गृह्णन्ति वनस्पतिम् ।

तत्[218] प्रयच्छन्ति संस्कर्तुरायुर्धीश्रीर्यशस्स्थितिम् ॥२६६॥

Offering prayer to the tree

Before collecting the tooth cleaning stick, the tree should be offered prayer as follows: "Oh tree ! Give me life and fame, power of speech, offsprings, cattle, wealth, spiritual power, wisdom and intellect." If the teeth cleaning stick is collected after offering the above-mentioned prayer, then the person is endowed with longevity, intellect, wealth, fame and stability in life.

[दन्तकाष्ठप्रयोगविधिर्गुणश्च]

द्वादशाङ्गुलं विप्राणां क्षत्रियाणां दशाङ्गुलम् ।

अष्टाङ्गुलं तु वैश्याणां शूद्राणां तु षडङ्गुलम् ॥२६७॥

दन्तकाष्ठं च गृह्णीयात्स्त्रीणां तच्चतुरङ्गुलम् ।

219

भक्षयेद्दन्तकाष्ठाग्रं दन्तमांसान्यपीडयन् ॥२६८॥

जिह्वानिलखनं कुर्यात्प्राङ्मुखो वा उदङ्मुखः ।

Method of Use of Tooth-cleaning Stick and Its Properties

The length of the tooth-cleaning stick should be twelve *aṅgulas* for *brāhmaṇas*, ten *aṅgulas* for *kṣatriyas*, eight *aṅgulas* for *vāiśyas*, six *aṅgulas* for *śūdras* and four *aṅgulas* for women. The tip of the tooth-cleaning stick should be chewed and brush made out of it so that its use does not cause any injury to the teeth and the gums. Thereafter, the tongue should be scraped facing towards the east or the north.

[गंडूषगुणाः]

अभावे दन्तकाष्ठस्य निषिद्धदिवसेषु च ॥२६९॥

अपां द्वादशगंडूषैर्मुखशुद्धिर्विधीयते ।

रसनादन्तजाः रोगाः वैरस्यमलसंभवाः ॥२७०॥

न भवन्ति मुखे तेन वैशद्यं लाघवं भवेत् ।

ततो गंडूषकरणं कफकण्डूमलापहम् ॥२७१॥

220

मुखप्रक्षालनं कार्यं पयसा शीतलेन च ।

रक्तपित्तास्यसंशोषनीलिकाव्यंगनाशनम् ॥२७२॥

Properties of Gargle

If the tooth-cleaning stick is not available and during such days, when the use of tooth-cleaning stick is prohibited, one should clean mouth by gargling with twelve handfuls of water. By doing so, there will be no disease either in the tongue or in the teeth, as a result of the bad taste and accumulation of excreta. The mouth becomes non-slime and light. By gargling, *kapha* gets eliminated and it subsides itching and also helps in the elimination of excreta. Thereafter, the face should be washed with cold water. It cures *rakta pitta* (a disease characterised by bleeding from different parts of the body), dryness of mouth, *nilikā* (blue moles) and *vyaṅga* (appearance of white spots in the face).

कुर्याद्वापि कटूष्णेन पयसास्यविशोधनम् ।
कफवातहरं स्निग्धं मुखदोषविनाशनम् ॥२७३॥

The mouth can also be cleaned with water which is pungent and hot. It eliminates *kapha* and *vāyu*. It causes unctuousness in the face and cures diseases of the mouth.

औषधं चात्र सेवेत सद्वैद्यप्रतिपादितम् ।
जातरोग[221]निवृत्यर्थमारोग्यबलवर्धनम् ॥२७४॥

In case of a disease of the mouth, one should act according to the advice of the wise physician. These medicines also help in the maintenance of health and promotion of strength.

[ताम्बूलभक्षणगुणाः]

ताम्बूलं भक्षयेत्पश्चाद्द्विजशेषं तु भोजनम्[222] ।
तीक्ष्णोष्णं कफवातघ्नं मुखदोषविनाशनम्[223] ॥२७५॥

Chewing of Betel leaf

After taking food, one should chew betel leaf which is sharp and hot and which alleviates *kapha* and *vāyu*. It also cures the diseases of the mouth.

[स्वकार्ये नियोजनम्]

ततोऽधिकारिणः सर्वे स्वाधिकारेषु योजितः ।

Performance of Duties

Thereafter, everybody should perform their duties for which they are employed and in which they are efficient.

[उद्वर्त्तनाभ्यङ्गगुणाः]

224
'ततश्चोद्वर्त्तनाभ्यंगं कारयेच्च यथेप्सितम् ॥२७६॥

उद्वर्त्तनं कफहरं मेदशुक्रादिवर्द्धनम् ।

श्रेष्ठं शोणितदं बल्यं कांतिकृद्दोषनाशनम्' ॥२७७॥

Properties of Unction and Massage

Thereafter, one should perform unction and massage as much as he desires. Unction alleviates *kapha* and promotes fat, semen etc. It is an excellent therapy for the increase of blood, promotion of strength and complexion and alleviation of *doṣas*.

[अभ्यङ्गः]

'अभ्यङ्गमाचरेद्यस्तु स जराश्रमवर्जितः ।

225
दृष्टिप्रसादपुष्ट्यायुः स्वास्थ्यत्वक्पाददार्ढ्यवान् ॥२७८॥'

अद्भिः संसिक्तमूलानां तरूणां पल्लवादयः ।

वर्धन्ते हि यथा नृणां स्नेहसंसिक्तधातवः ॥२७९॥

Massage

By the habitual use of massage, one can overcome ageing process and exertion of the body. Massage promotes eye-sight, happiness, nourishment, longevity and health. It cures the diseases of skin and produces sturdiness of the legs. Tender leaf etc., appear in a tree whose root is sprinkled with water. Similarly, *dhātus* (tissue elements) of a person increase in quantity when the body is massaged with oil.

[स्नानम्]

ततः स्नानं प्रकुर्वीत सुखोष्णेनैव वारिणा ।
तेन गात्राभिषेकस्तु भवत्येव बलावहः ॥२८०॥
अत्युष्णेनोत्तमाङ्गस्य बलहृत्केशचक्षुषाम् ।
स्नानस्यानन्तरं सम्यग्वस्त्रेण तनुमार्जनम् ॥२८१॥

Bath

Thereafter, one should take bath in luke-warm water. By the wash of the body with this water, the strength is increased. If the head is washed with very hot water, it takes away the strength and is harmful for the hair and the eyesight. After taking bath, one should properly clean the body with a piece of cloth.

[वस्त्रपरिधानम्]

कान्तिप्रदं शरीरस्य कंडूत्वग्दोषनाशनम् ।
शीतकाले तु कौषेयं काषायं घर्मवासरे ॥२८२॥

226

वर्षासु श्वेतवस्त्रं स्यादेवं वस्त्राणि धारयेत् ।

Wearing of Apparel

In Winter season, one should use silken cloth and in summer, one should use cloth impregnated with the juice of astringent trees. In rainy season, one should use white cloth. By doing so, there is promotion of complexion in the body. It also alleviates itching sensation and skin diseases.

227
'कौशेयं चित्रवस्त्रं वा रक्तवस्त्रं तथैव च ॥२८३॥

वातश्लेषमहरं नृणां शीतकाले प्रधारयेत् ।

मेध्यं सुशीतं पित्तघ्नं काषायं वस्त्रमुच्यते' ॥२८४॥

तद्धारयेद्धर्मकाले काषायं वस्त्रमुत्तमम् ।

Silken cloth, *citra vastra* (cloth with variegated colours) and *rakta vastra* (red coloured cloth), alleviate *vāyu* and *kapha* of human beings. Therefore, such type of cloth should be used during winter season, The *kāṣāya vastra* (cloth impregnated with the decoction of astringent trees) promotes intellect. It produces cooling effect and it alleviates *pitta*. Therefore, such type of cloth should be used during summer season.

शुक्लं च सुखदं चैव शीतातपनिवारणम् ॥२८५॥

न चोष्णं न च वा शीतं शुक्लं वस्त्रं च धारयेत् ।

The white cloth gives pleasure and prevents cold as well as heat. It is neither very hot nor very cold. Therefore, in rainy season, such white cloth should be used.

[उद्वर्तनम्]

गन्धनोद्वर्तनं चादौ ततो लेपं प्रकारयेत् ॥२८६॥

कुंकुमं चन्दनं चैव कृष्णागुरुविमिश्रितम् ।

उष्णभावमिदं श्रेष्ठं शीतकालेषु शोभनम् ॥२८७॥

228
'चंदनं चांबुनायुक्तं कर्पूरेण विमिश्रितम् ।

सुगंधं च सुशीतं च धर्मकाले सुशोभनम्' ॥२८८॥

चन्दनं [कुंकुमोपेतं][229] मृगनाभिसमायुतम् ।

न चोष्णं न च वा शीतं वर्षाकाले प्रशस्यते ॥२८९॥

Unction

First of all, there should be unction over the body with the paste of fragrant drugs. Thereafter, ointments prepared of saffron, sandal-wood and black variety of *aguru* should be smeared over the body. This ointment has heating property, and therefore, it is exceedingly useful in winter season. In summer season, the ointment prepared of sandal-wood, *aguru*, camphor which is fragrant and cooling, is very useful. During rainy season, the ointment prepared of sandal-wood, saffron and musk which is neither very hot nor very cold is useful.

कुलाचारं तु कुर्वीत सन्ध्योपासनमादृतः ।

सूर्योपस्तिं ततः कुर्यादिष्टदेवस्य चार्चनम् ॥२९०॥

दत्त्वा दानं च विप्रेभ्यो गृह्णीयात्तेभ्य आशिषम् ।

केशानां निचये कुर्यात्कस्तूर्याद्यैश्च[230] लेपनम् ॥२९१॥

One should perform the professional duties adopted traditionally along with *sandhyā*, *upāsanā*, prayer to sun and prayer to the tutelary deity. One should give *dāna* (donation or charity) to *Brāhmins* and get their blessings. In the hair, the paste prepared of musk etc., should be smeared.

[पुष्पधारणम्]

सुपुष्पाणि सुगन्धीनि नित्यं शीर्षे प्रधारयेत् ।

[231] क्लेदायाससमुद्भूतं स्वेददुर्गन्धिनाशनम् ॥२९२॥

चक्षुष्यं दाहशमनं सौमनस्यं च जायते ।

तीक्ष्णाप्रलुप्तकेतक्याः कोमलं धारयेद्दलम् ॥२९३॥

जातिपुष्पं च वैलेखा[232] जाम्बवं कुटजं तथा ।
पाटलं च बृहत्पुष्पं बकुलं चम्पकं तथा ॥२९४॥
श्रीखण्डं चैव गोल्लालं कस्तूर्या सह धारयेत् ।
मंदारं मरुवं चैव नीलोत्पलकुमुद्वकम् ॥२९५॥
रक्तोत्पलं यूथिकाञ्च कर्पूरैः सह धारयेत् ।
अस्नातैर्मल्लिकाधार्या सुस्नातैर्जातिबिल्वजम्[233] ॥२९६॥
अभ्यङ्गे केतकी धार्या धार्यं चोत्पलकं सदा ।
जातिकुन्दं च नैवारं[234] श्रीखण्डं बिल्वमल्लिकाम् ॥२९७॥
मकरन्देन संयुक्तं शिरसा धारयेन्नरः ।
सर्वाण्येतानि तुल्यानि रसतो वीर्यतस्तथा ॥२९८॥
त्रिदोषशमनायैव सर्वकाले प्रधारयेत् ।
केतकं[235] बकुलं पुष्पं श्रीखण्डं शतपत्रकम् ॥२९९॥
गोल्लालकं[236] चंपकं च वातश्लेष्महरं परम् ।
उष्णवीर्यं च तत्प्रोक्तं शीतकाले प्रधारयेत् ॥३००॥
श्रीवकं[237] मरुवं चैव नीलोत्पलसवत्सकौ ।
कुलकं पाटलं चैव श्रीखण्डं च तथैव च ॥३०१॥
नात्युष्णं न च वा शीतं सर्वदोषनिवर्हणम् ।
निर्मलं नेत्रदोषघ्नं वर्षाकाले प्रधारयेत् ॥३०२॥

Wearing of Flowers

Daily one should wear in his head fragrant flowers. This removes the foul smell caused by sweating, stickiness and exertion. This promotes eye sight, alleviates burning sensation and produces happiness. The soft petals of the *ketaki* which is cleaned of its sharp edged teeth, should be worn. Along with *kastūri*, one should use *jāti puṣpa*, *vailekhā*, flower of *jaṁbu*, *kuṭaja*, *pāṭala*, *bṛhat puṣpa*, *vakula*, *campaka*, *śrikhaṇḍa* and *gaullāla*. One should wear with camphor the flower of *mandāra*, *maruva*, *nilotpala*, *kumuda*, *raktotpala* and *yūthikā*. Without bath, one should wear *mallikā* and after bath, one should use the flower of *jāti* and *bilva*. During massage, one should wear *ketaki*. *Utpalla* flower can be worn any time. On the head, one should wear the flowers of *jāti*, *kunda*, *nivāra*, *śrikhaṇḍa*, *bilva* and *mallikā* along with *makaranda*. All these flowers are similar in taste and *virya* (potency). They alleviate all the three *doṣas* and therefore, they can be worn at all times. The flowers of *ketaki*, *vakula*, *śrikhaṇḍa*, *śata patra*, *gaullālaka* and *campaka* alleviate *vāyu and kapha*. They are hot in potency. Therefore, they should be used during the winter season. During rainy season, one should use the flowers of *śrivaka*, *maruva*, *nilotpala*, *vatsaka*, *kulaka*, *pāṭala* and *śrikhaṇḍa*. They are neither hot nor cold. They alleviate all the three *doṣas*. They are free from any dirt and they cure eye diseases.

षड्यामं जातिकुसुमं नैवालं द्विमुहूर्तकम्[238] ।
त्रिरात्रमुत्पलं चैव पञ्चरात्रं तु केतकी ॥३०३॥
"द्विरात्रं[239] शतपत्रं च अर्द्धरात्रं तु मल्लिका" ।
अहोरात्रं चंपकं तु यूथिकां द्विमुहूर्तकम् ॥३०४॥
श्रीखण्डमेकरात्रं तु बकुलं माधवी तथा ।
श्रीपर्णं यावदाहारं तावत्कालं तु धारयेत् ॥३०५॥
मंदारमरुवं चैव दामनं[240] च सुपाटलम्[241] ।
यावत्कालं भवेद्गंधं[242] तावत्कालं तु[243] धारयेत् ॥३०६॥

One should wear the flower of *jāti* for six *yāmas*, *naivāla* for two *muhūrtas*, *utpala* for three nights, *ketakī* for five nights, *śata-patra* for two nights, *mallikā* for half of the night, *campaka* for one day and night, *yūthikā for two muhūrtas*, *śrikhaṇḍa*, *vakula* and *mādhavi* for one night, and *śriparṇa* only till the taking of the food is over. One should wear *mandāra*, *maruva*, *dāmana* and *pāṭala* flowers till they have their fragrance.

त्रिदोषशमनी जाती महादाहविनाशिनी ।

The flower of *jāti* alleviates all the three *doṣas* and cures serious type of burning sensation.

244
सुगन्धं दोषशमनं नैवालीपुष्पमुच्यते ॥३०७॥

The flower of *naivāla* is fragrant and it alleviates *doṣas*.

245
'पित्तहृद्विशदं चैव चक्षुष्यं चोत्पलं स्मृतम् ।

The flower of *utpala* alleviates *pitta*, causes non-sliminess and promotes eye sight.

श्लेष्मवातप्रशमनं उष्णवीर्यं च निर्मलम् ॥३०८॥

पुष्पाणां प्रवरं चैव केतकीपुष्पमुच्यते ।'

The flower of *ketaki* alleviates *kapha* and *vāyu*. It is hot in potency. It is free from dirt and it is the best among the flowers.

ईषदुष्णं सुगन्धं च सुशीतं दृष्टिदायकम् ॥३०९॥

शिरोभ्रमविनाशार्हं शतपत्रं तु शोभनम् ।

The flower of *śata patra* is slightly hot, fragrant, exceedingly cooling (?) and promoter of eye sight. It is useful in curing the giddiness in the head.

246
"श्रधायं मल्लिकापुष्पं दृष्टिहानिकरं परम् ॥३१०॥

One should not wear the flower of *mallikā* (?) because it spoils the eye sight.

चंपकं वातशमनं चक्षुष्यं विशदं शुभम् ।

The flower of *campaka* alleviates *vāyu.* It promotes eye sight, causes non-sliminess and auspiciousness.

पाटलं च महच्छीतं श्लेष्मवातप्रवर्द्धनम् ॥३११॥

मन्दाग्निपित्तदोषघ्नं कर्णव्याधिविनाशनम् ।

पाटलं धारयेद्यस्तु सम्यक्वाससमन्वितम् ॥३१२॥

ज्वरमूर्च्छापिपासाघ्नमायुष्यं दाहनाशनम् ।

The flower of *pāṭala* is exceedingly cooling and it aggravates *kapha* as well as *vāyu.* If the flower of *pāṭala* which has appropriate fragrance is worn, it cures *mandāgni* (loss of power of digestion), diseases of *pitta* and ear diseases. It cures fever, fainting and morbid thirst. It promotes longevity and cures burning sensation.

हेमन्ते शिशिरे चैव शतपत्रं तु शोभनं" ॥३१३॥

वसन्ते केतकी धार्या[247] घर्मे नैवालमालती ।

प्रावृट्सु पाटलं धार्यं चंपकं शरदि स्मृतम् ॥३१४॥

In *hemanta* (early winter) and *śiśira* (late winter), the flower of *śata patra* is useful. In spring season, *ketakī* should be used. In summer season, *naivāla* and *mālati* flowers are useful. *Pāṭala* is useful in *prāvṛṭ* (beginning of rainy season) and *campaka* is useful in autumn.

[आभूषणम्]

भूषणैर्भूषयेदङ्गं यथा विभवसारतः ।

शुचि सौभाग्यसंतोषदायकं काञ्चनं स्मृतम् ॥३१५॥

रत्नादिभूषणानां च धारणं ग्रहतुष्टिकृत् ।

Ornaments

Depending upon the availability of wealth, one should wear different types of ornaments. Ornaments of gold produce purity, auspiciousness and a sense of satisfaction. Ornaments studded with gems and jewels, counteract the effects of planets in evil position.

धर्मसंग्रहणं कार्यं दीनदानोपवासकैः ॥३१६॥

स्वबन्धुपितृदेवानां ब्राह्मणानां च तर्पणम् ।

कार्यं यशस्यमायुष्यं स्वर्ग्यं पापहरं परम् ॥३१७॥

One should acquire virtues by charity to the poor, *upavāsa* (fasting) and *tarpaṇa* (offering water with incantations) for pleasing his relations, dead ancestors, the gods and *brāhmaṇas*. This *tarpaṇa* promotes fame and longevity. It is conducive to the attainment of heaven and it destroys sins.

ततो भोजनवेलायां कृताचारः सदात्मवान् ।

देवान् पितृन् समभ्यर्च्य कुर्यान्मङ्गलवीक्षणम् ॥३१८॥

Thereafter, during the time of food one should perform his rituals, remain self-controlled, offer prayer to the gods and ancestors and look to auspicious things.

लोकेऽस्मिन्मङ्गलान्यष्टौ ब्राह्मणो गोर्हुताशनः ।

हिरण्यं सर्पिरादित्यः आपो राजा तथाऽष्टमः ॥३१९॥

एतानि सततं पश्येन्नमस्येदर्चयेत्तथा ।

प्रदक्षिणं सदा नित्यमायुर्धर्ममनुत्तमम् ॥३२०॥

In this universe, eight things are considered to be auspicious. They are, *brāhmaṇa*, cow, fire, gold, ghee, sun, water and the king. One should always have the sight of these auspicious things and offer prayer to them. They should be circum-ambulated. By doing so daily, they excellently promote the longevity and the religious virtues.

पत्नीं विहितशृंगारां प्राप्य भोजनमण्डपम् ।

यथाचाग्निबलं वीक्ष्य कुर्याद्भोजनकं नरः ॥३२१॥

एक एव न भुञ्जीत यदीच्छेत्सिद्धिमात्मनः ।

द्वित्रिभिर्वहुभिः सार्द्धं भोजनं तु दिवानिशम् ॥३२२॥

ततश्चाभीष्टसिद्धिः स्यात्तुष्टिः काम्यं तु सम्पदः ।

ताम्बूलं भक्षयेत्पश्चाद्दत्त्वा विप्राय भोजनम् ॥३२३॥

मनसोहर्षणं श्रेष्ठं रतिदं मदकारम् ।

248 249

"मुखरोगकृमिहरं तांबूलं रुचिकारकम् ॥३२४॥"

The food should be served by the wife, who is well decorated with cosmetics. Food should be taken in *bhojana-maṇḍapa* (platform specially constructed for dining). A person should take food keeping in view his *agni bala* (power of digestion and metabolism). If one wants self-accomplishment, he should not take food alone. During day and night, he should take food along with two, three or many persons. This helps in the accomplishment of one's own desires. This gives satisfaction. This is desirable and this endows a person with wealth. After feeding *brāhmins*, one should offer them *tāmbūla* (betel leaves). This causes exhileration of the mind and it is an excellent drug for the promotion of sexual desire. This is intoxicating. This cures the diseases of mouth and destroys germs. It promotes appetite.

दिवास्वापं न कुर्वीत स यतो हि कफावहः ।

[250]'दिवा स्त्रीगमनं नृणामायुःक्षयकरं भवेत् ॥३२५॥

One should not sleep during day time because it aggravates *kapha*. Indulgence in sex with a woman during day time reduces the span of life.

धर्मशास्त्राणि सततं पुराणश्रवणं तथा ।

कारयेद्विधिना सम्यक् आत्मतत्त्वविवेचनम्' ॥३२६॥

One should invariably study religious scriptures and hear the recitation of *purāṇas*. According to the prescribed procedure, one should critically think of his own soul.

[251]'सुखार्थाः सर्वभूतानां यतः सर्वप्रवृत्तयः ।

सुखं च.न विना धर्मं तस्माद्धर्मपरो भवेत्' ॥३२७॥

[अष्टाङ्गहृदय : सूत्र२:२०]

All the activities in this world are meant for the happiness of the living beings and this happiness cannot be achieved without *dharma* (religious virtues). Therefore, one should keep himself busy in religious activities.

'हिंसास्तेयान्यथाकामं पैशून्यं[252] परुषानृतम्[253] ।'

[अष्टाङ्गहृदय : सूत्र२:२१]

दुर्गोष्टमहितचिन्ता परद्रव्यस्य चिन्तनम् ॥३२८॥

'पापकर्मेति दशधा कायवाङ्मानसैस्त्यजेत् ।

अवृत्तिव्याधिशोकार्तानानुवर्तेत शक्तितः ॥३२९॥'

[अष्टाङ्गहृदय : सूत्र२:२३]

The following are the ten types of sinful acts :

1. *Hiṁsā* (violence);
2. *Steya* (stealing);
3. *Anyathā kāma* (desire for unnatural things);
4. *Piśuna* (back-biting);
5. *Paruṣa* (use of strong words while quarrelling with others);
6. *Anṛta* (speaking lies);
7. *Durga* (inconsistency in the speech and action);
8. *Iṣṭa* (desire to enjoy other's achievements);
9. *Ahita cintā* (thinking ill of others); and
10. *Para dravya cintana* (thinking of taking away other's wealth).

These ten sinful acts should be avoided in body, speech and mind. According to his capacity, one should serve the unemployed persons, persons suffering from diseases and persons in grief.

भक्त्या सेवेत मित्राणि न सेवेताहिताञ्जनान् ।
[254] आत्मवत्सततं पश्येत् सर्वजन्तुपिपीलिकम् ।।३३०।।

One should deal with his friends affectionately. One should not have any dealing with harmful persons. One should look to all creatures, including ants like himself.

'उपकारप्रधानः स्यादपकारपरेऽप्यरौ ।'

[अष्टाङ्गहृदय : सूत्र२:२५]

[255] "काले हितं मितं ब्रूयान्नाहितं तु कदाचन ।।३३१।।

हिताभिलाषी सुमुखो भवेत्सकरुणो मृदुः [256] ।”

‘नैकः सुखी न सर्वत्र विश्रब्धो न च शङ्कितः ॥३३२॥

न कश्चिदात्मनः शत्रुं नात्मानं कस्यचिद्रिपुम् ।’

[अष्टाङ्गहृदय : सूत्र२:२७]

प्रकाशयेन्नापमानं [257] न चातिस्नेहतां व्रजेत् ॥३३३॥

न पीडयेदिन्द्रियाणि [258] नात्यर्थं लालयेद्बुधः ।

[259] परम्पराविरुद्धो यः त्रिवर्गस्तं समाचरेत् ॥३३४॥

[260] अनुयायात्प्रतिपदं सर्वधर्मेषु मध्यमम् ।

कृतरोमनखश्मश्रुशुद्धवेशधरो भवेत् ॥३३५॥

‘चैत्यपूज्यध्वजाशस्तच्छायाभस्मतुषाशुचीन् ।

नाक्रमेच्छर्करालोष्टवलिस्नानभुवो [261] न च ॥३३६॥

नदीं तरेन्न बाहुभ्यां [262] नाग्निस्कन्धमपि व्रजेत् ।

संदिग्धनावं वृक्षं च [263] नारोहेद्दुष्टयानकम् ॥३३७॥

नासंवृतमुखः कुर्यात्क्षुतिहास्यविजृम्भणम् ।

[264] “नासिकांन विकुष्णीयान्नाकस्माद्विलिखेद्भुवम् ॥३३८॥

नाङ्गैश्चेष्टेत विगुणं नासीतोत्कटकश्चिरम् ।

देहवाक्चेतसां चेष्टाः प्राक् श्रमाद्विनिवर्तयेत् ॥३३९॥”

[अष्टाङ्गहृदय : सूत्र२:३३-३७]

[265]
'अङ्गानि मोटयेन्नैव नासीतोत्कटुकस्थितिः ।'

[266]
'नोर्ध्वंजानुश्चिरं तिष्ठेत् नक्तं सेवेत न द्रुमम् ॥३४०॥

तथा चत्वरचैत्यान्तश्चतुष्पथसुरालयान् ।'

[अष्टाङ्गहृदय : सूत्र२:३७-३८]

[267]
शून्याटवीं शून्यगृहं श्मशानानि दिवाऽपि च [268] ॥३४१॥

त्यज्येद् दुराचारतांस्तु तुषारपरुषानिलान् ।

'कुलच्छायां नृपद्विष्टं [269] व्यालदंष्ट्रिविषाणिनः ॥३४२॥'

[अष्टाङ्गहृदय : सूत्र२:४१]

One should always try to be helpful to others, and if required, he should also help his enemy. In appropriate time, one should talk only useful things within limits. One should never talk things which are harmful to others. One should always be desirous of the well being of others. He should be pleasing, with compassion and soft. One should not try to be happy alone. One should not believe everybody. One should not be afraid of others. One should feel as if he has no enemy and he himself should not have animosity against others. One should not expose his own insults. One should not get exceedingly attached to anybody. One should not exceedingly strain the sense organs. The sense organs should not be pampered in excess. One should perform such actions which are not against the tradition and which help in the attainment of *trivarga* (religious virtues, wealth and salvation). In every step, one should follow others and be moderate in his approach. One should have trimmed hair, nail and beard. One should wear clean dress. One should not cross a *caitya* (a big tree at the end of the village which is considered to be auspicious and the abode of the gods), *pūjya* (respectable persons), *dhvaja* (auspicious flags), *aśasta chāyā* (shadow of inauspicious things), *bhasma* (heap of ash), *tuṣā* (heap of grain-chaff) and *aśuci* (heap of unclean garbage). One should not also cross the place of sand, gravels, sacrificed objects and bath. One should not make efforts to cross a river by swimming with his own arms. One should not go near strong fire. One should not climb over a fragile boat or tree and one should not use a dangerous vehicle. One should not sneeze, laugh or yawn without covering his face. One should not resort to itching the nostrils and one should not try to write something on the earth abruptly. One should not maintain bad postures with his limbs and one should not sit on a very unpleasant seat for a long time. One should withdraw from the physical, vocal and mental efforts before he gets adjusted. One should not strain his limbs and one should not sit in an unpleasant posture for a long time. One should not remain with his legs upwards for a long time. One should not reside under a tree at night. One should not sleep at night in a *catvāra* (platform specially constructed for purpose of rituals), under a *caitya* (big tree at the end of the village which is considered to be auspicious and which is considered to be the abode of the gods), *catuṣpatha* (cross-roads) and *surālaya* (temples). Even during day time, one should not remain in uninhabited forest, empty house or crematorium. One should avoid criminals, frost and strong wind. One should not sit in the shadow of the bank of rivers, one should not have any association with persons who are against the king and one should not have any dealing with wild animals, snakes and animals having horns.

सन्ध्यासु भोजनं स्वप्नं मैथुनाध्ययनं त्यजेत् ।

270
'गात्रवक्त्रनखैर्वाद्यं हस्तकेशावधूननम् ॥३४३॥'

[अष्टाङ्गहृदय : सूत्र२:४३]

271
'मद्यातिसक्तिं विश्रम्भस्वातन्त्र्ये स्त्रीषु च त्यजेत् ।'

[अष्टाङ्गहृदय : सूत्र२:४४]

शास्त्रं नृत्यं च गीतं च वाद्यं सेवेत च[272] क्षणात् ॥३४४॥

अत्यर्थं व्यसनं त्याज्यं[273] कायवाक्चेतसां दमः ।

स्वार्थंतुष्टि[274] परार्थेषु पर्याप्तमिति सद्व्रतम् ॥३४५॥

[अष्टाङ्गहृदय : सूत्र२:४६]

One should avoid taking food, sleep, sexual intercourse and study in the evenings. One should not produce sound with the help of the body, mouth or nails. One should not bite the hair or hands. One should not excessively indulge in alcohol. One should avoid liberal and secret dealings with ladies. In appropriate time, one should study religious scriptures, practise dance, sing songs and give musical performances. Excessively luxurious life should be avoided. One should have control over the body, the speech and the mind. One should take interest in the welfare of others.

These are the *sadvratas* (noble rituals) in their complete form.

निशि[275] स्वस्थमना तिष्ठेत् मौनी दण्डी सहायवान् ।

[अष्टाङ्गहृदय : सूत्र२:३३]

एवं दिनानि मे यान्तु चिन्तयेदिति सर्वदा ॥३४६॥

दुःखभाक् न भवत्येवं नित्यं संनिहितस्मृतिः ।

एवं कृत्स्नं दिनं नीत्वा [276]रात्रियामार्धकावधिः ॥३४७॥

दिवासंध्यां वर्जयित्वा सदा पर्वदिनानि च ।

रात्रौ व्यवायं कुर्वीत योषिता निजया सह ॥३४८॥

कुचीलां[277] च कुशीलां च विधवां च परस्त्रियम् ।

नारीं[278] नीचकुलोद्भूतां त्यजेत्सम्यग्विचक्षणः ॥३४९॥

वयोधिकां स्त्रियं गत्वा तरुणः स्थविरायते ।

[279] "वृद्धोपि तरुणीं गत्वा यौवनत्वमवाप्नुयात्" ॥३५०॥

ऋतुकाले तु सुरतमवश्यं कारयेद् बुधः ।

स्त्रीणां श्वासहतः पुंसो दुर्भगत्वं हि जायते ॥३५१॥

न ऋते[280] षोडशाद्वर्षात्तथाऽतिक्रान्तसप्ततेः ।

स्त्रियं कामयमानस्य जायते हि बलक्षयः ॥३५२॥

At night, one should remain in *svastha mana* (with introspection, or in a healthy mind). In case of any urgent work, one should move at night along with a staff and with persons accompanying. One should always think to spend the days in this manner. If one always keeps the above points in his mind, he will never suffer from miseries. He should lead the whole day and half of *yāma* (one *yāma*=three hours) of the night in the above manner.

For sexual intercourse, one should avoid day time and *sandhyā* (dawn and dusk). One should avoid sex during day time, *sandhyā* (dawn and dusk) and *parva dina* (days of rituals). One should indulge in sex only at night with his own wife. A wise man would always avoid a woman who has bad manners and conduct, who is a widow, who is another man's wife and who is born of a lower caste or clan. By indulging in sex with an older lady, even a youngman becomes older. Even an old man becomes youthful if he indulges in sex with a young girl. One should invariably perform sexual acts during *ṛtu kāla* (appropriate season and appropriate menstrual phase of the woman). If this is not performed, then this leads to the miseries of the man who gets afflicted by the sorrowful breath of the woman. One should not indulge in sex before he attains sixteenth year of age and after he becomes seventy years old. If this is done before or after that, then it results in diminution of strength.

त्र्यहाद्वसन्तशरदोः पक्षाद्वृष्टिनिदाघयोः ।

प्रकामं तु निषेवेत मैथुनं शिशिरागमे ॥३५३॥

शीते रात्रौ दिवा ग्रीष्मे प्रावृष्यासारगर्जिते ।

वसन्ते च दिवा रात्रौ शीलयेत्स्वस्त्रियं नरः ॥३५४॥

एकशायी द्विभुञ्जानोषण्मूत्री त्रिपुरीषकः ।

स्वल्पमैथुनकारी च शतं वर्षाणि जीवति ॥३५५॥

॥ इति दिनचर्या ॥

In spring and autumn one should have sexual intercourse on the third day; in rainy season and summer, it should be performed on the fifteenth day and in the beginning of winter season, one should perform it as much as he likes. One should perform sexual acts at night during winter season; in the day time during summer season; at the time of the roaring cloud in the rainy season and during both the day and night in the spring season, along with his own wife.

A person who performs sex acts only with one woman, (or sleeps only once during day and night), who eats food only twice a day, who passes urine six times a day and stool three times (the correct reading appears to be two times) a day and who performs less of sexual acts lives for one hundred years.

Thus, ends the description of regimens for the day and night.

अथ वयःपरीक्षा

"तत्र वयः संक्षेपेण त्रिविधम्—बालं, मध्यं, वृद्धमिति । तत्रोनषोडशवर्षाः बालाः ।[281] षोडशसप्तत्योरन्तरालं मध्यं वयः । तस्य विकल्पो—वृद्धिर्यौवनम्, सर्वसंपूर्णता ।[282] तत्र विंशतेर्वृद्धिः । आत्रिंशतो यौवनम् । आचत्वारिंशतः सर्वधात्विन्द्रियबल[वीर्यं] संपूर्णता" ॥३५६॥

Examination of the Age of the Person

In brief, age is divided into three categories, namely, *bāla* (young age), *madhya* (middle age) and *vṛddha* (old age). Before the attainment of sixteenth year of age a person is called *bāla* (young) and from sixteenth to seventieth year, he is called *madhya* (middle age). This middle age is again divided into three stages, namely, *vṛddhi* (growth), *yauvana* (youthfulness) and *sarva sampūrṇatā* (completion of all the growth); upto the twentieth year of age, it is the time of *vṛddhi* (growth); upto thirtieth year of age, it is *yauvana* (youth) and upto 40th year all the tissue elements and sense organs are full of strength and potency.

बाल्यं वृद्धिः छविर्मेधा त्वग्दृष्टि शुक्रविक्रमौ[283] ।
बुद्धिः कमन्द्रियं चैव जीवितं दशतो ह्रसेत्[284] ॥२५७॥

A happy life has the following ten aspects :

1. *Bâlya* (tenderness of age);
2. *Vṛddhi* (growth of the body);
3. *Chavi* (aura);
4. *Medhā* (intellect);
5. *Tvak* (softness of the skin);
6. *Dṛṣṭi* (eye sight);
7. *Śukra* (semen);
8. *Vikrama* (adventurous spirit);
9. *Buddhi* (wisdom); and
10. *Karmendriya* (excellence of motor organs).

[Reference : Verse no. 230 in Chapter-2]

'अग्निक्षारविरेकैस्तु बालवृद्धौ विवर्जयेत् ।

285
तत्साध्येषु विकारेषु मृद्वीं कुर्यात्क्रियां शनैः ॥३५८॥'

[सुश्रुत : सूत्र३५:३२]

॥ इति संक्षेपेण वयः परीक्षा ॥

To young and old persons, one should not administer *agni kriyā* (cauterisation therapy), *kṣāra kriyā* (alkali therapy) and *vireka* (emetic and purgation) therapies. When these persons get afflicted by diseases which can be cured only by the administration of such therapies, then these should be administered only in a mild form and gradually.

Thus, ends the description of examination of age in brief.

अथ बलपरीक्षा

यथा चोक्तं सुश्रुतेन यस्माद्बलवतः सर्वक्रियाप्रवृत्तिस्तस्माद्बलमेव प्रधानमधिकरणानाम् ॥३५९॥

[सुश्रुत : सूत्र३५:३५]

Examination of Strength

It is said in *Suśruta*, "Because a person endowed with strength performs all activities, therefore, the strength is the most important factor in the body."

'केचित् कृशाः प्राणवन्तः स्थूलाश्चाल्पबला नराः ।
तस्मात् स्थिरत्वं व्यायामैर्बलं वैद्यः प्रतर्कयेत् ॥३६०॥'

[सुश्रुत : सूत्र३५:३६]

There are some lean and thin persons who have great strength (endowed with life). There are many fatty persons who have less of strength. Therefore, a physician should critically examine the suitability and the strength of a person by his ability to perform *vyāyāma* (physical exercises or physical efforts).

'तच्च बलं किमुच्यते—तत्र रसादीनां[286] शुक्रान्तानां धातूनां यत् परं तेजस्तत्[287] खल्वोजस्तदेव बलमित्युच्यते, स्वशास्त्रसिद्धान्तात्[288] । तत्र बलेन स्थिरोपचितमांसता सर्वचेष्टास्वप्रतिघातः स्वरवर्णप्रसादो बाह्यानामाभ्यन्तराणां[289] च करणानामात्मकार्यप्रतिपत्तिर्भवति' ॥३६१॥

[सुश्रुत : सूत्र१५:१९-२०]

What is this *bala* (strength)? The excellent essence of the *dhātus* beginning from *rasa* and ending in *śukra* is called *ojas*. This *ojas* is also called *bala* in the context of the medical science. Because of the strength, there is stability and nourishment of the muscle tissues and the person remains undeterred in all efforts. He gets endowed with excellence of voice and complexion. His external sense organs and internal senses are capable of performing their activities with their full abilities.

अथ किमिदं तेजः? तेजोप्याग्नेयं, क्रमशः पच्यमानानां धातूनां अभिनिर्वृत्तमुदर-[290] स्नेहजातं वसाख्यं स्त्रीणां स विशेषतो भवति। तेन मार्दवसौकुमार्यमृद्वल्परोमतोत्साहदृष्टिस्थितिपक्तिकान्तिदीप्तयो भवन्ति ॥३६२॥

What is this *tejas* (essence) ? *Tejas* is *āgneya* (originated from *agni mahābhūta*). During gradual process of metabolism of the tissue elements, a substance called *vasā* is produced out of the fat accumulated in the abdomen. This is produced in excess in women. This is called *tejas* and because of this there is softness, tenderness, less number of soft hairs, exhilaration, eye sight, stability, power of digestion and metabolism, beauty and grace in them.

अथौजः किमुच्यते

'ओजः सोमात्मकं स्निग्धं शुक्लं शीतं स्थिरं सरम् ।
विविक्तं मृदु हृत्स्थं[291] च प्राणायतनमुत्तमम् ।
देहः सावयवस्तेन व्याप्तो भवति देहिनः ॥३६३॥'

[सुश्रुत : सूत्र१५:२१-२२]

What is this *ojas* ? *Ojas* is *somātmaka* (of the nature of *soma* or *jala mahābhūta*). It is unctuous, white, cold, stable, fluid, *vivikta* (which remains separated from others) and soft. It is located in the heart and it is one of the excellent sustainers of life. The body along with its limbs in the living beings are pervaded by this *ojas*.

अथ चरकः

"[292]भ्रमरैः पुष्पसारेभ्यो यथा संह्रियते मधु ।
[293]पाचकाद्यैस्तु सारस्थमोजः संह्रियते तथा" ॥३६४॥
'हृदि तिष्ठति यच्छुद्धं रक्तमीषत्सपीतकम् ।
ओजः शरीरे विख्यातं[294] तन्नाशान्म्रियते नरः ॥३६५॥'

[चरक : सूत्र१७:७४]

According to Caraka

As the bees collect honey from the essence of flowers, similarly *ojas* is collected from the essence of the tissue elements by the *agnis* (enzymes) like *pācaka* etc. The one which dwells in the heart and which is predominantly white and slightly reddish as well as yellowish in colour is known as *ojas* in the body. If the *ojas* is destroyed, the human being succumbs to death.

गुरु शीतं [295]मृदुस्निग्धं बहलं मधुरं स्थिरम् ।

प्रसन्नं [296]पिच्छिलं शुक्लमोजो दशगुणं स्मृतम् ॥३६६॥

[चरक : चिकित्सा२४:३१]

Ojas has ten attributes, viz., heaviness, coldness, softness, unctuousness, thickness, sweetness, stability, *prasanna* (freshness), sliminess and whiteness.

एवं चरकाचार्येण षड्रसं पीतं शुक्लं च द्विरूपमोजो वर्णितम् ॥३६७॥

Thus, according to *Caraka*, *ojas* which has six tastes, is of two types—one is of yellow colour and the other is white in colour.

कृष्णात्रेयोऽपि

व्यापदादि भवेच्छुक्ले नत्वारक्ते सपीतके ।

According to Kṛṣṇātreya

The defects like *vyāpat* etc., occur in the white variety of the *ojas* and not in the reddish yellow variety.

अत्र कारणम्

[297]अग्निषोमगुणत्वं च जगतः परिकीर्त्तितम् ॥३६८॥

तस्माद्विविधमोजः स्याच्छुक्लरक्तादिभेदतः ।

[298]"अतः शुक्ले तु संक्षीणे कष्टं प्राणान्तिकं भवेत् ॥३६९॥

रक्तवर्णस्य संक्षीणे देहः सोममयो भवेत्" ।

न जीवति ध्रुवं तस्माद्देही वा कृष्णशासनात् ।

रक्तपीतगुणैर्युक्तं परं स्याद् अष्टविन्दुकम् ॥३७०॥

The reason for that

The universe is known to have two attributes viz., *agni guṇa* (heating attribute) and *soma guṇa* (cooling attribute). Therefore, *ojas* is of two types—one is white and the other is yellowish red. If there is reduction in the quantity of the white variety of *ojas* then it leads to extremely serious and painful conditions. If the *ojas* having red colour is reduced in quantity then the body becomes full of water i.e., the patient succumbs to instantaneous death. According to *Kṛṣṇātreya*, the death of the person in this condition is certain. The yellow and red variety of *ojas* which is of superior type is eight drops in quantity.

अग्निवेशात्

'प्राकृतस्तु बलं श्लेष्मा विकृतो मल उच्यते ।

स चैवौजः स्मृतः काये स च पाप्मोपदिश्यते' ॥३७१॥

[चरक : सूत्र१७:११७]

According to Agniveśa

The *kapha* in its natural state promotes strength of the body in the form of *ojas*. When in morbid condition, it takes the form of excreta and causes miseries.

श्लेष्मा दशगुणैर्युक्तो गुरुशीतादिभिस्तथा ।

आमाशये संभवति श्लेष्मा मधुरशीतलः ॥३७२॥

Śleṣmā (*kapha*) has ten attributes viz, heaviness, coldness etc. The sweet and cold *śleṣmā* originates from the *āmāśaya* (stomach including small intestine).

ओजस्तु सप्तधातूद्भवसारः । कफस्तु रसमलः । अतएव सुश्रुतेन कफस्त्वोजस्थाने न गणितः । ओजस्तु कफाद्भिन्न एव ।

Ojas is the essence of all the seven types of tissue elements. *Kapha* is the *mala* (excreta) of *rasa*. Therefore, *Suśruta* has not described *kapha* as one of the locations of the *ojas*. *Ojas*, therefore, is different from *kapha*.

तत्र बलं त्रिविधं उत्तमाधममध्यममिति ॥३७३॥

Varieties of Strength

Bala (strength) is of three types viz., *uttama* (superior) *adhama* (inferior) and *madhyama* (moderate).

आत्रेयः

सहजं कालयुक्तिभ्यां कृतं च त्रिविधं बलम् ।

According to Ātreya

Bala (strength) is of three types viz., *sahaja bala* (hereditary strength), *kāla kṛta bala* (strength gained during different stages of life) and *yukti kṛta bala* (strength gained as a result of drugs, diet etc.)

शरीररसयोर्यत्तु सुवृतं सहजं हितम् ॥३७४॥

देहावस्थां तु जानीयात् द्विधा कालकृतं बलम् ।

विहाराहारयुक्तिभ्यां यत्तु देहकृतं बलम् ॥३७५॥

The *bala* which is produced as a result of the nature the *rasa* (plasma etc.) in the body is called *sahaja* and it is useful. The condition of the body during different stages of life determines two types of *bala* which is of the second category. The third category of *bala* is produced as a result of appropriate regimens and diet.

देहावस्थावयोपचयभेदेन, उपचयः कोऽर्थः? वयःसन्धिरिति । तच्चबलं केवलं रसविशेषात् त्रिविधम्, उत्तमाधममध्यमं इति ॥३७६॥

The term *dehāvasthā* used in the above verse connotes two types of *bala* as a result of *vayas* (age) and *upacaya*, that is, the transitional phase from one stage of life (age) to the other. The *bala* which is attained as a result of the specific nature of *rasa* (plasma etc.) only is divided into three categories, viz., superior type of strength, inferior type of strength and moderate type of strength.

तद्यथा

[299]अरोगोऽल्पजरो दक्षो ज्ञानविज्ञानवाञ्छुचिः ।
सुसंहतशरीरस्तु स्वस्थः सर्वगुणैर्युतः ॥३७७॥

For example

A person who is free from diseases, who has low ageing process, who is skilful in his profession, who is proficient in spiritual and materialistic (scientific) knowledge, who is clean and who has compact body, is called *svastha* or a healthy person (with all these attributes).

सुसहतदेहलक्षरणम्

अग्निवेशात्

समभक्तविभक्तास्थिश्लिष्टाश्च दृढसन्धयः ।
विभक्तमांसं बलिनं शरीरं स्यात्सुसंहतम् ॥३७८॥
देहेषु संहतः श्रेष्ठं मध्यमं नातिसंहतः ।
जघन्येषु शरीरेषु जघन्यं लक्षयेद्बलम् ॥३७९॥
दारुणं वीक्ष्य रक्तं वा शोकं प्राप्याथवा भयम् ।
यस्तु प्राप्नोति मूर्छां च [300]मरणं रोगमाशु वा ॥३८०॥
सुमहत्यपि देहेऽल्पसत्त्वः परमदुर्बलः ।

Characteristic Features of Compact Body According to Agniveśa

A person who has properly apportioned and properly separated bones, whose joints are well-knit and sturdy, whose muscles are well divided and whose body is strong, is called *susaṁhata* (compact). Among the physiques the compact ones are the best. Those which are not very compact are of moderate nature and those which are not at all compact are the worst. The third category of physique has the inferior type of strength. If a person faints, dies, or succumbs to diseases while witnessing serious type of bleeding or while facing serious type of grief or fearful situation, he is to be considered as a very weak person—both mentally and physically even though he is possessed of a big physique.

महाव्याधिपरीतस्य बहुदोषस्य देहिनः ।
बलमास्थापयेद्वैद्यः[301] शनैर्दोषान् विनिर्हरेत् ॥३८१॥

A physician should restore the strength and gradually eliminate the *doṣas* of a patient who is suffering from serious type of disease and whose body is afflicted with a lot of vitiated *doṣas*.

"तथा च[302]

दुर्बलस्य बलान्दोषानल्पानल्पान् पुनः पुनः ।
बलमाप्याययेद्वैद्यः शनैर्दोषान्विनिर्हरेत्" ॥३८२॥

In a weak person having excessively vitiated *doṣas*, the physician should restore strength and eliminate *doṣas* gradually—little by little.

सुश्रुतः

'त्रयो दोषा बलस्योक्ता व्यापद्विस्रंसनक्षयाः ।
विश्लेषसादौ गात्राणां दोषविस्रंसनं श्रमः ॥३८३॥

अप्राचुर्यं क्रियाणां च बलविस्रंसलक्षणम् ।
गुरुत्वं स्तब्धताऽङ्गेषु ग्लानिर्वर्णस्य भेदनम् ॥३८४॥
तन्द्रा निद्रा वातशोफो बलव्यापदि लक्षणम् ।
मूर्छा मांसक्षयो मोहः प्रलापोऽज्ञानमेव च ॥३८५॥
पूर्वोक्तानि च लिङ्गानि मरणं च बलक्षये' ।

[सुश्रुत : सूत्र१५:२५-२८]

According io Suśruta

There are three types of derangements in *bala* (*ojas* or strength) namely, *vyāpat*, *visraṁsana* and *kṣaya*. Looseness and prostration of the body, vitiation of *doṣas*, exertion and inability to perform much of work—these are the signs and symptoms of *visraṁsana* type of derangement in the *bala* (*ojas*). The *vyāpat* type of derangement of *bala* is characterised by heaviness and numbness of the body, *glāni* (a feeling as if covered with a wet cloth), discolouration, drowsiness, excessive sleep and oedema of of the body caused by *vāyu*. The signs and symptoms of the third type of derangement of *bala*, namely, *kṣaya*, are fainting, wasting of muscles, stupour, delirium, unconciousness, manifestation of the signs and symptoms already described in respect of *vyāpat* and *visraṁsana* types of derangement and even death.

यथा दोषबलं चापि कुर्याच्चात्र प्रतिक्रियाम् ॥३८६॥
शोकेर्ष्याक्रोधदैन्यं च व्यायाम सुरतं तथा ।
स्त्रीणां संदर्शनं वापि वर्जयेत्साहसादिकम् ॥३८७॥
भजेद्रसायनं काम्यं तथा वाजीकरं शुभम् ।
क्षयोक्तं च क्रमं सेव्यं जीर्णज्वरहरं तथा ॥३८८॥
नानाविधानि तैलानि वातरोगहराणि च ।

Depending upon the quantum and the variety of vitiated *doṣas* and the strength of the patient, one should prescribe therapies for the treatment of these conditions. The patient should avoid grief, jealousy, anger, timidity, exercise, sexual act including vision of ladies and exhibition of the strength of one's capacity. One should take the desirable rejuvenation therapy and aphrodisiacs. For the treatment of these conditions, one should adopt the line of treatment suggested for *kṣaya* (tuberculosis) and *jīrṇa jvara* (chronic fever). Different types of medicated oils which are used for the alleviation of *vāyu* are useful in this condition.

303

सत्त्वमपि च द्विविधं भीरुत्वं च सहिष्णुत्वम् ॥३८९॥

तत्र सहिष्णौ तीक्ष्णामिरितरेष्वाश्वास्य रोगिणम्, मृद्वीं कुर्यात्प्रयत्नादिति वैद्यकशा-

स्त्रसिद्धान्तः ॥३९०॥

॥इति बलपरीक्षा॥

Examination of Sattva

Sattva is of two types namely, *bhīrutva* (cowardice) and *sahiṣṇutva* (having power of tolerance). A person having the latter type of *sattva* can be administered sharp (strong) therapies. Patient of the former category should be given only mild therapies, after giving consolation to him. Such patients, according to the medical doctrine, need more of efforts.

Thus, ends the description of the examination of *bala*.

[अथ सात्म्यम्]

सात्म्यं चतुर्विधं प्रोक्तं देहदेशर्तुरोगजम् ।

अनुशेते तु यद्देहं सौहित्याद्देहसात्म्यं तत् ॥३९१॥

ऋतुसात्म्यं स्निग्धोष्णं हेमन्ते कटुकतिक्तरूक्षाणि ।

शिशिरान्ते शस्यन्ते ग्रीष्मे सुखशीतमधुराणि ॥३९२॥

Examination of Sātmya

Sātmya (wholesomeness) is of four types namely, *deha sātmya* (wholesomeness for the body), *deśa sātmya* (wholesomeness for the locality), *ṛtu sātmya* (wholesomeness for the seasons) and *roga-sātmya* (wholesomeness of the disease). Things which when taken habitually are useful for the body are called *deha sātmya*. Unctuous and hot things are wholesome for *hemanta* (early part of winter). Pungent, bitter and ununctuous substances are wholesome at the end of *śiśira* (latter part of winter). Pleasing, cooling and sweet things are useful and are wholesome for summer. These are called *ṛtu sātmya*.

व्याधेः सात्म्यं विद्याज्ज्वरस्य पेयाविरेचनम् ।
छर्दैः स्वेदं नस्यं धूमो व्याधौ च स्यात्प्रतिश्याये ॥३९३॥

In fever, administration of *peyā* (thin gruel) and purgation are wholesome. Fomentation therapy is wholesome for a patient suffering from vomiting. For a patient suffering from *pratiśyāya* (chronic cold), inhalation therapy and smoking are wholesome. These are the examples of *vyādhi* (*roga*) *sātmya*.

मात्रायोगात् क्रियादेशकालावस्थादिभेदतः
304
न जायन्ते हि द्रव्यस्य विनाभ्यासाद्गुणागुणाः ॥३९४॥

मात्रया सेवितं मद्यं हन्ति रोगांस्तदुद्भवान् ।
निषेव्यमाणं तिलशो विषमप्यमृतायते ॥३९५॥

305
भजेते विषरूपत्वं तुल्यांशे मधुसर्पिषी ।
क्षारोम्लरसयोगेन मधुरी भवति क्षणात् ॥३९६॥

पूगताम्बूलसंयोगं गन्धवर्णरसोद्भवं ।
कोद्रवो हन्त्यसृक्पित्तं करोत्येष विदाहिभिः ॥३९७॥

306

कुष्ठं तत्कालपि[?]तिलो हन्ति भल्लातकैः सह ।

गुडः कर्त्ताऽग्निसादस्य हर्ताशु त्वभयादिभिः ॥३९८॥

सक्तवो वातला रूक्षाः पीतास्ते तर्पयन्ति च ।

आर्द्रकाज्जायते शुंठी संस्कारेण लघीयसी ॥३९९॥

307

"भृष्टः क्षणोऽपि पृथुको रक्तशालेर्लघोर्गुरुः ।

शालिः पिष्टो गरीयस्तु गोधूमादपि गच्छति ॥४००॥

संग्राहिणीर्लघुर्मुद्गः कुल्माषो भेदनो गुरुः ।"

While administering a drug, one should keep in view the dosage, the nature of the recipe, the therapeutic effects, the nature of the locality and the time, the stage of the disease etc. However, the good or bad effects of a substance cannot be ascertained without using it habitually for sufficient time. If alcohol is taken i limited quantity, then it cures diseases caused by alcoholism. If poison is taken in the quantity of a *tila* (size of a sesamum seed) then it works like ambrosia. When honey and ghee are taken together in equal quantity, they work like a poison in the body. Combination of alkalies and sour things produces sweetness instantaneously. Addition of *pūga* (areca nut) to *tāmbūla* (betal leaf) helps in the manifestation of good smell, colour and taste. *Kodrava* cures *rakta pitta* (a disease characterised by bleeding from different parts of the body). But, when *kodrava* is mixed with other substances having *vidāhi* property (which produce burning sensation) then it causes *rakta pitta* itself. *Tila* (?) produces *kuṣṭha* (obstinate skin diseases including leprosy). But when given along with *bhallātaka*, it cures *kuṣṭha*. *Guḍa* (jaggery) causes *agni māndya* (suppression of the power of digestion). But, when given alongwith *abhayā* etc., *guḍa* cures *agni māndya*. Different types of *saktu* (roasted corn flour) are aggravators of *vāyu* and they are ununctuous. But when taken in the form of a drink by adding water, it produces nourishing effect. *Śuṇṭhī* (dry ginger) is prepared out of *ārdraka* (green ginger). But the former is lighter than the latter because of the processing. *Pṛthukā* is prepared by frying and pounding the red variety of *śāli* rice. By this processing, the former becomes heavier than the latter. *Śāli* is light for digestion. But the pastry prepared of it is heavier even in comparison to *godhūma*. *Mudga* is constipative and light by nature. But *kulmāṣa* (a preparation of *mudga* by adding other grains) is purgative and heavy.

भूमि सात्म्यं दधि क्षीरं करीरं मधुरादिषु[308] ॥४०१॥
क्षीरं प्राच्येषु[309] मत्स्यास्तु सैन्धवे भस्मकेषु च ।
तैलाम्लकन्दमूलादि मालवे कोंकणे पुनः ॥४०२॥
पेयामंथ उदीच्येषु गोधूमोऽवन्तिभूमिषु ।
इत्याद्या देशसात्म्याश्च,

Curd, milk, *karīra* and sweet things are wholesome in specific localities. Milk is wholesome in the eastern part of the country. Fish is wholesome in Sindhu and Bhasmaka. Oil, sour things, rhizomes and roots are wholesome for people inhabiting Mālava and Koṅkaṇa. In the north, *peyā* (thin gruel) and *mantha* (thick gruel) are wholesome. *Godhūma* (wheat) is wholesome in the land of Avanti. These are examples of *deśa sātmya*.

देहसात्म्यमथोच्यते ॥४०३।
देहसात्म्यं दधिक्षीरं मद्यं मांसं तु कस्यचित् ।
पेया यूषो रसोऽन्नस्य[310] गोधूमाद्याश्च कस्यचित् ॥४०४॥

Now begins the description of *deha sātmya*. For some persons, curd, milk, alcohol, and meat are wholesome. For the body of some other persons, *peyā* (thin gruel), *yūṣa* (vegetable soup), *rasa* (meat soup), *anna* (cereals), *godhūma* (wheat) etc., are wholesome.

सात्म्यं ह्याशु बलं धत्ते नातिदोषं च बाधते[311] ।
स्रंसनं सत्पयो गव्यं भवति ग्राहि कस्यचित् ॥४०५॥

Wholesome things produce strength instantaneously and they do not vitiate *doṣas* in excess. Cows milk which generally works as a laxative, may cause constipation in some persons.

पयः स्वादुरसं शीतं विपरीतं ततो दधि ।
कालेन जायते तस्मात्क्षीरवच्च पुनर्घृतम् ॥४०६॥
तक्रं ग्राहि कषायाम्लमम्लमेव तु भेदनम् ।
रसायनं काकमाची सद्यः पर्युषितं विषम् ॥४०७॥
मूलकं दोषजिद्बालं विपरीतं तु कन्दवत् ।

Milk has sweet taste and it is cooling. But curd which is prepared out of the milk, has opposite qualities. Ghee which is produced out of milk has, however, properties similar to the latter. Butter-milk which is astringent and sour, works as a constipative. But when it becomes exceedingly sour, it work as a laxative. Freshly collected *kākamāci* causes rejuvenation, but when it becomes stale, it works like a poison. Tender radish alleviates all the *doṣas*, but when it is over-matured, it aggravates all of them like other rhizomes.

छर्दिहृद्रोगगुल्मान्ते वमनं च चिकित्सितम् ॥४०८॥
निषिद्धमपि निर्दिष्टं बस्तिरर्शसि[313] कुष्ठिते ।

For the cure of *chardi* (vomiting), *hṛd roga* (heart disease) and *gulma* (phantom tumour), emetic therapy is prescribed. Enema therapy is normally contra-indicated in *arśas* (piles) and *kuṣṭha* (obstinate skin diseases including leprosy). But, in certain conditions, enema therapy is useful in these diseases also.

ज्वरे तुल्यर्तुदोषत्वं[313] प्रमेहे तुल्यदूष्यता ॥४०९॥
रक्तगुल्मे पुराणत्वं सुखसाध्यत्वहेतवः[314] ।

Similarity in the nature of the season and the *doṣa* makes *jvara* (fever) easily curable. In the same way, similarity of *dūṣya* (*dhātus* or tissue elements) make *prameha* (obstinate urinary disorders including diabetes) easily curable. *Rakta gulma* becomes easily curable only when it attains the chronic stage.

315

अपथ्यं पथ्यमप्यन्नं निशायां चैव रोगिणाम् ॥४१०॥

अहिताः सक्तवः शुष्का हितास्ते तु प्रमेहिणः ।

For a patient the wholesome food becomes harmful if taken at night. *Saktu* (roasted corn flour) is generally harmful if taken in dry form; but it is useful for a patient suffering from *prameha* (obstinate urinary disorders including diabetes).

316

एवं विज्ञाय सद्वैद्यस्ततो भावान्परीक्षयेत् ॥४११॥

॥इति सात्म्यलक्षणम्॥

A wise physician should always keep the above points in view and then examine different aspects of the patient and the therapies.

Thus, ends the description of the characteristic features of *sātmya* (wholesomeness).

इति श्रीमहाराजाधिराज-श्रीटोडरमल्लविरचिते टोडरानंदे आयुर्वेदसौख्ये पञ्चात्मकद्रव्यलक्षणं पाचनादि पृथग्द्रव्योदाहरणं रस-वीर्य-विपाक-प्रभावलक्षणं ऋतुचर्यावयबलसात्म्यपरीक्षाकथनं नाम तृतीयो हर्षः ॥४१२॥

Thus, ends the third Chapter of *Āyurveda saukhyaṁ* in *Ṭoḍarānanda* composed by the Great king Ṭoḍara malla, which deals with the following topics :

1. Characteristic features of substances dominated by five *mahābhūtas*;

2. Description of *pācana* etc., along with examples;

3. Description of *rasa* (taste), *virya* (potency), *vipāka* (taste that emerges after digestion) and *prabhāva* (specific action);

4. Regimens for different types of seasons; and

5. Examination of age, strength, wholesomeness etc.

NOTES AND REFERENCES

1. 'वल्लभीनां' इति द्वितीयपुस्तके पाठः ।
2. 'संस्तूयमानं' इति प्रथमषष्ठपुस्तकयोः पाठः ।
3. 'भुवि' इति षष्ठपुस्तकपाठोऽसङ्गतः ।
4. 'तनोत्विदं' इति द्वितीयपुस्तकपाठः ।
5. '०भूपैः' इति द्वितीयपुस्तके पाठः ।
6. 'सा' इति प्रथमपञ्चमपुस्तकयोः पाठः ।
7. 'स्वेदजान्युद्भिजानि' षष्ठवर्जसर्वपुस्तकपाठः, स तु अपपाठ एव ।
8. द्रष्टव्यम्—सुश्रुत : सूत्र१:२८-३० ।
9. 'पुनर्द्विविध उच्यते' इति प्रथमपुस्तके पाठः ।
10. 'चोद्भिजं' इति आदर्शपुस्तकेषु पाठः ।
11. द्रष्टव्यम्—चरक : चिकित्सा १:१:३-४ ।
12. श्लोकार्धोऽयं प्रथमपञ्चमपुस्तकयोर्नोपलभ्यते ।
13. 'हि तत्' इति षष्ठपुस्तके पाठः ।
14. द्रष्टव्यम्—सुश्रुत : सूत्र१:३२ ।
    चरक : सूत्र१:७०-७१ ।
15. 'कपालाद्यस्तथाऽन्यश्च' इति प्रथमपञ्चपुस्तकयोः पाठः ।
16. द्रष्टव्यम्—चरक : सूत्र१:७१-७४ ।
    सुश्रुत : सूत्र१:२९-३१ ।
17. 'क्षाराः' इति द्वितीयषष्ठपुस्तकयोः पाठः ।

18. द्रष्टव्यम्—चरक : सूत्र१:६८-७६।
सुश्रुत : सूत्र१:३०।
19. 'कोष्ठमन्त्राणि' इति षष्ठपुस्तके पाठः।
20. 'वर्णानि' इति द्वितीयपुस्तके पाठः।
21. 'स्नेहमभिष्यन्द' इति द्वितीयषष्ठपुस्तकयोः पाठः।
22. 'सनीलं' इति षष्ठपुस्तकपाठः।
23. 'विवरम्लानि' इति षष्ठपुस्तक पाठः।
24. 'करहाटफलादिकम्' इति द्रव्यगुणविज्ञानम् पाठः।
25. 'भवेद्दाह' इति द्वितीयपुस्तके पाठः।
26. '०दन्ती' इति द्रव्यगुणविज्ञानम् पाठः।
27. 'यदुक्तं' इति प्रथमपंचमषष्ठपुस्तकानां पाठः।
28. 'तथा' इति षष्ठपुस्तके पाठः।
29. 'लङ्घने पाचने' इति प्रथमपुस्तके पाठः।
30. 'कफजुष्टानां' इति पञ्चमपुस्तके पाठः।
31. श्लोकार्धोऽयं द्वितीयषष्ठपुस्तकयोः न दृश्यते।
32. 'सामान्यसपथानुगान्' इति षष्ठपुस्तके पाठः।
33. 'पाचको' इति षष्ठपुस्तके पाठः।
34. 'सवृद्धास्ते' इति द्वितीयपुस्तके पाठः।
35. 'सुखादिगुण' इति षष्ठपुस्तके पाठः।
36. 'तथाथधातुसंश्लिष्टाः' इति द्वितीयपुस्तके पाठः।
37. 'साम्यान् नो दूषयत्यपि' इति षष्ठपुस्तके पाठः।
38. 'शमनं———रक्षणात्' पाठोऽयं द्वितीयपुस्तके नोपलभ्यते।
39. 'विनासंशोधनद्रव्यैस्तत्संशोधनमुच्यते' इति षष्ठपुस्तके पाठः।
40. 'यद्विद्रावतिरेचकः' इति प्रथमपुस्तके पाठः।
'यात्यधः' इति च द्वितीयपुस्तके।
41. 'यद्विरुद्धं' इति षष्ठपुस्तके पाठः।

42. 'ह्तिम्' इति पञ्चमपुस्तके पाठः।
43. 'यच्छिष्टां स्तु छेदनं बलात्' इति षष्ठपुस्तके पाठः।
44. 'हि तम्' इति प्रथमद्वितीयपुस्तकयोः पाठः।
45. 'तु' इति प्रथमपुस्तके पाठः।
46. 'यौस्यात्क्षुब्धा' इति द्वितीयपुस्तके पाठः।
47. 'विशेद्यत्' इति प्रथमपञ्चमपुस्तकयोः पाठः।
48. 'सुभान्' इति प्रथमपुस्तके पाठः।
49. 'श्लेष्मि च तं मतम्' इति षष्ठपुस्तके पाठः।
50. 'दोषाज्जातस्थान्यत्करोति' इति द्वितीयपुस्तके पाठः।
'दोषान् स्त्रोतोस्थान्यः करोति' इति प्रथमपुस्तके पाठः।
51. 'ज्ञेयो मदकारी सुरादिकम्' इति द्वितीयपुस्तके पाठः।
52. 'छेदनं———सुरादिकम्' पाठोऽयं द्वितीयषष्ठपुस्तकयोर्नास्ति।
53. 'माखास्तालमूली' इति प्रथमपुस्तके पाठः।
54. 'नरः' इति षष्ठपुस्तके पाठः।
55. अत्र द्वितीयपुस्तकस्य त्रुटितत्वात् चतुर्थचरणो नास्ति।
56. 'आश्रयानामसंख्यानां' इति आदर्शपुस्तकेषु पाठः।
57. 'षड् द्रव्यमिश्रिता ज्ञेया मलाः पाकवलावह्वाः' इति द्वितीयपुस्तके पाठः।
58. 'सलिलस्यातिरेकजः' इति द्वितीयपुस्तके पाठः।
59. 'मुखनासाक्षितोददाहार्त्तिसंश्रुवै' इति प्रथमपुस्तके पाठः।
60. 'रसस्तु विश्लेषी वैशद्याह्लादशोषणैः' इति द्वितीयपुस्तके पाठः।
61. 'नो देयाः' इति द्वितीयपुस्तके पाठः।
62. 'प्रायो चक्षुष्यं सैन्धवादृते' इति आदर्शपुस्तकेषु पाठः।
63. 'स्तम्भनमभयां विना' इति द्वितीयपुस्तके पाठः।
64. 'पटो' इति आकरे पाठः।
65. 'परमं' इति आकरे पाठः।
66. षष्ठपुस्तके श्लोकोऽयं नावलोक्यते।

67. 'अथ' इति द्वितीयपुस्तके पाठः ।

68. 'व्यवायी च विकाशी च सरगुणस्यैव' इति द्वितीयपुस्तके पाठः ।

69. 'तैक्ष्ण्यौष्ण्यलघुताश्चैव' इत्याकरे पाठः ।

70. 'श्लेष्मना:' इति षष्ठपुस्तके पाठः ।

71. 'ये रसाः———तत्कर्मकारिणः' श्लोकोऽयं द्वितीयपुस्तके नोपलभ्यते ।

72. 'विदाहमानं यदम्लपित्तं भजत्यपि' इति षष्ठपुस्तके पाठः ।

73. 'आग्नेयत्वास्थूणाष्वान्यां' इति पञ्चमपुस्तके पाठः ।

74. 'पाक्यो' इति प्रथमपुस्तके पाठः ।

75. 'विदग्धोऽपि स्तरपाके' इति षष्ठपुस्तके पाठः ।

76. द्रष्टव्यम्—सुश्रुत : सूत्र४०:१० ।

77. 'पाकेषु कफशुक्रानिलापहः' इति द्वितीयपुस्तके पाठः ।

78. 'चन्दनः' इति द्वितीयपुस्तके पाठः ।

79. 'नागरास्तथा' इति द्वितीयपुस्तके पाठः ।

80. द्रष्टव्यम्—सुश्रुत : सूत्र ४०:१०।

81. द्रष्टव्यम्—अष्टाङ्गहृदय : सूत्र९:२० ।

82. 'सात्मये' इति प्रथमद्वितीयषष्ठपुस्तकेषु पाठः ।

83. 'क्षारमूलकः' इति द्वितीयषष्ठपुस्तकयोः पाठः ।

84. समस्तेषु आदर्शपुस्तकेषु 'आममूलकम्' इति पठितम् । तत्तु न सम्यक् । आममूलकम् नाम बालमूलकम् तत्तु त्रिदोषघ्नत्वे भूयसः उक्तम् बृद्धमूलकं तु त्रिदोषकरम् । अत्र तु मूलकशब्देन वृद्धमूलकं ग्राह्यम् ।

85. 'मण्यौषधीणां...प्रभावस्तत्रकारणम्' पाठोऽयं द्वितीयषष्ठपुस्तकयोः नोपलभ्यते ।

86. 'विशवं' इति द्वितीयषष्ठपुस्तकयोः पाठः ।

87. '०प्रतिभागं' इति षष्ठपुस्तके पाठः ।

88. 'कालसम्वत्सरः' इति पञ्चमपुस्तके पाठः ।

89. द्रष्टव्यम्—चरक : विमान८:१२५ ।

90. 'वर्षे' इति प्रथमपुस्तके पाठः ।
'वर्षो' इति पञ्चमपुस्तके पाठः ।

91. 'ऋतुसंबन्धि वर्षः' इति प्रथमद्वितीयपञ्चमपुस्तकेषु पाठः ।

92. 'भवेत्' इति प्रथमपञ्चमपुस्तकयोः पाठः ।

93. 'च' इति आकरे पाठः ।

94. 'तस्मिन् ह्यत्यर्थतीक्ष्णोष्णरूक्षा' इति आकरे पाठः ।

95. 'शांतता ये' इति आदर्शपुस्तकेषु पाठः ।

96. 'यदोद्भवः' इति द्वितीयपुस्तके पाठः ।

97. 'क्लेदयत्युच्चै' इति षष्ठपुस्तके पाठः ।

98. 'चापि' द्वितीयपुस्तके पाठः ।

99. द्रष्टव्यम्—अष्टाङ्गसंग्रह : सूत्र४:८ ।

100. 'चयप्रकोपप्रशमा' इति आकरे पाठः ।

101. 'च' इति सर्वादर्शपुस्तकेषु पाठः ।

102. 'गजाजमहिषवाजिवाहसशूकराः' इति षष्ठपुस्तके पाठः ।

103. 'केदारानीरधान्योद्वला' इति षष्ठपुस्तके पाठः ।

104. 'प्रवरोऽनलः' इति प्रथमपुस्तके पाठः ।

105. 'अथ षड्रससंभाव्यं' इति द्वितीयपुस्तके पाठः ।

106. 'मस्तकाभ्यङ्गशोषणक्वचिन्नोद्वर्त्तयेत्तनुम्' इति द्वितीयपुस्तके पाठः ।

107. '०शेषेणक्वचिल्लोद्वर्त्तयेत्तनुम्' इति षष्ठपुस्तके पाठः ।

108. 'श्रोत्रविधानतः' इति षष्ठपुस्तके पाठः ।

109. 'दृष्टिकोद्धर्षणं' इति प्रथमपुस्तके पाठः ।

110. 'सत्यभावेन' इति प्रथमपुस्तके पाठः ।

111. 'लघूष्णभंवरसेव्यं' इति प्रथमपुस्तके पाठः ।
'लघूष्ममधः संसेव्यं' इति षष्ठपुस्तके पाठः ।

112. 'कामं' इति प्रथमपुस्तके पाठः ।

113. 'न' इति पञ्चमपुस्तके पाठः ।

114. 'धूमकुङ्कुमयोवनैः' इति द्वितीयपुस्तके पाठः।

115. 'वाग्भटात्———जायते' पाठोऽयं प्रथमद्वितीयपञ्चमपुस्तकेषु नोपलभ्यते।

116. 'अंगारतापसंतृप्तगर्भभूवेश्मशायिनः' इति षष्ठपुस्तके पाठः।

117. 'उष्णस्वभावैर्मृदुभिः' इति षष्ठपुस्तके पाठः।

118. द्रष्टव्यम्—चरक : सूत्र ६:२१।

119. 'शिशिरे च विशेषतं' इति षष्ठपुस्तके पाठः।

120. 'बहुलशिशिरवातां' इति षष्ठपुस्तके पाठः।

121. 'शुष्कसस्यैस्तु' इति द्वितीयपुस्तके पाठः।

122. 'कोलधूपप्रलेपितान्' इति षष्ठपुस्तके पाठः।

123. 'चातिगौल्पान्नं' इति प्रथमपुस्तके पाठः।

124. 'सादृकार्द्रा तु संधाना' इति षष्ठपुस्तके पाठः।

125. 'सुसैन्धवा' इति प्रथमपुस्तके पाठः।

126. 'मलयमारुततुल्यगुणान्वितं' इति षष्ठपुस्तके पाठः।

127. 'कुसुभोमलाः' इति षष्ठपुस्तके पाठः।

128. '०रूक्षोष्णभोजनैः' इति द्वितीयपुस्तके पाठः।

129. 'पुराणयवगोधूमक्षौद्रजांगलस्वल्पभुक्' इति षष्ठपुस्तके पाठः।

130. 'गमयेत्सुधी' इति द्वितीयपुस्तके पाठः।

131. 'नेकतोमुखः' इति षष्ठपुस्तके पाठः।

132. 'शान्तचक्रांकयुगलाः' इति षष्ठपुस्तके पाठः।

133. 'मारुतावान्र्ताः' इति प्रथमपुस्तके पाठः।

134. 'पत्राञ्चल' इति षष्ठपुस्तके पाठः।

135. 'श्रमनिवर्हणाः' इति प्रथमपुस्तके पाठः।

136. 'राजखाडं' इति षष्ठपुस्तके पाठः।

137. 'सदृका' इति प्रथमपुस्तके पाठः।

138. द्रष्टव्यम्—अष्टाङ्गहृदय : सूत्र३:२९।

139. 'सुगन्धिहितपानीयसिच्यमाना पटान्तिके' इति द्वितीयपुस्तके पाठः।

140. 'शव्याढकी' इति प्रथमपुस्तके पाठः ।

141. 'सशितोपलं' इति प्रथमपुस्तके पाठः ।

142. 'नालिकेलोदकानि च' इति षष्ठपुस्तके पाठः ।

143. '०सत्प्रवरार्द्रक०' इति द्वितीयपुस्तके पाठः ।

144. 'देशो' इति पञ्चमपुस्तके पाठः ।

145. 'स्वल्यका' इति प्रथमपुस्तके पाठः ।

146. 'इन्द्रगोपकठिराजितां' इति षष्ठपुस्तके पाठः ।

147. 'इन्द्रगोपकविराजाराजितां' इति पञ्चमपुस्तके पाठः ।

148. 'वहु' इति प्रथमपुस्तके पाठः ।

149. 'सन्' इति षष्ठपुस्तके पाठः ।

150. 'पूपाना' इति षष्ठपुस्तके पाठः ।

151. 'गर्ज्जनमेघकरीद्रकं दलदलीसस्यावृतास्तथा श्यामला' इति षष्ठपुस्तके पाठः ।

152. 'देशिनां' इति द्वितीयपुस्तके पाठः ।

153. 'देहशीतता' इति द्वितीयपुस्तके पाठः ।

154. 'तरुण्यश्चाल्पवीजास्तु चौषध्योऽपि' इति आदर्शपुस्तकेषु पाठः ।

155. द्रष्टव्यम्—सुश्रुत : सूत्र६:११ डल्हण टीका ।

156. 'जाङ्गलान् रसान्' इति प्रथमपुस्तके पाठः ।

157. 'अभिन्नवटाकांश्चापि सुभिन्नांश्च प्रलेहयेत्' इति द्वितीयपुस्तके पाठः ।

158. 'पुकाक्षं' इति षष्ठपुस्तके पाठः ।

159. 'सोपदंषां निषेवेतं' इति द्वितीयपुस्तके पाठः ।

160. 'च' इति षष्ठपुस्तके पाठः ।

161. 'ह्यल्पस्वनाः सारसा' इति प्रथमपुस्तके पाठः ।

162. 'समा तु भूः' इति आदर्शपुस्तिकासु पाठः ।

163. 'बामसप्ताह्व०' इति प्रथमपुस्तके पाठः ।

164. 'भूर्निम्नोन्नतसमेतु' इति षष्ठपुस्तके पाठः ।

165. द्रष्टव्यम्—सुश्रुत : सूत्र६:३६ डल्हण टीका ।

166. 'सन्नीतं' इति षष्ठपुस्तके पाठः ।

167. 'तप्तानां संचितं' इति आदर्शपुस्तकेषु पाठः ।

168. 'वृष्ट्या' इति आदर्शपुस्तकेषु अधिकः पाठः ।

169. 'कषायं मधुरं तिक्तं विशेषेणोल्वणोत्तरम्' इति द्वितीयपुस्तके पाठः ।

170. 'च' इति आदर्शपुस्तकेषु अधिकः पाठः ।

171. 'क्षुधितोयं रसादिषु' इति द्वितीयषष्ठपुस्तकयोः पाठः ।

172. 'द्रव्येषु मुद्गशाल्यादि प्रदेयं मधु जांगलम्' इति द्वितीयषष्ठपुस्तकयोः पाठः ।

173. 'हितमुष्णोदकं सदा' इति षष्ठपुस्तके पाठः ।

174. 'दप्यहोरात्रमगस्तेन पवित्रितम्' इति द्वितीयपुस्तके पाठः ।

175. 'सरोऽच्छं' इति द्वितीयपुस्तके पाठः ।
'सरोऽत्थं' इति षष्ठपुस्तके पाठः ।

176. 'तीक्ष्णमध्यदिवा०' इति सर्वादर्शपुस्तकेषु पाठः ।

177. 'चरेच्चर्यां' इति द्वितीयपुस्तके पाठः ।

178. 'नित्यं सेवेत' इति प्रथमपुस्तके पाठः ।

179. 'प्राविडासारगर्जिते' इति षष्ठपुस्तके पाठः ।

180. 'नित्यमन्त्राद्यैः स चतुर्विधः' इति द्वितीयपुस्तके पाठः ।

181. 'चतुर्थकः' इति द्वितीयपुस्तके पाठः ।

182. 'हीनताः' इति द्वितीयपुस्तके पाठः ।

183. 'तत्रान्नपाने हीने' इति द्वितीयपुस्तके पाठः ।

184. 'परिविनिश्चितम्' इति द्वितीयषष्ठपुस्तकयोः पाठः ।

185. 'चाशुसम्भवाः' इति प्रथमपुस्तके पाठः ।

186. 'प्रयोजनम्' इति द्वितीयपुस्तके पाठः ।

187. 'गुरु' इति प्रथमपुस्तके पाठः ।
'गुणं' इति षष्ठपुस्तके पाठः ।

188. 'दुष्टाविलक्षणाः' इति षष्ठपुस्तके पाठः ।

'दुष्टविलक्षणैः' इति प्रथमपुस्तके पाठः ।

189. 'प्रवर्तयेत्' इति प्रथमपुस्तके पाठः ।

190. 'जीवीनं' इति षष्ठपुस्तके पाठः ।

191. 'कालदेशाङ्गनाशनाः' इति द्वितीयषष्ठपुस्तकयोः पाठः ।

192. 'ग्रहणाच्छत्र-संस्थान०' इति द्वितीयपुस्तके पाठः ।

193. 'प्रमानजनवैकृतौ' इति प्रथमपुस्तके पाठः ।

194. 'घर्मवर्षासुलक्षणम्' इति द्वितीयपुस्तके पाठः ।

195. 'तृणोलुपलतागुल्मजातव्रततिसंकुलः' इति द्वितीयपुस्तकेः पाठः ।

196. 'संक्षुच्च' इति आदर्शपुस्तिकासु पाठः ।

197. 'इति' इति षष्ठपुस्तके पाठः ।

198. 'दीपादीनां' इति आदर्शपुस्तकेषु पाठः ।

199. 'वचोत्पन्तिः' इति प्रथमपुस्तके पाठः ।

200. 'प्रसादश्च' इति द्वितीयपुस्तके पाठः ।

201. 'कृमिक्लेदं पैच्छिल्येश्चोप्यपद्रुतम्' इति द्वितीयपुस्तके पाठः ।

202. 'न ह्यारोग्यकरं' इति द्वितीयपुस्तके पाठः ।

203. 'वित्याजितः' इति प्रथमपुस्तके पाठः ।

204. 'सर्वैश्चोद्भिदोगणः' इति प्रथमपुस्तके पाठः ।

205. 'दुः परिहार्यत्वात्पूर्वपूर्वं' इति षष्ठपुस्तके पाठः ।

206. 'सभ्यगृतु' इति द्वितीयपुस्तके पाठः।

207. 'विषवृक्षापहारिण्यो०' इति प्रथमपञ्चमपुस्तकयोः पाठः ।

208. 'वेह्वरोगा' इति षष्ठपुस्तके पाठः ।

209. 'युत' इति षष्ठपुस्तके पाठः ।

210. 'शुभदेशे' इति षष्ठपुस्तके पाठः ।

211. 'च वर्तते' इति षष्ठपुस्तके पाठः ।

212. 'सकला' इति षष्ठपुस्तके पाठः ।

213. 'हीनमिथ्यातिमात्रिकः' इति द्वितीयपुस्तके पाठः ।

214. 'दिशोधनम्' इति प्रथमपुस्तके पाठः ।

215. 'क्षीरितिक्तकेषायाणां' इति षष्ठपुस्तके पाठः ।

216. 'कनिष्ठिकाग्रसमस्थौल्यं' इति प्रथमपुस्तके पाठः ।

217. 'क्षीरवृक्षस्यशोभनम्' इति षष्ठपुस्तके पाठः ।

218. 'ताः' इति द्वितीयपुस्तके पाठः ।

219. 'दन्तमांसान्येपीडयेत्' इति षष्ठपुस्तके पाठः ।

220. 'कुर्यात्' इति षष्ठपुस्तके पाठः ।

221. 'जातरोगनिवृत्यर्थमाग्येयं बलवर्धनम्' इति द्वितीयपुस्तके पाठः ।

222. 'शोभनं' इति प्रथमपुस्तके पाठः ।

223 'मुखवैशद्यकारकम्' इति प्रथमपुस्तके पाठः ।

224. 'ततश्चोद्वर्त्तनाभ्यंगं———कांतिकृद्दोषनाशनं' पाठोऽयं द्वितीयषष्ठपुस्तकयोः नोपलभ्यते ।

225. 'ग्रभ्यङ्गमाचरेन्नित्यं स जराश्रमवातहा ।
दृष्टिप्रसादपुष्ट्यायुः स्वप्नसुत्वक्त्वदार्ढ्यकृत्' । इति ग्राकरे पाठः (ग्रष्टाङ्गहृदय : सूत्र२:८) ।

226. 'शीतं पित्तघ्नं कषायं वस्त्रमुच्यते' इति द्वितीयषष्ठपुस्तकयोः पाठः ।

227. 'कौशेयं———वस्त्रमुच्यते' इति प्रथमपञ्चमपुस्तकयोः ग्रधिकः पाठः ।

228. 'चन्दनं———सुशोभनं' श्लोकोऽयं द्वितीयपुस्तके नोपलभ्यते ।

229. 'घुस्टणोपेतं' इति सर्वपुस्तकेषु पाठः ।

230. 'कुर्यात्कस्तूर्याद्यैस्तु' इति प्रथमपुस्तके पाठः ।

231. 'स्वेदायाससमुद्भूतं' इति द्वितीयपुस्तके पाठः ।

232. 'वेलेया' इति षष्ठपुस्तके पाठः ।

233. 'सुस्नातैर्जातिवैल्वजं' इति षष्ठपुस्तके पाठः ।

234. क. 'नैमालं' इति पञ्चमपुस्तके पाठः ।

ख. 'नैजालं' इति प्रथमपुस्तके पाठः ।

ग. 'नैवालं' इति षष्ठपुस्तके पाठः ।

235. 'केतकं' इति षष्ठपुस्तके पाठः ।

236. 'गोल्लालवं' इति षष्ठपुस्तके पाठः ।

237. 'श्रीपर्णं' इति षष्ठपुस्तके पाठः ।

238. 'द्विमुहूर्तिकम्' इति पञ्चमपुस्तके पाठः ।

239. 'द्विरात्रं———मल्लिका' पाठोऽयं प्रथमपञ्चमपुस्तकयोः अधिकमुपलभ्यते ।

240. 'दमनं' इति षष्ठपुस्तके पाठः ।

241. 'सुखावहम्' इति द्वितीयपुस्तके पाठः ।

242. 'भजेद्गंधं' इति प्रथमपुस्तके पाठः ।

243. 'प्रधारयेत्' इति प्रथमपुस्तके पाठः ।

244. 'गौलाल्लं' इति प्रथमपुस्तके पाठः ।

245. 'पित्तहृद्विशदं———केतकी पुष्पमुच्यते' पाठोऽयं षष्ठपुस्तके नोपलभ्यते ।

246. 'अधार्यं———शतपत्रं तु शोभनं' पाठोऽयं द्वितीयषष्ठपुस्तकयोः नोपलभ्यते ।

247. 'चोक्ता' इति षष्ठपुस्तके पाठः ।

248. 'मुखरोगक्रमिहरं————रुचिकारकं' पाठोऽयं द्वितीयषस्ठपुस्तकयोः नोपलभ्यते ।

249. 'त्वविकारकं' इति प्रथमपुस्तके पाठः ।

250. 'दिवास्त्रीगमनं————आत्मतत्वविवेचनं' पाठोऽयं द्वितीयषष्ठपुस्तकयोः नोपलभ्यते ।

251. 'सुखार्थाः सर्वभूतानां मताः सर्वाः प्रवृत्तयः ।
सुखं च न विना धर्मात्तस्माद्धर्मपरो भवेत्' । इति आकरे पाठः ।

252. 'पैशून्यं' इति आकरे पाठः ।

253 'परुषानृते' इति आकरे पाठः ।

254. 'पश्येदपि कीटजन्तुपिपीलिकम्' इति आकरे पाठः ।

255. 'ब्रूयान्नहितं' इति द्वितीयपुस्तके पाठः ।

256. द्रष्टव्यम्—अष्टाङ्गहृदय : सूत्र२:२६ ।

257. 'न च निः स्नेहतां प्रभो' इति आकरे पाठः ।

258. 'न चैतान्यतिलालयेत्' इति आकरे पाठः।

259. 'परम्पराविरुद्धः' इति पाठः सम्यक् प्रतिभाति।

260. 'अनुभूयात्प्रतिपदं' इति द्वितीयपुस्तके पाठः।

261. 'अपि च' इति आदर्शपुस्तकेषु पाठः।

262. 'नाग्निस्कन्धमभिव्रजेत्' इति आकरे पाठः।

263. 'नारोहेदुष्टयानवत्' इति आकरे पाठः।

264. 'नासिकां———श्रमाद्विनिवर्तयेत्' इति षष्ठपुस्तके अधिकं पाठः।

265. 'अंगानि———स्थितिः' पाठोऽयं द्वितीयषष्ठपुस्तकयोः नोपलभ्यते।

266. 'नोर्ध्वजानुश्चिरं———सुरालयान्' पाठोऽयं द्वितीयपुस्तके नोपलभ्यते।

267. 'सूनाटवी' इति आकरे पाठः।

268. 'न' इति आकरे पाठः।

269. 'नृपद्वेषी' इति आदर्शपुस्तकेषु पाठः।

270. 'गात्रवक्त्रनखैर्वाद्यं———त्यजेत्' पाठोऽयं द्वितीयपुस्तके नोपलभ्यते।

271. 'विश्रम्भस्वातन्त्रयं विशेषात्' इति षष्ठपुस्तके पाठः।
'विश्रंभं स्वातंत्र्यं' इति प्रथमपुस्तके पाठः।

272. 'तत्' इति षष्ठपुस्तके पाठः।

273. 'आर्दसंतानता त्यागः' इति आकरे पाठः।

274. 'स्वार्थबुद्धिः' इति आकरे पाठः।

275. 'निशि चात्ययिके कार्ये दण्डी मौली सहायवान्' इति आकरे पाठः।

276. 'रात्रियामार्द्धकाविधि' इति द्वितीयपुस्तके पाठः।

277. 'कुचोलां' इति षष्ठपुस्तके पाठः।
'कुचिलां' इति पञ्चमपुस्तके पाठः।

278. 'नारीणां च कुलोद्भूतां' इति षष्ठपुस्तके पाठः।

279. 'वृद्धोपि ———वाप्नुयात्' पाठोऽयं द्वितीयपुस्तके नोपलभ्यते।

280. 'तेवै' इति पञ्चमपुस्तके पाठः।

281. 'तस्याधिक' इति द्वितीयपुस्तके पाठः।

282. द्रष्टव्यम्—सुश्रुत : सूत्र३५:२६।

283. 'शुक्रविक्रमौ' इति द्वितीयपुस्तके पाठः ।

284. 'हसेत्' इति पञ्चमपुस्तके पाठः ।

285. 'कुर्यात्क्रियामिमाम्' इति द्वितीयपुस्तके पाठः ।

286. 'तत्ररसादीनां——बलमित्युच्यते' पाठोऽयं प्रथमपुस्तके नोपलभ्यते ।

287. 'तेजस्तदोजस्तदेव बलमुच्यते' इति द्वितीयपुस्तके पाठः ।

288. 'स्वसिद्धिन्तानबलक्ष्य' इति द्वितीयपुस्तके पाठः ।

289. 'बाह्यानामात्मकार्यजातानां शक्तिर्बलम्' इति द्वितीयपुस्तके पाठः ।

290. 'अभिनिर्वृतमुदरस्थस्नेहजातं' इति प्रथमपुस्तके पाठः ।

291. 'मृत्सनं' इति आकरे पाठः ।

292. 'भ्रमरैः फलपुष्पेभ्यो यथा संभ्रियते मधु ।
तद्वदोजः स्वकर्मभ्यो गुणैः संभ्रियते नृणाम्' । इति आकरे पाठः ।

293. 'पावकाद्यैस्तु' इति द्वितीयपुस्तके पाठः ।

294. 'संख्यातं तन्नाशन्ना विनश्यति' इति आकरे पाठः ।

295. 'मृदुश्लक्ष्णं' इति आकरे पाठः ।

296. 'स्निग्धमोजो' इति आकरे पाठः ।

297. 'अग्निषोमगुरुत्वं' इति द्वितीयपुस्तके पाठः ।

298. 'अतः——सोमभयो भवेत्' पाठोऽयं प्रथमपञ्चमपुस्तकयोः नोपलभ्यते ।

299. 'अल्पज्वरो' इति द्वितीयपुस्तके पाठः ।

300. 'मूर्छायमरणं' इति द्वितीयपुस्तके पाठः ।

301. 'बलमाप्याययेद्वैद्य' इति प्रथमपुस्तके पाठः ।

302. 'तथा च——शनैर्दोषान्विनिर्हरेत्' पाठोऽयं पञ्चमपुस्तके अधिकमुपलभ्यते ।

303. 'सहिष्णुता' इति द्वितीयपुस्तके पाठः ।

304. 'ज्ञायन्ते' इति द्वितीयपुस्तके पाठः ।

305. 'भजते' इति द्वितीयपुस्तके पाठः ।

306. 'तत्कार्यपि' इति प्रथमपुस्तके पाठः । उभयत्र तु छन्दोभङ्गः संजातः ।

307. 'भृष्टः———भेदनो गुरुः' पाठोऽयं द्वितीयषष्ठपुस्तकयोः नोपलभ्यते ।

308. 'मधुराशिषु' इति द्वितीयपुस्तके पाठः।
'मथुवाशिषु' इति पञ्चमपुस्तके पाठः।

309. 'सात्म्यास्तु' इति षष्ठपुस्तके पाठः।

310. 'रसोन्यस्य' इति प्रथमपुस्तके पाठः।

311. 'धावति' इति द्वितीयपुस्तके पाठः।

312. 'वस्तिरर्शांसि' इति द्वितीयपुस्तके पाठः।

313. 'त्वल्पर्तु' इति द्वितीयपुस्तके पाठः।

314. 'हेतवे' इति द्वितीयपुस्तके पाठः।

315. 'नेत्र' इति प्रथमपुस्तके पाठः।

316. 'भोगान्यपिक्षयेत्' इति षष्ठपुस्तके पाठः।

CHAPTER 4

वेणुं क्वणन् ब्रह्मारसं वितन्वन्प्राक्क्रीडताव्यान्नृपतिं सगोपैः ।

श्रीटोडरेन्द्रं जनरक्षणार्थं वेदान्तवेद्यो भुवि वल्लभेशः ॥१॥

Lord Kṛṣṇa who transmitted the knowledge of Brahman while singing with flute prior to his play, who is the knower of essence of the Vedas and who is the supporter of his disciples and retinues, may, along with cow-herd boys, bless Śrī Ṭoḍarendra for the protection of people in this world.

[There appears to be some mistakes in this invocation.]

पञ्चात्मकं पञ्चसु वर्तमानं षडाश्रयं षड्गुणयोगयुक्तम् ।

तत्सप्तधातु त्रिमलं द्वियोनिं चतुर्विधाहारमयं शरीरम् ॥२॥

The *śarira* (body) is *pañcātmaka* (composed of five *mahābhūtas*). It is maintained by the activities of five types of sensory and motor organs. It is sustained by the food having six tastes and is produced by the attributes of these six categories of diet. It comprises seven types of *dhātus* (tissue elements) and three types of *malas* (waste products). According to sex it is of two types. It is pervaded by four categories of diet.

पञ्चात्मकं गुणं पूर्वं कथितम् ॥३॥

Mahābhautic composition of the body has already been described earlier (vide Chapter 3:6).

पंचसुवर्त्तमानम्, यथा

व्योमादिपंचकं स्वेषु विषयेषु प्रवर्तते ।
शब्दं च वाचा वचनं पाणिना दानमेव च ॥४॥
पद्भ्यां विहरणं चेति पायुनोत्सर्गमेव च ।
उपस्थेनानन्द इति पंचसु वर्त्तमानम् ॥५॥

The five types of sensory organs help in the maintenance of the body by receiving their objects viz., sound, touch, vision, taste and smell. The five types of motor organs which help in the maintenance of the body are as follows :

1. Tongue to produce voice and speech;
2. Hands to donate (give things to others);
3. Legs to walk;
4. Anus for elimination of waste products; and
5. Genital organ for sexual enjoyment.

शब्दं कोऽर्थः? श्रवणम् ॥६॥

The term *śabda* used in the above verse means *śravaṇa* or hearing (?).

षडाश्रयं यथा

षड्रसा मधुराद्यास्तु केवला मिश्रितास्तथा ।

एतन्मयाहारपरं षडाश्रयमिति स्मृतम् ॥७॥

The body is sustained by the food having six tastes like sweet, sour, saline, pungent, bitter and astringent. They are present in the food either individually or in a mixed form.

एतेषां गुणसंयोगाच्छुक्रं तत्संभवं ततः ।

तेन षड्गुणयोगेन युक्तमित्यभिधीयते ॥८॥

Śukra (semen) is the output of the conglomeration of the attributes of all these six tastes. Therefore, the body, which is produced of *śukra* (semen), is called the product of the attributes of these six tastes combined together.

विण्मूत्रं स्वेद एवेति मलत्रयं दोषात्मकं ।

Stool, urine and sweat—these are the three waste products, and they, by nature, are harmful.

लिङ्गाङ्कं च भगाङ्कं च द्वियोनीति निगद्यते ॥९॥

The two types of sex are characterised by the presence of the male genital organ and the female genital organ.

आहारचतुष्टयम्

भक्ष्यं भोज्यं लेह्यं पेयं इत्याहारचतुष्टयम् ।

Āhāra catuṣṭaya

The diet which pervades the body is of four categories viz., *bhakṣya* (chewable), *bhojya* (eatable), *lehya* (which are taken by licking) and *peya* (drinkable).

तत्र कृष्णात्रेयः

"[1]यदन्नं देहधात्वोजोबलवर्णादिपोषणम् ।

तत्राग्निर्हेतु एवेति न ह्यपक्वाद्रसायनम् ॥१०॥"

According to Kṛṣṇātreya

The food which nourishes the tissue elements of the body, *dhātus*, *ojas*, strength, complexion etc., does so by the help of *agni*. Rejuvenation does not take place by undigested food products.

तत्र भालुकिः

'नाभिमध्ये शरीरस्य विज्ञेयं सोममण्डलम् ।
सोममण्डलमध्यस्थं विद्यात् सूर्य[2]स्य मण्डलम् ॥११॥
प्रदीपवत्तत्र नृ[3]णां स्थितो मध्ये हुताशनः ।
['देहिनां भोजनं भुक्तं नानाव्यञ्जनसंस्कृतम्'[4]] ॥१२॥
[5]'जरायुमध्ये प्रच्छन्नः काचकोशस्थदीपवत् ।'
सूर्यो दिवि यथा ति[6]ष्ठंस्तेजोयुक्तैर्गभस्तिभिः ॥१३॥
विशोषयति सर्वाणि [7]पल्वलानि सरांसि च ।
तद्वच्छरीरिणां भुक्तं जाठरो नाभिसंस्थितः ।
मयूखैः क्षिप्रमादत्ते [8]नानाव्यञ्जनसंस्कृतम्[9] ॥१४॥'

[आयुर्वेदीयक्रियाशारीर : पृष्ठ६७६]

According to Bhāluki

Inside the umbilicus there is a circle of *soma* (moon). Inside the circle of *soma* there is the circle of *sūrya* (sun). In human beings, inside the circle of *sūrya*, *agni* is present in the shape of a lamp. It helps in the digestion of the food taken along with various vegetable preparations. The *agni* in the form of a lamp is covered with a shell of glass as the embryo is covered with amniotic membrane. As the sun, located in the sky, absorbs water from all the wells and ponds with the help of its hot rays, similarly *agni* located in the umbilical region helps in the immediate digestion of food taken along with various vegetable dishes by the help of its rays.

योगप्रदीपादग्निप्रमाणं लिख्यते

स्थूलकायेषु सत्त्वेषु यवमात्रं प्रमाणतः ।
ह्रस्वकायेषु सत्त्वेषु तिलमात्रं प्रमाणतः ॥१५॥
कृमिकीटपतङ्गेषु बालमात्रं प्रतिष्ठते ।

Quantity of Agni according to Yoga pradīpa

In animals having big body the size of *agni* is like that of a *yava* (grain of barley). In animals having small body *agni* is of the size of a *tila* (seed of sesame). In worms, insects and locusts it is of the size of the tip of the hair.

तस्योपरि स्थितं दैवात्तृष्णाच्छादनकं तिलम् ॥१६॥

An organ called *tṛṣṇācchādanaka* or *tila* is appropriately located above the location of *agni*.

धातूनां सप्तसप्तानां भूतानां पञ्च पञ्च च ।
त्रयोदशभवन्त्येते सह जाठरवह्निना ॥१७॥

Agnis are of thirteen categories. Each of the seven *dhātus* and five *mahābhūtas* has its own *agni* and the thirteenth one is called *jāṭharāgni*.

अथ सुश्रुतः

10

अत्र जिज्ञास्यं किं पित्तव्यतिरेकादन्योऽग्निरित्याहोस्वित् पित्तमेवाग्निरिति? ॥१८॥

[11] तत्रोच्यते

न खलु पित्तव्यतिरेकादन्योऽग्निरुपलभ्यते, [12] 'आग्नेयत्वात् पित्ते दहनपचनादिष्वभि-
वर्तमानेऽग्निवदुपचारः क्रियतेऽन्तरग्निरिति;' क्षीणे ह्यग्निगुणे तत्समानद्रव्योप-
योगात्, आगमाच्च पश्यामो न खलु पित्तव्यतिरेकादन्योऽग्निरिति ॥१९॥

[सुश्रुत : सूत्र २१:९]

According to Suśruta

Whether *agni* has separate existence from *pitta* or it is the same as *pitta*? In this connection it is said, *agni* has no separate existence from *pitta*. The *pitta* is *āgneya* (permeated with the attributes of *agni*) and it causes burning, digestion etc. Therefore *pitta* is treated secondarily as *antarāgni*. When the attributes of *agni* are reduced in *pitta* then similar substances are administered for increasing it.

Further, scriptural testimony is in favour of the identity between the *agni* and the *pitta*. Therefore, *agni* has no separate existence from *pitta*.

डल्हणः

ननु यदि पित्ताग्न्योरभेदस्तत्कथं घृतं पित्तशमनं वह्निदीपनम्, अजापयश्च
मत्स्यादयश्च पित्तवृद्धिं कुर्वन्ति न चाग्निदीप्तिकराः, दिवास्वप्नश्च ॥२०॥

[डल्हण : सुश्रुत : सूत्र२१:९]

According to Dalhaṇa

If *pitta* and *agni* are identical then why *ghee* which alleviates *pitta* causes stimulation of *agni*? The milk of goat, fish etc. increases the quantity of *pitta*. But they do not stimulate *agni*. The same is the case with sleep during day time.

तथा च

13
क्रोधशोकश्रमकृतः शरीरोष्मा शिरोगतः ।
पित्तं च केशान् पचति पलितं तेन जायते ॥२१॥

[सुश्रुत : निदान १३:३७]

It is also said

Because of anger, grief and exhaustion the heat of the body goes to the head and being associated with *pitta* it causes grey colour of the hair as a result of which *palita* (premature greying of hair) is caused.

अत्रापि शरीरोष्मा अग्निः ॥२२॥

In the above verse the term "*śarīroṣmā*" means *agni*.

अग्निर्भिन्नगुणैर्ज्ञेयः पित्तमग्निगुणैस्तथा ।
द्रवं स्निग्धमधोगञ्च पित्तं वह्निरतोऽन्यथा ॥२३॥

Agni has different attributes, and *pitta* has also got different attributes. *Pitta* is *drava* (liquid), *snigdha* (unctuous) and *adhoga* (which moves downwards). But *agni* has opposite qualities.

अन्यान्यपि पित्ताग्निभेदप्रतिपादकानि वाक्यानि सन्ति, तानीह विस्तरभयान्न दर्शितानि । यत् पुनरिहाग्निपित्तयोरभेदकथनं कृतं, तद्रसवीर्यादिगुणोपाधियुक्तस्य पित्तस्य चिकित्साद्वारेणाग्नेश्चिकित्सा कार्य्येति दर्शनार्थम्, अन्यथा रसादिगुणोपाधिरहितस्य वह्नेश्चिकित्सा कर्त्तुं नो पार्य्यत इति ॥२४॥

[डल्हण : सुश्रुतः सूत्र२१:६]

There are many other quotations in which *pitta* and *agni* are treated as different. These elaborate descriptions are not being furnished here. When *pitta* is not treated as different from *agni*, this is done largely with a view to indicating that *pitta* has attributes like *rasa* (taste), *vīrya* (potency) etc., and through its treatment, *agni* (which has no such attributes) can be corrected. Otherwise, the treatment of erratic *agni* which has no attributes like *rasa* etc., is impossible.

[अग्निः]

वैश्वानरः

तस्मात्तेजोमयं पित्तं पित्तोष्मा यश्च शक्तिमान् ।

समं चरति कुक्षिस्थः सर्वतो धमनीमुखैः ॥२५॥

14

स कायाग्निः स कायोष्मा सम्यकाश्रय जीवनम् ।

अनन्यगतिरित्येष देहे कायाग्निरुच्यते ॥२६॥

Agni

According to Vaiśvānara

Therefore, *pitta* is *tejomaya* (fully pervaded by *agni*) and it is the heat of *pitta* which is powerful. Along with *pitta*, *agni* moves in the *kukṣi* (lower abdomen) and through all the openings of channels of circulation. This is called *kāyāgni* or *kāyoṣmā*. This *kāyāgni* is also known as the *samyagāśraya* (proper substratum), *jīvana* (life) and *ananya gati* (invariable dependant) of the body.

वसिष्ठः

15

पञ्चभूतात्मके देहे आहारः पाञ्चभौतिकः ।

16

विपक्वः पञ्चधा सम्यक् गुणान्स्वान्स्वान्प्रवर्द्धयेत् ॥२७॥

According to Vaśiṣṭha

The body is composed of five types of *mahābhūtas*. The diet is also composed of these five *mahābhūtas*. The diet, after digestion, is divided into these five groups to nourish the respective attributes of the body.

अविदग्धः कफं, पित्तं विदग्धः, पवनं पुनः ।
सम्यग्विपक्को निःसार आहारः परिवर्धयेत् ॥२८॥[17]

[सुश्रुत : सूत्र४६:५२६-५२७]

Before digestion of food, *kapha* is produced, during digestion *pitta* is produced and after the digestion is over *vāyu* is produced. Thereafter, the residue of the food which is without any essence is eliminated.

अन्नं कालेऽभ्यवहृतं कोष्ठे प्राणानिलाहृतम् ।
'द्रवैर्विभिन्नसङ्घातं नीतं स्नेहेन मार्दवम् ॥२९॥
सन्धुक्षितः समानेन पचत्यामाशयस्थितम् ।
[औदर्योऽग्निर्यथा बाह्यः स्थालीस्थं तोयतण्डुलम्] ॥३०॥
आदौ षड्रसमप्यन्नं मधुरीभूतमीरयेत् ।
फेनीभूतं कफं, यातं विदाहादम्लतां ततः ॥३१॥
पित्तमामाशयात्कुर्याच्च्यवमानं, च्युतं पुनः ।
अग्निना शोषितं पक्वं पिण्डितं कटुमारुतम् ॥३२॥'

[अष्टाङ्गहृदय : शारीर३:५५-५८]

The food taken in appropriate time is taken to the *koṣṭha* (gastro-intestinal tract) by the help of *prāṇa vāyu*. There, it gets disintegrated by the liquid secretions and it becomes soft by the unctuous secretions which are produced by the stimulation of *samāna vāyu*. The diet located in *āmāśaya* (stomach including small intestine) gets digested on the analogy of the cooking of rice mixed with water and placed in a vessel on the external fire. In the beginning of the digestion, the food consisting of six tastes becomes sweet, and thus, produces *kapha* of foamy nature. In the second stage, because of the *vidāha* (burning) it becomes sour, and during this process when the food leaves *āmāśaya, pitta* is produced. After it has left *āmāśaya* the watery portion from the residue gets absorbed by the process of digestion and it takes the shape of *piṇḍa* (formed solid mass). During this process, pungent *māruta* (wind) is produced.

'भौमाप्याग्नेयवायव्याः पञ्चोष्माणः सनाभसाः ।

पञ्चाहारगुणान्स्वान् स्वान् पार्थिवादीन् पचन्त्यनु ॥३३॥

यथास्वं ते च पुष्णन्ति पक्त्वा भूतगुणान् पृथक् ।

पार्थिवाः पार्थिवानेव शेषा शेषांश्च देहगान् ॥३४॥'

[अष्टाङ्गहृदय : शारीर३:५९-६०]

Thereafter, the five *bhūtāgnis* viz., *bhaumāgni, āpyāgni, āgneyāgni, vāyavyāgni* and *nābhasāgni* digest the five groups of attributes of the food. These attributes, after metabolic transformation of their *bhautic* nature separately, nourish those of the *dhātus*. The *pārthiva* attribute of the food nourish the *pārthiva* attribute of the *dhātus*. In the same way remaining attributes are nourished.

कोऽर्थः? [18] औषधि गुर्वादिगुणव्यतिरिक्तान् आप्यादिमहाभूतगुणान्देहगानित्यर्थः ॥३५॥

By implication, apart from the attributes like *guru* (heaviness) etc., of the drugs, these *agnis* help in the metabolic transformation of the attributes of the *mahābhūtas* like *jala* etc. in the body.

'केचिदाहुरहोरात्रात्षडहादपरे, परे ।

मासेन याति शुक्रत्वं [19] रसः पाकक्रमेण हि ॥३६॥

[अष्टाङ्गहृदय : शारीर ३:६५-६६]

According to some scholars, the *rasa* (end product of the gastro-intestinal digestion) by the process of *pāka* (metabolism) takes one day and one night (24 hours) to become *śukra.* According to some others, it takes about six days. Some others however, hold the view that this process takes one month for the transformation of *rasa* to *śukra.*

20
सुश्रुतात्

स खलु त्रीणि त्रीणि कलासहस्राणि एकैकशो धातवोऽवतिष्ठन्ते ।

कलादशभागश्च ॥३७॥

Ăccording to Suśruta

Rasa remains in each *dhātu* for 3010 *kalās* (one hour = 25 *kalās*).

'अष्टादशसहस्राणि सङ्ख्या ह्यस्मिन् समुच्चये ।

कलानां नवतिश्चोक्ता स्वतन्त्रपरतन्त्रयोः ॥३८॥

[सुश्रुत : सूत्र १४:१५]

For the transformation of *rasa* to *śukra* it takes 18090 *kalās* in total. This is accepted in this and other medical texts.

'रस' गतौ धातुः अहरहर्गच्छतीत्यतो रसः ॥३६॥

[सुश्रुत : सूत्र१४:१३]

The term *rasa* is derived from the root '*rasa*' which means "to go". Therefore, the *dhātu* which always moves is called *rasa.*

वाजीकराण्यौषधयस्तथा क्षीरादिकं च यत् ।

स्वलक्षणगुणोत्कर्षाच्छुक्रं शीघ्रं विरेचयेत् ।

यथा विरेचनद्रव्यं रेचयन्ति तथैव च[21] ॥४०॥

Aphrodisiac drugs, milk etc., help in the ejaculation of semen by virtue of the excellence of their own attributes. This happens on the analogy of the purgative action of purgative drugs.

[धातुः]

'रसासृङ्मांसमेदोऽस्थिमज्जशुक्राणि धातवः ।'

[अष्टाङ्गहृदय : सूत्र१:१३]

Dhātu

Rasa (plasma and other liquid elements of the body), *rakta* (hemoglobin fraction of the blood), *māṁsa* (muscle tissue), *medas* (fat tissue), *asthi* (bone tissue), *majjā* (bone marrow) and *śukra* (sperm including ovum)—these are the seven *dhātus*.

शरीरं धारयन्त्येते धात्वाधाराश्च सर्वशः ॥४१॥

They sustain the body, and the entire body is composed of these *dhātus* (tissue elements).

[धातुकर्म]

'प्रीणनं जीवनं लेपः स्नेहो धारणपूरणे ।

गर्भोत्पादश्च धातूनां कर्माणि क्रमशो विदुः[22] ॥४२॥'

[अष्टाङ्गहृदय : सूत्र११:४]

Functions of Dhātus

Priṇana (nourishment), *jīvana* (life), *lepa* (coverage), *sneha* (oleation), *dhāraṇa* (formation of basic matrix), *pūraṇa* (filling up) and *garbhotpāda* (procreation)—these are the functions of the seven *dhātus* respectively.

ननु यदि रसादयः परिणमन्ति रक्तानुभावेन तर्हि पूर्वेषामुत्सादः स्यात् । सत्यपि परिणामे किञ्चित्तिष्ठति इति चेत्तर्हि पूर्वेषामल्पता स्यात् उत्तरेषां बाहुल्यमिति । नैतदस्ति । मलस्थूलाणुभागविशेषेण त्रिधा परिणामो भवति ॥४३॥

If *rasa* etc., get transformed into *rakta* etc., then this should result in the complete non-existence of the preceding *dhātus*, If it is argued that they are not completely transformed but a portion of it remains as the predecessor *dhātu*, even then, the preceding *dhātu* will get reduced in quantity and the successor *dhātu* will become excess in quantity. Therefore, this argument does not hold good. These *dhātus* are actually divided into three parts viz., *mala* (excreta), *sthūla* (gross element) and *aṇu* (the subtle element) before they actually get metabolised.

23
तत्र चरकः

स्थूलाण्वंशमलै सर्व्वे भिद्यन्ते धातवस्त्रिधा ।

स्वः स्थूलोंऽशः परं सूक्ष्मस्तन्मलः याति तन्मलः ॥४४॥

According to Caraka

All the *dhātus* are divided into three parts viz. *sthūla* (gross part), *aṇu* (subtle part) and *mala* (excreta). The gross part of the *dhātu* remains in the body matrix of the *dhātu*. The subtle part gets transformed into the successor *dhātu* and the *mala* becomes the excreta of the concerned *dhātu*.

अन्नात्पानात्पच्यमानात् विण्मूत्रं मलः, सारो रसः । रसादग्निपक्वान्मलः कफः, स्थूलो भागः रसः, सूक्ष्मभागो रक्तम् । रक्तादग्निपक्वान्मलः पित्तं, स्थूलो भागः शोणितम्, अणुभागस्तु मांसमिति । ततोऽपि आत्मपावकपच्यमानान्मलः मुखनासाकर्णाक्षिप्रजननादिस्रोतोमलः, स्थूलो भागो मांसं, सूक्ष्मो मेदः । ततोऽपि निजवह्निपच्यमानात् स्वेदो मलः, स्थूलोंऽशो मेदः, एवं सूक्ष्मभागोऽस्थिः । ततो

पच्यमानात् मलः केशलोमश्मश्रूणि, स्थूलोऽस्थि, सूक्ष्मस्तु मज्जा । ततोऽपि निजवह्निपच्यमानात् श्रवणपुरीषत्वगादिषु स्नेहः, स्थूलो भागो मज्जा, सूक्ष्मः शुक्रः । ततः पच्यमानादपि मलो न विद्यते । स्थूलो भागः शुक्र एव ॥४५॥

After the digestion of food and drinks, stool and urine come out as excreta and the essence of food and drinks is transformed as *rasa* (chyle, plasma etc). When *rasa* is acted upon by the *rasa dhātvagni*, its excreta come out as *kapha*, the gross part remains in the matrix of *rasa* and the subtle part of it is transformed into *rakta* (hemoglobin fraction of blood). When *rakta* is acted upon by the *rakta dhātvagni*, its excreta come out as *pitta*, the gross part remains in the matrix of *rakta* and the subtle part of it is transformed into *māṁsa* (muscle tissue). When *māṁsa* is acted upon by the *maṁsa dhātvagni*, then its waste products come out in the form of excreta from the mouth, nose, ears, eyes, genital organ and such other channels. Its gross part remains in the matrix of *māṁsa* and the subtle part of it is transformed into *medas* (fat tissue). When *medas* is acted upon by *medo dhātvagni*, then the excreta comes out as sweat. Its gross part remains in the matrix of *medas* and its subtle part is transformed into *asthi* (bone tissue). When the *asthi* is acted upon by the *asthi dhātvagni* then the excreta come out as the *keśa* (big hair), *loman* (small hair) and *śmāśru* (hair of beard). Its gross part remains in the matrix of *asthi* and its subtle part is transformed into *majjā*. When *majjā* is acted upon by the *majjā dhātvagni*, the excreta come out as the fatty substance in the ear, stool, skin etc., the gross part remains in the matrix of *majjā* and the subtle part of it is transformed into *śukra* (sperm and ovum). When *śukra* is acted upon by the *śukra dhātvagni*, it does not result in the production of any excreta. Its gross part remains as *śukra*.

तद्यथा

अग्निभिः पच्यमानेषु मलाः षट्सु[24] रसादिषु ।
न शुक्रे पच्यमानेषु हेमनीवाक्षये मलः[25] ॥४६॥

The preceding six *dhātus* produce *malas* (excreta) when they are acted upon by their respective *dhātvagnis*. This does not happen in the case of the seventh *dhātu* i.e. *śukra*. This is on the analogy of pure gold which when exposed to fire, does not produce any excreta.

ततोऽपि पच्यमानान्मलस्तेजोभूतं ओज इत्येके ॥४७॥

According to some scholars, as a result of the interaction between *śukra* and its *dhātvagni*, *ojas* which is full of *tejas* (energy) comes out as excreta.

तद्यथा

कफः पित्तं मलाः खेषु प्रस्वेदो नखरोम च ।
कर्णविट्चक्षुषः स्नेहो धातूनां क्रमशो मलाः[26] ॥४८॥

[अष्टाङ्गहृदय : शारीर३:६३-६४]

It is said

The following are the excreta of the preceding six *dhātus* seriatim :

1. *Kapha*;
2. *Pitta*;
3. Excreta in the openings of the body;
4. Sweat;
5. Nail and hair; and
6. Fat of the ears, stool and eyes.

अत्रोच्यते

'ओजस्तु सर्वभूतानां सारः सुश्रुतकीर्तितः ।
यस्यक्षयेन नियतं मरणं तत्कथं[27] मलः ॥४९॥

According to Suśruta *ojas* represents, the essence of all the *dhātus* (tissue elements). Reduction of its quantity certainly results in death. Then how can it be a *mala* (excreta) ?

तस्मादोजो भिन्न एव । श्मश्रुशुक्रमल इत्येके । [28]तन्नास्मत् सम्मतम् ।

श्मश्रुहीनस्यापि शुक्रदर्शनात् । तत्र मुष्को [29]पुंभावसंज्ञत्वमिति वचनात् ।

[30]अश्मश्रुकाणामण्डयोरेवासम्भवात् क्षितावेवमल इति जैय्यटः ।

Therefore, *ojas* is different from the *mala* of *śukra.* According to some, *śmaśru* is the excreta or waste product of *śukra.* We do not agree with this view because, *śukra* is also found in persons who have no beard. Testicles are considered to be the indicator of male sex. It is impossible for persons to have testicles if they do not have beard. On the basis of this argument Jaiyyaṭa has included beard as the *mala* (the waste product) of *śukra.*

युवानं पिडिका नृणां जायन्ते शुक्रतस्तथा । ते [31]केचिदपि शुक्रतेजोष्मणाकृत्वायुवान-

पिडिका [32]जायन्ते [33]शुक्रमलाः ॥५०॥

Yuvāna piḍikā (pimples in the face) in men appear because of *śukra.* According to some scholars these pimples appear as a result of *tejas* (heat) of the *śukra.* Therefore, according to them these pimples are the *mala* (waste product) of *śukra.*

[34]अग्निवेशात्

रोम्णां कोट्यस्तु पञ्चाशच्चतस्रः कोट्य एव च ।

सप्तषष्ठिस्तथा लक्षाः [35]सार्धकोटयस्तथैव च ॥५१॥

संख्यात इत्यर्थः ॥५२॥

त्रयोलक्षास्तु विज्ञेयाः श्मश्रुकेशाः शरीरिणाम् ।

According to Agniveśa

Romās (small hairs) are fifty four and half crores and sixty-seven lakhs in number. The hairs of the beard are three lakhs in number.

36
ततो हीना स्मृता योषा हीनकूर्चा मता बुधैः ॥५३॥

खलतिर्नभवेत्स्त्रीणां यस्मात्तल्लिख्यतेऽधुना ।

अत्यन्तसुकुमाराणां रजो दुष्टं स्रवन्ति च ॥५४॥

37
अव्यायामरताः यस्मात्तस्मान्न खलतिः स्त्रियः ।

वायुः पित्तं शमं याति व्यायामपरिवर्जनात् ।

रजः स्रवत्यतः शुद्धिर्जायते सा न जायते ॥५५॥

॥इति विदेहसंहितायाम्॥

According to Videha Saṁhitā

In ladies the number of hairs is less than what is stated above. Therefore, they are called *hīnakūrcā* (having less of hairs).

Now we shall write the reasons for which baldness does not appear in ladies. They are very tender and the waste products of their body come out through their menstrual secretion. They do not indulge in exercise. Therefore, ladies do not suffer from baldness. Avoidance of exercise alleviates *vāyu* and *pitta*. Because of menstrual secretion their body becomes clean. Therefore, they do not get baldness.

अथौपधेनवात्, चिकित्सासारसंग्रहात्

रसाद्रक्तं विसदृशात्[38] कथं देहेऽभिजायते[39] ।

रसस्य च न रागोऽस्ति स[40] कथं याति रक्तताम् ॥५६॥

[41] द्रवाद्रक्तात् स्थिरं मांसं कथं तज्जायते नृणाम् ।

द्रवधातोः स्थिरान्मांसान्मेदसः संभवः कथम् ॥५७॥

श्लक्ष्णाभ्यां मांसमेदोभ्यां खरत्वं कथमस्थिषु ।

खरेष्वस्थिषु मज्जा च केन स्निग्धो मृदुस्तथा ॥५८॥

मज्ज्ञश्च परिणामेन यदि शुक्रं प्रवर्तते ।

सर्वदेहगतं शुक्रं प्रवदन्ति मनीषिणः ।

तथाऽस्थिमध्यमज्ज्ञश्च[42] शुक्रं भवति[43] देहिनाम् ॥५९॥

[चरक : चिकित्सा १५:२२-२६]

छिद्रं न दृश्यतेऽस्थ्नां च तन्नि:सरति[44] वा कथम् ।

कीदृशौ रजबीर्यौ च प्रोत्तमौ गर्भकारकौ ॥६०॥

बालानां शुक्रमस्तीति न वास्तीति वद प्रभो ।

[45] स एवमुक्तः शिष्येण गुरुः प्रोवाच उत्तरम् ॥६१॥

[46] संसिद्धास्तेजसाह्यापः शरीरस्थेन देहिनाम् ।

अव्यापन्ना प्रसन्नेन रक्तमित्यभिधीयते ॥६२॥

According to Aupadhenava tantra and Cikitsā sāra saṁgra ha

Rakta looks different from *rasa*. How the former is produced from the latter in the body ? There is no colour in *rasa*. How does it become red ? *Rakta* is liquid in nature. How is *māṁsa* which is solid in nature is produced out of this *rakta* ? How *medas* which is liquid in nature is produced out of solid *māṁsa* ? *Asthi* is rough by nature. How is it produced out of *maṁsa* and *medas* which are smooth in nature ? How *majjā* which is unctuous and soft is produced inside the rough bones ?" It is stated that *śukra* is produced by the transformation of *majjā*. *Śukra* according to scholars pervades the entire body where as *majjā* is located inside the bones. Then how is it possible that the *śukra* is produced out of the *mājjā* ? No hole is found in the bones. Then how semen comes out of these bones ? What type of *rajas* (ovum) and *vīrya* (sperm) are suitable for conception ? Do children have semen or not ? These questions were put by the disciples. Thereafter, the preceptor replied, "The unpolluted *ap dhātu* (watery elements) of living creatures gets metabolised by the unafflicted *tejas* (enzymes) of the body as a result of which *rakta* is produced.

[47]ततः सुश्रुतः [48]रसरक्तयोरभेदं दर्शयन्नाह

[49]'रसादेवस्त्रिया रक्तं रजः संज्ञं प्रवर्त्तते ॥६३॥

[सुश्रुत : सूत्र१४:६]

[50]प्रवृत्तस्य रक्तस्य ऋतुजं रजः संज्ञमुच्यते इत्यर्थः ॥६४॥

[डल्हण : सुश्रुत : सूत्र१४:७]

रक्तार्त्तवयोः सौम्यरससम्भूतयोरपि स्वभावाद्भेदं दर्शयन्नाह

"आर्त्तवं शोणितमाग्नेयं, शुक्रं सौम्यमितिकृत्वा अग्निषोमीयो गर्भो भवति ।

तस्मादार्त्तवस्याग्नेयत्वमुक्तम्, तत्तस्यापि कथं नाग्नेयत्वं भवति। तयोः स्वभाव-

[51]भेदात् ॥६५॥"

The difference between Rasa and Rakta according to Suśruta

The menstrual blood in ladies is produced from out of *rasa*.

The blood that comes out during menstrual period is called *rajas*. Both *rakta* (ordinary blood) and *ārttava* (menstrual blood) are produced from *rasa* which is *saumya* in nature. Even then there is difference between them. The *ārttava śoṇita* (menstrual blood including ovum) is *āgneya* (having heating nature) and *śukra* (semen including sperm) is *saumya* (having cooling nature). Embryo is formed by their combination, and therefore, the nature of embryo is *agniṣomīya* (both heating and cooling). There is a difference in their nature.

तत्राह

'आर्त्तवशोणितं त्वाग्नेयमिति । आर्त्तवञ्चतच्छोणितञ्चेति आर्त्तवशोणितम् । तु शब्दोऽत्रावधारणे[52] ॥६६॥'

[डल्हणः सुश्रुत : सूत्र१४:८]

रक्तं पुनः

उष्णं[53] शीतञ्च मधुरं स्निग्धं रक्तं च वर्णतः ।
शोणितं गुरु विस्रं स्याद्विदाहश्चास्य पित्तवत् ॥६७॥

It is said

The menstrual blood is invariablly *āgneya* (having heating property). *Rakta* (ordinary blood) is both *uṣṇa* and *sīta* (hot and cold). It is sweet, unctuous, red in colour, heavy and *visra* (foul smelling). Like *pitta* it also causes *vidāha* (burning sensation).

तथा च वृद्धात्रेयात्

अत्रापि च महाप्राज्ञ जिज्ञासा वर्त्ततेऽपरा ।
रक्तमेव रजः स्त्रीणां[54] किंवा रक्तं विना रजः ॥६८॥
इति तस्य वचः श्रुत्वा प्रोवाच ऋषिपुंगवः ।

ऋतुसंबन्धजं रक्तमार्त्तवं प्रोच्यते बुधैः ॥६९॥

स्त्रीणां गर्भाशये वायुर्यद्रक्तं लभते शनैः ।

55
चत्वारो जलयो मासाच्यवर्त्ते योनिमार्गतः ॥७०॥

स्तुतावशेषं तत्प्रस्थं रज इत्युच्यते बुधैः ।

स्तुतावशेषमथवा यदि तिष्ठति वाधिकम् ॥७१॥

56
तदाशु शुक्रस्य संसर्गी जायते मलवर्जितम् ।

यथा मलिनखंडस्य मलं च हरते बलात् ।

क्षीरं क्षारस्तथा विदुर्गर्भं आर्त्तवशुद्धिकृत् ॥७२॥

According to Vṛddhātreya

Oh ! Great Wiseman, there is another query about it. In women whether the *rajas* (menstrual blood) is the same as *rakta* (ordinary blood) or they are different ? The great sage replied, "The blood that flows during the menstrual period is called *ārttava*. It gets accumulated in the uterus and because of *vāyu*, it flows through the genital tract for 4 days every month. After the flow, about one *prastha* (768 ml.) of it remains inside the body which is called *rajas*. Sometimes this quantity is more or less than what is already stated. This gets purified when it comes into contact with the semen. As a piece of jaggery which is originally full of impurities becomes clean by the addition of *kṣīra* (milk) and *kṣāra* (alkalies), similarly, *ārttava* (menstrual blood) becomes pure after the pregnancy.

57
सुश्रुतः

अन्नं चतुर्विधं सम्यक्पाचितं पाचकाग्निना ।

मासेन याति शुक्रत्वं तद्वत्स्त्रीणां रजो भवेत् ॥७३॥

According to Suśruta

Four categories of food properly digested by the *pācakāgni*, become *śukra* in one month's time. The same thing happens about the *rajas* or *ārttava* (ovum) in the women.

'अत्रार्त्तवशब्दोऽयं शुक्रे वर्त्तते। न तु रजसि। रजोहि रसाद्रक्तवत्सप्तमेऽहनि जायते। अथवा यद्ययमार्त्तवशब्दः शुक्रे न वर्त्तते तदा स्त्रीणां शुक्रस्याभावात् षड्धातुत्वं भवति। तस्मादार्त्तवशब्दश्चात्र शुक्रे प्रवर्त्तते। स्त्रीणां शुक्रमप्यस्तीति वृद्धवाहडः[58] ॥७४॥

The term *ārttava* (?) used above means the *śukra* and not *rajas* or menstrual blood. Like *rakta* (ordinary blood), *rajas* (menstrual blood) is also produced from *rasa* (chyle or plasma) on the seventh day. If the term '*ārttava*' does not mean *śukra* in the women, then they will be devoid of one *dhātu* and will have only six *dhātus* in their body which is not correct. Therefore, the term '*ārttava*' used above means *śukra* (ovum in woman). According to *Vṛddha Vāhaḍa* women also have *śukra*.

स्त्रियोऽपि स्रवन्त्येव शुक्रं पुंसां समागमे ।
तन्न गर्भोपकारी स्यादतो नात्रैव कथ्यते।[59] इति ॥७५॥

During the intercourse with men, women also ejaculate *śukra*. But this *śukra* of women does not take part in conception because of which it is not described here.

रजस्तु

मासेनोपचितं काले धमनीभ्यां तदार्तवम् ।
इषद्विगन्धि कृष्णं च वायुर्योनिमुखं नयेत् ॥७६॥

तद्वर्षाद्द्वादशादूर्ध्वं याति पंचाशतः क्षयम्[60] ।

विस्रता द्रवता रागः स्यन्दनं लघुता तथा ।

भूम्यादीनां गुणाः ह्येते दृश्यन्ते[61] चात्र शोणिते ॥७७॥

[सुश्रुत : सूत्र१४:६]

Rajas

The menstrual blood which keeps accumulating in the vessels for one month is taken to genital tract by the *vāyu*. It has a slightly foul smell and it is black in colour. Menstruation starts after 14th year of age and menopause takes place when the lady is 50 years of age.

The *visratā* (foul smell), *dravatā* (liquid nature), *rāga* (colouration), *syandana* (flowing property) and *laghutā* (lightness) present in the blood represent the attributes of five *mahābhūtas* viz., *bhūmi* etc.

'पञ्चत्वमुपपन्नस्य देहे रक्तं न दृश्यते[62] ।

तस्माद्रक्तं जीव इति पूर्वाचार्यैर्निवेदितम्[63] ॥७८॥

In a dead body blood is not found. Therefore, scholars of the yore have described *rakta* (blood) as *jīva* (life).

वाय्वग्नितेजसा रक्तमूष्मणा चापि संयुतम् ।

विशोष्यमाणं भूयस्तु संयुक्तं याति मांसताम् ॥७९॥

यथाग्नितेजसा युक्तो वायु स्रोतांसि दारयेत् ।

अनुप्रविश्य पिशितं पेशीर्निभज्यते तथा ॥८०॥

When *rakta* gets associated with the energy of *vāyu*and *agni* and heat, it gets dried up and becomes compact to form the muscle tissue. As channels get perforated by *vāyu* when it becomes associated with the energy of *agni*, similarly the *māṁsa dhātu* gets divided into various muscles.

सुश्रुतः

यथा बिसमृणालानि विवर्द्धन्ते समन्ततः ।

भूमौ पङ्कोदकस्थानि तथा मांसे सिरादयः ॥८१॥

[सुश्रुत : शारीर४:६]

64

According to Suśruta

As the lotus stalks grow in different directions while remaining together in the mud and water, similarly vessels etc., spread into different directions from the muscles.

"श्लेष्माणं तु समाश्रित्य मांसस्नेहाभिसंयुतम् ।

स्थिरतां प्राप्य शौक्ल्यं च मेदो देहे प्रजायते ॥८२॥

This *māṁsa dhātu* then gets pervaded with *kapha*. This gets mixed with the unctuous fraction of *māṁsa*, and thus, gets stability and becomes white in colour resulting in the production of *medas*.

पृथिव्यग्निजलादीनां संयातः श्लेष्मणाऽवृतः ।

खरत्वं प्रकरोत्यस्य जायतेऽस्थि ततो नृणाम् ॥८३॥

करोति तत्र सौषिर्यमस्थ्नां मध्ये समीरणः ।

मेदसा तानि पूर्यन्ते स्नेहो मज्जा ततः स्मृतः ॥८४॥

तस्मान्मज्जा ततः स्नेहं शुक्रं संजायते ततः ।

वाय्वाकाशादिभिर्भावैः सौषिर्यं जायतेऽस्थिषु ॥८५॥

येन स्रवति तच्छुक्रं नवकुम्भादिवोदकम् ।

स्त्रोतोभिः स्यन्दते देहात्समन्ताच्छुक्रवाहिभिः ॥८६॥

This *medo dhātu* then gets pervaded by the *mahābhūtas* like *pṛthvi*, *agni* and *jala* and it becomes surrounded with *kapha* which causes roughness resulting in the production of *asthi*. Vaccum or porosity inside the bones is caused by *vāyu* and these vacant spaces get filled up by fatty substance and its unctuous portion or essence is called *majjā*. The unctuous portion or essence of *majjā* is called *śukra*. Because of the predominence of *vāyu* and *ākāśa mahābhūtas*, bones become porous and through these pores, there is exudation of *śukra* as water exudates from a fresh earthen jar. It percolates through all the *śukra vāhi srotas* (channels of circulation of *śukra*) and gets ejaculated from the whole of the body.

हर्षेणोदीरितं रागात्संकल्पाच्च मनोभावात् ।
बस्तौ सन्धेर्विनिर्याति स्थलान्निम्नादिवोदकम्[65] ।।८७।।

Because of attachment, determination and pleasant mood, *śukra* (semen) gets excited leading to its elimination through the junction between the opening of the seminal vesicle and the urinary tract as the water flows from a higher to a lower place.

वशिष्ठः

कोरकस्थो यथा गन्धः अस्ति नास्तीति वा बुधैः ।
न वक्तुं शक्यते तद्वद्बालानां शुक्रसंभवः ।।८८।।
तत्सतां वापि[66] भावानां सौक्ष्म्यात् एवोपलभ्यते ।
प्रपुष्टदलकिञ्जल्कसंभूते च सुलक्षणम्[67] ।।८९।।

According to Vaśiṣṭha

Even for a wise person, it becomes difficult to ascertain if there is fragrance in a bud or not. Similarly, it is impossible to say if semen is present in a child or not. Certain factors, even if they are present, are not observable because of their subtle nature. The fragrance of a flower can be observed only when its petals and stamens have appeared.

"[68]यथा पयसि सर्पिस्याद्यथा चेक्षौ रसो भवेत् ।

तिलमध्ये यथा तैलं तथा शुक्रं शरीरिणाम् ॥६०॥

द्व्यङ्गुलं दक्षिणे पार्श्वे बस्तिद्वारस्य चाप्यधः ।

मूत्रस्रोतः [69]पथे शुक्रं पुरुषस्य प्रवर्त्तते ॥६१॥

[सुश्रुत : शारीर४:२२]

As the ghee is present in the milk, as juice is present in the sugar-cane and as oil is present in sesamum seed, similarly, semen is present in living beings. At a distance of two *aṅgulas* (one *aṅgula* = half an inch) towards the right side below the opening of urinary bladder, in the urinary tract, the semen of the man gets ejaculated.

अग्निवेशात्

चतुर्विधं षट्प्रभवं शुक्रं गर्भत्वमृच्छति ।

रसेभ्यः प्रभवोऽथास्य षड्भ्यः षट्प्रभवं ततः ॥६२॥

सान्द्रता गौरवं स्थैर्यं मधुगन्धं च पार्थिवम् ।

[70]माधुर्यं द्रवता स्नैग्ध्यमाप्यमस्याथ मार्दवम् ॥६३॥

तेजोऽवयवसंयोगादुष्णं कायोष्मणा च यत् ।

वातात्मको[71]ऽपि [72]सर्गश्च तस्माच्छुक्रं चतुष्पदम् ॥६४॥

According to Agniveśa

Śukra which has four categories of attributes and which is the outcome of six types of food, is responsible for conception. It is produced from the food having six types of tastes. Therefore, semen is called *ṣaṭ-prabhava* (product of six). The density, heaviness, stability and honey like smell in semen are the attributes of *pṛthvī mahābhūta.* Sweetness, liquidity, unctousness and softness in semen are the attributes of *ap mahābhūta.* Semen is hot which represents the *tejas mahābhūta.* This heat is imparted to semen by the *kāyāgni.* The ejaculation of semen takes place because of the attributes of *vāyu mahābhūta.* Therefore, semen is stated to be *catuṣpāda* (having four limbs).

कट्वम्लपाकाः यदुक्ताः शुक्रघ्नाः पाकसंग्रहे ।
कषायकटुपट्वम्लं शुक्रं षट्प्रभवं कथम् ॥६५॥
उक्तः सर्वरसाभ्यासो धातूपचयसात्म्यकृत् ।
न तथैकरसाभ्यासः शुक्रं षट्प्रभवं ततः ॥६६॥

While describing *vipakās*, it has been stated that substances having *kaṭu* (pungent) and *amla* (sour) *vipākas* reduce *śukra.* Similarly, astringent, pungent, saline and sour tastes also reduce *śukra.* If it is so then how it is said that *śukra* is *ṣaṭprabhava* (product of six tastes) ? It has been stated that habitual intake of all the tastes causes nourishment of *dhātus* and it is wholesome. Similar effect is not achieved by the habitual intake of only one taste. Therefore, *śukra* is *ṣaṭ prabhava* (product of six tastes).

वसिष्ठः

शुक्रशोणितसंयोगो यन्निमेषेण जायते ।
तदा[73] पञ्चात्मसंयुक्तः[74] आत्मप्रकृतिभिर्पुनः[75] ।
अङ्गप्रत्यङ्गसहितो विभुश्चैवावतिष्ठते ॥६७॥

According to Vasiṣṭha

When there is union of *śukra* (sperm) and *śoṇita* (ovum), at the same moment the all pervading Soul along with its *aṅga pratyaṅga* (parts and sub-parts) and *pañcātman* (five *vāyus* or subtle *mahābhūtas*) gets located there by virtue of its own nature.

सुश्रुतः

क्षेत्रज्ञो वेदयिता स्प्रष्टा घ्राता द्रष्टा श्रोता [रसयिता पुरुषः स्रष्टा गन्ता धाता][76] वक्ता यः कोऽसावित्येवमादिभिः पर्यायवाचकैर्नामभिरभिधीयते दैवसंयोगादक्षयो-ऽव्ययोऽचिन्त्यो भूतात्मना सहान्वक्षं सत्त्वरजस्तमोभिर्दैवासुरैरपरैश्च भावैर्वायुना-ऽभिप्रेर्यमाणो गर्भाशयमनुप्रविश्यावतिष्ठते ॥६८॥

[सुश्रुत शारीर ३:४]

According to Suśruta

The universal soul who has synonyms like *kṣetrajña* (knower of body), *vedayitā* (one which produces sensation), *spraṣṭā* (one which perceives the sense of touch), *ghrātā* (one which perceives the sense of smell), *draṣṭā* (one who sees), *rasayita* (one who tastes), *sraṣṭā* (one who creates), *gantā* (one who goes), *dhātā* (one who sustains), *vaktā* (one who speaks) etc., by *daiva saṁyoga* (providential cause) gets united with the *bhūtātman* (individual soul) which latter is *akṣaya* (which does not undergo diminution), *avyaya* (which is non-expendible) and *acintya* (which is unthinkable). This union, endowed with the attributes of *sattva*, *rajas* and *tamas* and the characteristic features of *deva* (the gods), *asura* (demons) and similar other objects, gets carried by *vāyu* to enter and stay inside the womb.

तत्र गर्भस्य खलु संभवतः पूर्वं शिरः संभवतीत्याह शौनकः, शिरोमूलत्वात् प्रधानेन्द्रियाणां; हृदयमिति कृतवीर्यो[77], बुद्धेर्मनसश्च स्थानत्वात्; नाभिरिति पाराशर्यः, ततो हि वर्धते देहो देहिनः, [पाणिपादमिति मार्कण्डेयः, तन्मूल-त्वाच्चेष्टाया गर्भस्य; मध्यशरीरमिति सुभूतिर्गौतमः, तन्निबद्धत्वात् सर्वगात्रसं-भवस्य।][78] तत्तु न सम्यक्, सर्वाण्यङ्गप्रत्यङ्गानि युगपत् संभवन्तीत्याह धन्वन्तरिः,

[गर्भस्य सूक्ष्मत्वान्नोपलभ्यन्ते] वंशाङ्कुरवच्चूतफलवच्च ॥९९॥[79]

[सुश्रुत : शारीर ३:३२]

According to Śaunaka when the embryo is formed, its head appears in the beginning because head is the root of all the sensory organs. According to Kṛtavīrya, it is the heart which appears in the beginning because it is the location of both the intellect and the mind. According to Pārāśarya, the *nābhi* (umbilicus) appears in the beginning, because from the umbilicus the growth of the body takes place. According to Mārkaṇḍeya, the hands and the legs appear first, because the activity of the foetus are based on these limbs. According to Subhūti Gautama, the trunk of the body appears in the beginning, because all the limbs of the body are connected with it. According to Dhanvatanri, these views are not correct. All the limbs and organs of the foetus appear simultaneously. Because of their subtility they are not distinctly recognisable, in the beginning, in the foetus like the bud of the bamboo tree, or like a small mango fruit.

जीवप्रमाणमाह वैष्णवागमे

'बालाग्रशतभागस्य शतधा कल्पितस्य च ।

भागो जीवः स विज्ञेयः स चानन्त्याय कल्पते ॥१००॥

आहाराचारचेष्टाभिर्यादृशीभिः समन्वितौ ।

दम्पती समुपेयातां तयोः पुत्रोऽपि तादृशः ॥१०१॥[80]

Size of Jiva, according to Vaiṣṇavāgama

If the tip of the hair is made to one hundred parts and one part of it is divided into hundred sub-parts again, one such sub-part represents the size of *Jiva*, which is responsible for eternal bliss. Whatever diet, regimen or activities the couple adopt during intercourse their offspring bears similar characteristics.

चरकात्

'सर्पिः शाल्योदनं क्षीरं शर्करा पायसं पुमान् ।

भक्षयेन्मासमात्रं तु ब्रह्मचर्यरतः सदा ॥१०२॥

स्त्रीणामपि विशेषेण कार्योऽसौ विधिरुत्तमः ।

अथवा तैलमाषाद्यैः[81] पैत्तिकैस्ता उपाचरेत् ॥१०३॥'

According to Caraka

The man should take food containing ghee, *śāli* rice, milk, sugar and *pāyasa* (milk preparation) for one month and observe celebacy during this period. Thereafter, he should have sexual intercourse with a view to procreating offspring. These wholesome regimens should specially be adopted by the woman. In the alternative, they should be given *paittika* (which aggravate of *pitta*) food consisting of *taila* (gingili oil), *māṣa* etc.

तत्र कारणम्

त्र्यहं यावत्प्रवृत्तिं च कुरुते शोणितं स्त्रियः ।

निरुपद्रवा प्रसूयेता[82]पत्यं तस्यास्तु निरुजम् ॥१०४॥

The reason

In the woman, menstrual blood flows for three days. By adopting these regimens, they deliver the child without any complication or pain.

तस्मात्त्रि[83]दिनमारभ्य भवेदाचार[84]वर्जिता ।

निर्वाते वेश्मनि स्थित्वा जनैश्च परिवर्जिते ॥१०५॥

मृत्पात्रे करपर्णेषु हविष्याहारभोजिनी ।

क्षैरेयं यावकं स्तोकं भूयः सौहित्यकारकम् ॥१०६॥

त्रिरात्रं दर्भतल्पस्थां कामिनीं रक्षयेत्पुमान् ।

From the beginning of these three days, she should avoid *ācāra* (routine house hold activities) and reside in a lonely house free from wind. She should take *haviṣya* (only one meal of *sāttvika* articles) either in an earthen plate, or by hand or in leaves. She should take a little more of *kṣaireya* (milk preparation) and *yāvaka* (gruel). For three nights she should sleep on the bed prepared of *darbha* grass and should not meet her husband.

'अशुद्धे[85] प्रवर्तितेऽस्त्रे यदि गच्छति मूढधीः' ॥१०७॥

दोषयुक्तोस्याद्बहुलो न बीजं गर्भधारकम् ।

यदि गर्भः प्रजायेत व्यंगोन्मत्तोऽल्पजीवितः[86] ।

भवेत्तस्मान्नगच्छेत न पश्येत्तु कदाचन ॥१०८॥

During the menstrual bleeding the body of the woman is impure. Only an unwise man enters into sexual intercourse with such woman. This has many harmful effects and coitus during this period does not result in conception. If at all there is conception the offspring suffers from *vyaṅga* (a type of skin disease or defective limbs) and *unmatta* (insanity). Such children get a very short span of life. Therefore, the man should never cohabit with or even look at such a woman.

[गर्भसामग्री]

ऋतुक्षेत्राम्बुबीजानां सामग्र्यादङ्कुरो यथा ।

[सुश्रुत : शारीर२:३६]

'पुष्टिश्रीरायुर्लभेत तथैव गर्भगो[87] ध्रुवम्[88] ॥१०९॥'

Composition of the Foetus

As germination takes place in the presence of *ṛtu* (appropriate season), *kṣetra* (suitable ground), *ambu* (water or moisture and *bija* (suitable seed), similarly, in the presence of these four factors the embryo grows. Such an embryo gets endowed with nourishment, auspiciousness and longevity.

शशासृक्प्रतिमं यच्च[89] यद्वा लाक्षारसोपमम् ।

तदार्त्तवं प्रशंसन्ति यद्वासो[90] न विरञ्जयेत्[91] ॥११०॥'

[सुश्रुत : शारीर२:१७]

The menstrual blood which is like the blood of rabit or like *lākṣā rasa* (liquid preparation of lac) and which does not stain the cloth is of excellent quality.

अदृष्टार्त्तवोऽप्यस्तीत्येके[92] भाषन्ते ॥१११॥

[सुश्रुत : शारीर३:६]

According to some scholars, there are ladies who do not menstruate (but they are fertile).

पीनप्रसन्नवदनां प्रक्लिन्नात्ममुखद्विजाम् ।

नरकामां प्रियकथां स्रस्तकुक्ष्यक्षिमूर्धजाम् ॥११२॥

स्फुरद्भुजकुचश्रोणिनाभ्यूरुजघनस्फिचाम् ।

हर्षौत्सुक्यपरां चापि विद्यादृतुमतीमिति ॥११३॥

नियतं दिवसेऽतीते सङ्कुचत्यम्बुजं यथा ।

ऋतौ व्यतीते नार्यास्तु योनिः संव्रियते तथा ॥११४॥

[सुश्रुत : शारीर३:७-९]

A *ṛtumati* (fertile) woman exhibits the following characteristic features :

1. Her face becomes plump and there is expression of happiness;
2. There will be stickiness in her mouth and teeth;
3. She likes the association of men;
4. She talks sweetly;
5. There is looseness in her lower abdomen, eyes and hair of the head;
6. There is twitching sensation in the upper limbs, breasts, hips, umbilicus, thighs, calf region and buttock; and
7. There is excess of excitement and anxiety.

As a lotus flower becomes closed at the end of the day, similarly the *yoni* (uterus or genital tract) becomes closed after the expiry of the period of fertility.

ततः पुष्पेक्षणादेव कल्याणध्यायिनी त्र्यहम् ।

[अष्टाङ्गहृदय : शारीर१:२३]

चतुर्थेऽह्नि ततः स्नाता शुक्लमाल्याम्बरा शुचिः ॥११५॥

इच्छन्ती भर्तृसदृशं पुत्रं पश्येत्पुरः पतिम् ।

[अष्टाङ्गहृदय : शारीर१:२५-२६]

Therefore, immediately after the beginning of menstruation, for three days, the woman should resort to wholesome regimen (described in verse numbers 105 to 107 above). Thereafter, on the fourth day, she should take bath. She should observe purity and wear white garlands and clothes. The woman desires a son having the characteristic features of her husband. Therefore, immediately after purificatory bath, she should first of all meet (see) her husband.

प्राग्दक्षिणेन पादेन शय्यां मौहूर्तिकाज्ञया ।

आरोहेत् स्त्री तु वामेन तस्य दक्षिणपार्श्वतः ॥११६॥[93]

[अष्टाङ्गहृदय : शारीर१:३१-३२]

According to the instruction of the astrologer the man should climb over the bed through his right leg in the beginning. Thereafter, the woman should go to the bed first by her left leg through the right side of the man.

अग्निवेशात्

अतः शुक्लवाससौ स्रग्विणौ सुमनसावन्योन्यमभिकामौ सम्वेसतामिति ब्रूयात् । स्नानात् प्रभृति पुण्येष्वहःसु संवसेयाताम् पुत्रकामौ न च न्युब्जां पार्श्वगतां वा सेवेत ।'[94] ॥११७॥

[चरक : शारीर८:५-६]

According to Agniveśa

After the purificatory bath, both of them should be instructed to wear white apparel and garlands and with happiness of mind and having attraction for each other, they should enter into cohabitation during auspicious days if they desire to have a son. During cohabitation, the woman should not assume a prone posture nor should she be in her sides.

तत्र कारणम्

न्युब्जायां वातो बलवान्भवेत्स योनिं पीडयति । पार्श्वगतायां दक्षिणपार्श्वे श्लेष्मा, स च्युतः पिदधाति गर्भाशयं; वामे पार्श्वे पित्तं, तदस्याः पीडितं विदहति रक्तं शुक्रं च; तस्मादुत्ताना बीजं गृह्णीयादिति ॥११८॥

[चरक : शारीर८:६]

The reason for that

If she maintains a prone posture during cohabitation, then *vāta* gets aggravated and afflicts her uterus. If she remains in her right side during cohabitation, then *kapha* which remains in that side, gets displaced and blocks the uterus. Left side in the abode of *pitta*. If pressure is put on that side during cohabitation then the ovum and the sperm get burnt up. Therefore, the woman should receive seed while lying in her back side.

[95]
सुश्रुतः

'चतुर्थी स्यात्सुते षष्ठीत्वष्टमीदशमी तथा ।
कन्यार्थिनः पञ्चमी स्यात्सप्तम्येकादशीतिथिः ॥११९॥
युग्मासु तु पुमान्प्रोक्तः अयुग्मे कन्यका भवेत् ।
त्रयोदशी निन्दिता स्यान्नगच्छेत्तत्र बुद्धिमान्[96] ॥१२०॥

According to Suśruta

For a male child, cohabitation should be performed on fourth, sixth, eighth or tenth days from the date of onset of menstruation. For a female child, this should be performed on fifth, seventh and eleventh days. Cohabitation on the even days after the date of onset of menstruation bears a male offspring and on odd days a female offspring. Cohabitation on the thirteenth day of the day of onset of menstruation is prohibited because it is harmful (lit. despisable).

विदेहः

अयुग्मे दिवसे त्वासां रजश्चाजस्री[97] भवेत् ।
संयोगं[98] तत्र यो गच्छेद्ध्रुवं कन्या प्रसूयते ॥१२१॥

युग्मेषु[99] तु ततः स्त्रीणां रजः स्वल्पतरं भवेत् ।

संयोगं तत्र यो गच्छेद्ध्रुवं[100] पुत्रं प्रसूयते ॥१२२॥

According to Videha

On odd days after the date of onset of menstruation, the ovum in the woman becomes *ajaptari* (more effective). Therefore, cohabitation on those days, bears a female offspring. On even days, on the other hand, the ovum in the woman becomes proportionately *alpa* (less in quantity or less effective). Therefore, cohabitation on these days certainly bears a male offspring.

अत्र युग्मायुग्मतिथिषु शुक्ररजो वृद्धौ दैवहेतुः ॥१२३॥

The increase in the *śukra* (sperm) and *rajas* (ovum) in the even and odd days is effected by providential cause.

तत्र वैखानसः[101]

यथा बहुलपक्षेषु[102] मातुलुङ्गोऽधिकायते[103] ।

न तथा जायते शुक्ले स्वभावश्चात्र कारणम् ॥१२४॥

According to Vaikhānasa

In *bahula pakṣa* (dark fortnight) more of *mātuluṅga* fruits appear in the tree. This does not happen in *śukla pakṣa* (bright fortnight). *Svabhāva* (nature) is the cause of this variation.

योगशरीरे[104]

मैथुनं च ततः कुर्याद्यामादूर्ध्वं पुनः पुनः ।

"ब्रह्माबृहस्पतिर्विष्णुः सोमसूर्यौ तथाऽश्विनौ ॥१२५॥

भगोऽथ मित्रावरुणौ वीरं ददतु मे सुतम् ।

गर्भं देहि[105] सिमीवाली[106]" इमं मंत्रं तथा जपेत् ।

गर्भाधानेषु ये मन्त्रास्तान् तान् कृत्वाऽथ मंत्रयेत्[107] ॥१२६॥

According to Yoga śarīra

One should enter into cohabitation after the expiry of the first three hours of the night and thereafter, it should be repeated again and again. During cohabitation, one should recite the following *mantra* : "Oh ! *Brahma*, *Bṛhaspati*, *Viṣṇu*, *Soma*, *Sūrya*, the *Aśvins*, *Bhaga* and *Mitrāvaruṇau*, give me a brave son. Oh ! *Simīvālī*, give me a progeny."

The various *mantras* prescribed for *garbhādhāna* should be recited during cohabitation.

सुश्रुतः

'नारी रजोऽधिकेंऽशे स्यान्नरः शुक्राधिकेंऽशके ।

उभयोः समसंख्यायां जायते षंडसंज्ञकः ॥१२७॥

According to Suśruta

If there is more of *rajas* (ovum) the offspring becomes a female and if there is more of *śukra* (sperm) there will be a male offspring. If both the *rajas* (ovum) and *śukra* (sperm) are equal in quantity (strength or number) then the offspring becomes *ṣaṇḍa* (eunuch).

तत्राधिकस्यापेक्षिकत्वात्प्रमाणमुच्यते शुक्रशोणितयोः[108] यथा योगप्रदीपे

त्रयोविंशद्रजोभागाः शुक्रभागाश्चतुर्दशः ।

गर्भसंजनने काले पुंस्त्रियोः संभवन्ति हि ॥१२८॥

The quantity of *śukra* and *śoṇita* described above is a relative term. One is more or less with reference to the other.

According to Yoga pradīpa

If during conception, the *rajas* is of 23 parts and *śukra* is of 14 parts, then this leads to the procreation of male and female offsprings respectively.

गोपुरः

शुक्रप्रमाणं प्रसृतिः रजः प्रसृति षोडशः ।
कथं चात्र प्रमाणस्य विवेको जायते किल ॥१२९॥
अह्निश्चतुर्थे प्रसृतिस्तिष्ठेच्छुद्धमथार्त्तवम् ।
बालानां वातिरक्तं च स्वच्छं स्निग्धं घनं तथा ॥१३०॥

According to Gopura

The quantity of *śukra* is one *prasṛti* (96 milli litre). The quantity of *rajas* is 16 *prasṛtis*. How to determine the quantity of these elements ? During the fourth day after the date of onset of menstruation, one *prasṛti* of *ārtava* remains inside body of the woman. In young girls this quantity is more. This *ārtava* is clean, unctuous and compact.

सुश्रुतः

घृतकुंभो यथैवाग्निमाश्रितः सुविलीयते ।
विसर्पत्यार्त्तवं नार्यास्तथा पुंसां समागमे ॥१३१॥

[सुश्रुत : शारीर२:३६]

According to Suśruta

As the ghee inside a jar melts when it is exposed to the heat of the fire, similarly, when a woman comes into contact with a man, her *ārtava* gets ejaculated.

110

संशुद्धं शुक्रसंयोगात्तथादृष्टस्य शासनात् ।

शुद्धं गर्भाशयं प्राप्य पुरुषो जायते ध्रुवम् ॥१३२॥

There would certainly be a male offspring if the pure *rajas* in the womb of the woman comes in contact with the pure *śukra*. Of course, *adṛṣṭa* (unseen factor) has a control over this event.

अथ सर्वाङ्गसुन्दरटीकायाम् स्त्रीपुरुषयोर्विसृष्टिकालसमयः

स्त्रीपुंसयोः समायोगे यद्यादौ विसृजेत्पुमान् ।

शुक्रं ततः पुमान्वीरो जायते बलवान् दृढः ॥१३३॥

अथ चेद्वनिता पूर्वं विसृजेद्रक्तसंयुतम् ।

111

'ततो रूपान्विता कन्या जायते दृढसंहतेति ॥१३४॥

अतएव च पुंगर्भाः केचित्किचिन्मातृसदृशा दृश्यन्ते स्त्रीगर्भाश्च केचित्किचित्पितृसदृशा दृश्यन्ते ॥१३५॥

[सर्वाङ्गसुन्दरटीकाः अष्टाङ्गहृदय : शारीर१:५]

The time of ejaculation of the Woman and Man, according to Sarvāṅga sundara Commentary

When the woman and the man enter into cohabitation, if there is ejaculation of semen of the man in the beginning, then this results in the procreation of a male offspring who will be brave, strong and sturdy. If however, there is ejaculation of *rakta* (ovum) of the woman in the beginning, then there will be a female offspring, who will be beautiful, sturdy and compact. Therefore, at times, a male child has the characteristic features of the mother and a female child has the characteristic features of the father.

स्त्रीरुपुषयोरेकदैव यदा भवति तदा षंढो जायते ॥१३६॥'

स्त्रीपुंसयोर्विसृष्टिश्चेदेकदैव भवेद्यदा ।

षंढास्तदा प्रजायन्ते इति मे निश्चिता मतिः ॥१३७॥

तयो रत्युत्सुकाक्रांता पूर्वं हि विसृजेच्च यः ।

तद्रूपं जनयेद्गर्भं नान्यथा सम्प्रपद्यते ॥१३८॥

If the ejaculation of both the man and the woman takes place simultaneously, then the offspring will be *ṣaṇḍa* (eunuch). I am certain in my mind about it i.e. *ṣaṇḍa* (eunuch) is procreated if there is ejaculation of both the woman and the man at the same time. The offspring bears the similarity to the man or the woman who ejaculates in the beginning during sexual intercourse.

स्यन्दनं च विसृष्टिश्च शुक्रस्य क्षरणं तथा ।

क्लिन्नता केवलं स्यन्दात् विसृष्टं मधुना शुभा ।

112

अन्तेत्वाक्षिप्तवेगायाः विसृष्टिर्नरवत्स्मृता ॥१३९॥

Syandana (melting), *visṛṣṭi* (elimination) and *kṣaraṇa* (external ejaculation) — these are the three characteristic features of semen. If there is only *syandana* (melting) then this produces stickiness. If there is *visṛṣṭi* (elimination) then this gives pleasant feeling. *Kṣaraṇa* (ejaculation) is the terminating point of the sexual urge. [The meaning of these verses is not clear.]

अथ सुश्रुतः

शङ्खनाभ्याकृतिर्योनिस्त्र्यावर्ता सा प्रकीर्तिता ।

113

तस्यास्तृतीये त्वावर्ते गर्भशय्या प्रवर्त्तते ॥१४०॥

यथा रोहितमत्स्यस्य मुखं भवति रूपतः ।

114
तत्संस्थानं तथा रूपं गर्भाधारं विदुर्बुधाः ॥१४१॥

[सुश्रुत : शारीर५:४३-४४]

According to Suśruta

The *yoni* (uterus) or genital tract, is like a conch shell and it has three whirls. In the third whirl is located the bed of the womb. In shape the uterus looks like the mouth of a *rohita* fish. The womb resembles its mouth both in shape and colour, according to experts on the subject.

अग्निवेशात्

115
गर्भस्तु खलु मातुः पृष्ठाभिमुख ऊर्ध्वशिराः सङ्कुच्याङ्गान्यास्तेऽन्तःकुक्षौ ॥१४२॥

[चरक : शारीर६:२२]

According to Agniveśa

The foetus lies in the uterus with its face towards the back of the mother, head upwards and limbs folded.

रत्नाकरात्

अध्यास्ते संकुचद्गात्रो गर्भो दक्षिणपार्श्वतः ।
116
वामपार्श्वगता नारी क्लीवं मध्याश्रितं मतम् ।
यद्यदत्र हितं तस्य प्रतिलोमे विपर्ययः ॥१४३॥

According to Ratnākara

A male foetus remains in the right side of the womb of the mother with its body folded. A female foetus remains in the left side of the mother and a *klīva* (eunuch) remains in the centre. She should be given regimens which are useful to her during the period of pregnancy. If the regimens of opposite nature are adopted then they will produce harmful effects.

117
अथ सद्योगृहीतगर्भलिङ्गानि

'ततस्तृप्तिः परो हर्षो गात्रसादो हृदि व्यथा ।

पुष्पस्यादर्शनं सादो मूर्च्छा छर्दिरकामतः ॥१४४॥

प्रसेकः पाण्डुता ग्लानिः रोमराजीप्रकाशनम् ।

118
आश्लेषगन्धविकृतिर्भवेत्कृष्णमुखौ स्तनौ ॥१४५॥

योनेः प्रस्फुरणं निद्रा तन्द्रातोदौ क्लमस्तथा ।

विदाहो गुरुता देहे श्रद्धा च विविधात्मिका ।

119
अपातः शुक्ररजसो गर्भे सद्यःस्थिते भवेत्' ॥१४६॥

Characteristic features of a freshly conceived Mother

The following are the characteristic features of a freshly conceived woman :

1. There will be a sense of satisfaction, excellent excitement, a feeling of prostration in the body and pain in the cardiac region;
2. There will be absence of menstrual flow;
3. There will be weakness, fainting and vomiting without any perceptible cause;
4. There will be salivation, anemic look and *glāni* (a feeling as if covered with a wet cloth or exhaustion without efforts);
5. There will be appearance of small hairs in different parts of the body;
6. There will be more of spitting and foul smell;
7. The nipples of the breast wil lbe black in colour;
8. There will be throbbing sensation in the genital tract;
9. There will be excessive sleep, drowsiness, pain and mental exhaustion;
10. There will be burning sensation and heaviness in the body;

11. There will be different types of likings; and

12. The *śukra* and *rajas* will not get eliminated from the genital tract.

अथ भोजः

गर्भो रुणाद्धि स्रोतांसि रजःशुक्रवहानि वै ।
रक्ताज्जरायुर्भवति नाडी चैव रसात्मिका ॥१४७॥
सा नाडी गर्भमाप्नोति तथा गर्भस्य वर्धनम् ।
यद्यदश्नाति मातास्य भोजनं च चतुर्विधम् ॥१४८॥
तस्मादन्नाद्रसीभूतं वीर्यं यत्संप्रवर्त्तते ।
भागः शरीरं पुष्णाति स्तन्यं भागेन वर्धते ॥१४९॥
गर्भं पुष्यति भागेन वर्धते च यथाक्रमम् ।
गर्भं कुल्ये च केदारे [120] नाडी प्रीणाति तर्पति ॥१५०॥

According to Bhoja

The embryo obstructs the channels of circulation of *rajas* and *śukra* [The appropriate reading appears to be *rasa*]. By the *rakta* placenta is formed and the umbilical chord is formed by the *rasa*. That umbilical chord gets connected with the embryo and helps in its growth. The essence of the four types of food eaten by the mother becomes *rasa* (chyle). This *rasa* is divided into three parts—one part helps in the nourishment of the body of the mother; the second part is utilised for the promotion of breast-milk while from the third part the foetus gets nourishment. As a field gets irrigated by small canals, similarly, through the umbilical chord the foetus gets nourishment.

तथा च कृष्णात्रेयात्

दैवाद्गृहीतगर्भाणां रजो भागास्त्रिधा भवेत् ।

स्तनयोः पीनतां स्तन्यमेको भागः प्रयच्छति ॥१५१॥

द्वितीयः स्वबलेनैव गर्भगं पोषयत्यपि ।

ततः परं पोषयति गर्भिणीं च ततो न हि ॥१५२॥

रजः प्रवर्त्तते[121] स्त्रीणां अथवार्त्तववाहिनाम् ।

स्त्रोतांस्यस्या हि रुध्यन्ते मार्गाः गर्भेण वा ध्रुवम् ॥१५३॥

According to Kṛṣṇātreya

When a woman conceives by providential cause, the *rajas* (the blood which is meant for menstruation) gets divided into three parts. One of it increases the plumpness of the breasts and helps in the accumulation of milk in them. The second part, by its strength, goes to the foetus to provide nourishment. The third part provides nourishment to the pregnant woman. Therefore, there is no menstrual flow in a pregnant woman. The channels which carry menstrual blood get certainly obstructed by the foetus.

यो भार्यायामृतौ मोहादंगनेव प्रवर्त्तते ।

तस्य स्त्रीचेष्टिताकारो जायते षंडसंज्ञकः ॥१५४॥

ऋतौ पुरुषवद्वापि प्रवर्तेताङ्गना यदि ।

ततः[122] कन्या यदि भवेत्सा भवेन्नरचेष्टिता ॥१५५॥

If a man, because of his ignorance, behaves like a woman during cohabitation at the time of fertility, then the offspring becomes a *ṣaṇḍa* (eunuch) who behaves like a woman. If during the period of fertility the woman acts like a man and if there is a female offspring, then she behaves like a man.

कललस्थो यदा वायुर्गर्भे कुप्यति हेतुतः ।

शुक्ररक्तांशवैषम्यात्साम्ये वा कललांशयोः ॥१५६॥

श्वमार्जारवराहाणां वायुः कर्मवशानुगः ।

123

बली विचुम्बत्कललं करोति बहुपुत्रताम् ॥१५७॥

When the *vāyu* located in *kalala* (jelly like embryo) gets aggravated by certain causes, then the portions of *śukra* (sperm) and *rajas* (ovum) inside the *kalala* (jelly like embryo) which are either in disproportionate quantity or in proper proportion get afflicted. This results in the procreation of foetus in the shape of a dog, a cat or a pig. As a result of the *karma* (past actions) the powerful *vāyu* divides the *kalala* into several parts resulting in the procreation of many sons.

सुश्रुतः

124

द्वे नार्यौ तु वृषयन्त्यौ कामाधिक्यात्कथंचन ।

'मुञ्चत्यौ शुक्रमन्योन्यमनस्थिस्तत्र जायते ॥१५८॥'

[सुश्रुत : शारीर२:४७]

According to Suśruta

If because of excessive sexual desire, two excited females enter into sexual intercourse and enjaculate *śukra* (?) then the offspring produced as a result of the coitus becomes devoid of any bone.

अग्निवेशः

शोकोपवास रूक्षान्नवेगसंधारणादिभिः ।

गर्भिण्याः कुपितो वायुः गर्भस्थो वितथो भवेत् ॥१५९॥

125

हीनाधिकाङ्गाः वधिराः जडकुब्जाः सवामनाः ।

126

खंजाः द्विशीर्षाः कुणपाः जायन्ते वातवैकृतात् ॥१६०॥

According to Agniveśa

Because of grief, fasting, intake of ununctuous food, suppression of the natural urges etc., of a pregnant woman, *vāyu* gets aggravated to afflict the foetus. As a result of this aggravation of *vāyu*, at times, the child has less or more of limbs. It becomes deaf, dumb, hunch back, dwarf, *khañja* (inability to move because of the affliction of the two lower limbs), having two heads or *kuṇapa* (producing smell of dead body or having deformity of limbs).

सुश्रुतः

सर्पवृश्चिककूष्माण्डविकृताकृतयश्च ये ।
गर्भा एवंविधाश्चान्ये ज्ञेयाः पापकृतो भृशम् ॥१६१॥
गर्भो वातप्रकोपेण दौहृदे वाऽवमानिते ।
भवेत् कुब्जः कुणिः पङ्गुर्मूको मिन्मिण एव वा ॥१६२॥ 127

[सुश्रुत : शारीर२:५०-५१]

According to Suśruta

As a result of serious types of sinful acts, the foetus takes the shape of a snake, a scorpion, a *kūṣmāṇḍa* (pumpkin) or such other types of morbid shapes. If there is aggravation of *vāyu* in the foetus and if proper regimens are not given during the bi-cardiac stage of the mother then the child becomes *kubja* (hunch back), *kuṇi* (deformity of limbs), *paṅgu* (inability to move), *mūka* (dumb) and *minmina* (speaking indistinctly through the nose).

"उत्तुशशिरवयः सत्वं रजः शितमोज्ञौतर्कशितभौमो एतैंतरान्मनः स्वा प्रकृति प्रयच्छतिरसन्वरजशा मया । यस्यांशे भास्करस्तादृक् वलिनासदृशा मूर्त्तिः बुद्धा चा जातिकुलदेशान् । इति सारावल्याम् ।"

[There are many mistakes in this paragraph, hence not translated]

मार्कण्डेयपुराणात्

नारिकेलीफलं यद्वत्सकोशं वृद्धिमृच्छति ।

तद्वत्प्रयात्यसौ वृद्धि सकोशोऽधोमुखस्थितः ॥१६३॥

According to Mārkaṇḍeya Purāṇa

As a fruit of coconut grows with its outer shell (*kośa*), similarly, the embryo grows inside a *kośa* (amniotic membrane). The embryo remains inside this amniotic membrane with its face downwards.

ग्रन्थान्तरात् सुश्रुताच्च

'कललं चैकरात्रेण पञ्चरात्रेण बुद्बुदम् ।
शोणितं दशरात्रेण मांसपेशी चतुर्दशे ॥१६४॥
घनो मासे द्वितीये च पंचधा संप्ररोहति ।
शिरोंसं सक्थिनी वाहू वाय्वग्निसमुदीरितम् ॥१६५॥
मासे तृतीये युगपत्सर्वाङ्गावयवोद्भवः ।
तस्मिन्नेव तृतीये तु नाभ्यां नाडी प्रवर्त्तते ।
यथा' सम्पोष्यते गर्भः केदार इव कुल्यया ॥१६६॥ [128]

From other Medical Texts and According to Suśruta

Within one night of the conception there is *kalala* (jelly like formation). Within five nights it takes the shape of *budbuda* (jelly having bubbles). Within ten nights it takes the shape of blood. In fourteen nights it takes the shape of a muscle. In two months, the embryo becomes compact and grows in five different directions. During this period, because of the effect of *vāyu* and *agni*, the head, sheulder, lower limbs and the upper limbs are formed. In the third month, all the limbs and the organs of the body appear simultaneously. During this third month, the umbilical chord appears in the umbilicus of the foetus. It is with the help of this umbilical chord that the foetus gets nourishment as a field gets irrigated by the canals.

वृद्धात्रेयात्

नाडी चाप्यायनी नाम नाभ्यां तस्य निबध्यते ।
स्त्रीणां तथोरुदेशे सा निवद्धा चैव जायते ॥१६७॥

चतुर्विधान्नपानोत्थो रसस्तस्याप्ययानुगः ।
गर्भं संपोषयेन्नित्यं तेन वृद्धिर्भवेद्ध्रुवम् ।
यावन्ननाडी संभवति तावद्वृद्धिः कथं भवेत् ॥१६८॥

According to Vṛdhātreya

The umbilical chord which is known as "*āpyāyani*" (which provides nourishment) gets connected to the umbilicus of the foetus. This chord also gets connected to the *uru* (thighs or lower abdomen) of the woman. The *rasa* which is produced out of the four types of eatables in the woman passes through this chord for the nourishment of the foetus. This results in the growth of the foetus. The question that may arise here is how the nourishment of the foetus takes place before this chord appears ?

[The reply is not furnished. Perhaps the quotation is incomplete because of the callgraphic omission.]

[मासानुमासिकगर्भाकारः तथा वृद्धिः]

तत्राह

वापनार्थे धान्यबीजं भाण्डस्थं जलसेचनात् ।
129
साध्यांकुरक्रमं प्राप्य पश्चात् क्षेत्रादियोगतः ॥१६९॥

यथा स्वरूपमाप्नोति तथा कालेन गर्भगः ।
130
तृतीयमासजा भावाश्चतुर्थे चाल्पबुद्धयः ॥१७०॥

आमपक्वाशयौ बस्तिकुक्षिवृक्कौयकृद्गुदम् ।
प्लीहान्त्रहृदयं चास्य जायते मासि पञ्चमे ॥१७१॥

द्विहृदा तु भवेत्तत्र तस्माद्दौहृदिनी भवेत् ।

131

दापयेत् वांछितं चास्यै तस्याः श्रद्धां न हापयेत् ॥१७२॥

मूकं वा मिन्मिनं यस्माज्जनयेद्विकृताकृतिम् ।

षष्ठे रसवहानाड्यो जायन्ते हृदि संस्थिताः ॥१७३॥

Growth of the Embryo-Month-wise

It is said in this connection

The seeds of corns and grains which are kept for sowing in a jar get germinated by the sprinkling of water. Thereafter, when placed (sown) on the ground, they acquire the shape of the plant Similarly, the embryo grows in appropriate time and gets endowed with the characteristics of the third month. During the fourth month there is slight development of intellect. During the fifth month *āmāśaya* (stomach), *pakvāśaya* (colon), *vasti* (urinary bladder), *kukṣi* (pelvis), *vṛkkau* (kidneys), *yakṛt* (liver), *guda* (rectum), *plīhan* (spleen), *antra* (small intestine) and *hṛdaya* (heart) appear in the embryo. During this month, the pregnant woman possesses two hearts—one of her own and the second of the foetus. Therefore, she is called *dauhṛdinī* (having two hearts). Whatever she desires during this period should be provided to her and her desires should not be denied. If her desires are not satisfied then she procreates *mūka* (dumb), *minmina* (speaking indistinctly through nose) and malformed child. During these six months vessels carrying *rasa* (plasma) appear in the heart of the embryo.

अत्र पाराशरः

कर्णौ तु भवतश्छिद्रौ षण्मासाभ्यन्तरेण हि ।

शिरा स्नाय्वस्थिपर्वाणी केशरोमनखत्वचः ॥१७४॥

सप्तमे मासि जायन्ते चेतना चास्य वर्धते ।
सम्प्राप्ते चाष्टमे मासे मैथुनं परिवर्जयेत् ॥१७५॥
यदि गच्छति दुर्मेधा काममोहादचेतनः ।
विपद्यते तदागर्भः पतते चात्र नान्यथा ॥१७६॥

According to Pārāśara

During the sixth month, holes appear in the ears of the embryo. During the seventh month vessels, ligaments, bones, phalanges, hair in head, small hairs, nail and skin appear in the embryo. The embryo becomes more conscious during this month. When the eighth month is reached, sexual intercourse should not be performed. If because of ignorance, cohabitation is performed because of passionate desire by an unwise person, the foetus gets afflicted and there will be miscarriage. The foetus will not survive by such act of cohabitation.

आत्रेयात्

सप्तधातुभवः सारश्चाष्टमे हृदयं प्रति ।
[132] 'समायाति ततो बालः कृष्णश्यामसमेचकः ।'
संभवेद्धातुपाकत्वात्तत्र जातो न जीवति ॥१७७॥

According to Ātreya

The *ojas* which is the essence of seven categories of tissue elements migrates to the heart of the foetus. As a result of this, the child becomes *kṛṣṇa* (black), *śyāma* (bluish black) or *mecaka* (greasy black). All these happen as a result of *dhātu pāka* (metabolic transformation of tissue elements). The foetus born during this period does not survive.

सुश्रुतः

133
'अष्टमेऽस्थिरी भवत्योजः, तत्र जातश्चेन्न जीवेन्निरोज-

स्त्वान्नैर्ऋतभागत्वाच्च, ततो बलिं मांसौदनमस्मै दापयेत् ॥१७८॥

[सुश्रुत : शारीर३:३०]

According to Suśruta

During the eighth month of pregnancy, there is unstability in the *ojas*. If there is delivery during this period, the child does not survive because of the absence of *ojas* in it and also because of the affliction from the *nairṛta* (south-west direction). Therefore, in suc, events *bali* (sacrificial offerings) of *māṁsaudana* (a food preparation in which meat and rice are cooked together) should be offered.

134
'एकाहे विनिवृत्ते तु यस्तु मासेऽष्टमे शिशुः ।

135
नवमे दशमे वापि जायते निरुपद्रवः ॥१७९॥'

Even one day after the eighth month i.e. in the ninth month or during the tenth month of pregnancy, the normal delivery takes place without any complication.

136
वसिष्ठः

अथवा नवमे मासे परिपक्वः स जायते ।

दशमे मासि सम्प्राप्ते घृणिस्तस्योपजायते ॥१८०॥

137
अकीर्त्ति नरकं ह्येतद्विण्मूत्रस्योपसेविनाम् ।

यदि दैवाद्वहिर्यामि स्मरामि मधुसूदनम् ॥१८१॥

यथात्र पुनरावेशं न प्राप्नोमि कदाचन ।

वर्षैकं वा द्विवर्षं वा वर्षत्रयमथापि वा ।

संतिष्ठते कर्मफलं भुक्त्वा पश्चाच्च निष्क्रमेत् ॥१८२॥

According to Vaśiṣṭha

During the ninth month of pregnancy, the foetus gets matured. During the tenth month the foetus develops *ghṛṇi* (hateful disposition). He feels the residence in the mother's womb as the placement in the hell because of the presence of stool and urine there. He feels, "if I get a chance to get out of it then I shall pray lord Madhusūdana so that I shall never be required to come to the mother's womb, again". In this condition the foetus might remain inside the womb for one, two or even three years experiencing *karma phala* (the results of the past actions), and thereafter, it comes out of the womb.

तत्र चतुर्थमासमारभ्य गुरुगात्रताकार्श्यतापादशोफच्छर्दिबलवर्णहानिक्लान्तमना भवति गर्भिणी । तत्कस्य हेतोः? ॥१८३॥

What is the reason for the appearance of signs and symptoms like heaviness in the body, emaciation, oedema in feet, vomiting, loss of strength and complexion and prostration from fourth month onwards in the pregnant woman ?

तत्र आत्रेयः

गर्भेणोत्पीडिता दोषास्तस्मिन्हृदयमाश्रिताः ॥१८४॥

According to Ātreya

Doṣas located in the heart get pressed by the foetus to produce such signs and symptoms.

138

विदाहलक्षणम् कृष्णात्रेयाल्लिख्यते

पाणिपादांसमूलेषु विविधश्चातिजायते

संतापास्त्वथ खल्ली च विदाह प्रोच्यते बुधैः ॥१८५॥

Vidāha according to Kṛṣṇātreya

Excess of *santāpa* (heating sensation) and *khalli* (cramps) in the hands, legs and shoulder joint is called *vidāha* by the Wise-man.

आत्रेयः

कण्ड्वादिवूपशान्त्यर्थं नवनीतं हितं मतम् ।

139

अन्तर्दाहेश्चोपयोगः कट्वम्लमधुरौषधैः ॥१८६॥

सिद्धं तथाम्ललवणं भोजनं चापि दापयेत् ।

According to Ātreya

Navanita (butter) should be used for the alleviation of itching etc. In *antardāha* (burning sensation inside the body) butter should be used after boiling with pungent, sour and sweet drugs. In this condition, food ingredients having sour and saline tastes are useful.

कंडू विदाहं छर्दि च हृल्लासं श्वयथुं तथा ।

140

जृम्भां प्रसेकं कुर्वन्ति विदाहेन पचत्यपि ॥१८७॥

During this period signs and symptoms like itching, burning sensation, vomiting, nausea, oedema, yawning and salivation appear in the pregnant woman and there is burning sensation during the digestion of food.

अग्निवेशः

141

'चतुर्थे मासि स्थिरत्वमापद्यते गर्भः ।' पञ्चमे मासि गर्भस्य मांसशोणितं षष्ठमासे

142

स्थिरत्वमापद्यते गर्भः । तस्मात्तदा गर्भिणी गुरुगात्रत्वमापद्यते ॥१८८॥

According to Agniveśa

During the fourth month there is stability in the foetus. During the fifth month flesh and blood appear in the embryo. During the sixth month there is again stability in the foetus. Therefore, since that period, there is heaviness in the body of the pregnant woman.

कृष्णात्रेयः

चतुर्थे मासि गर्भस्य केशाः जायन्ते ।

तस्माच्छर्दिर्जायते ॥१८९॥

According to Kṛṣṇātreya

During the fourth month, hair appears in the foetus. There fore, there will be vomiting in the pregnant woman.

माहेन्द्रवारुणाध्याये सत्त्वाश्चात्र प्रकीर्तिताः ।

तस्मिन्मध्ये गर्भगस्य येन सत्त्वमयः पुमान् ॥१९०॥

तदात्मके[143] च तत्सत्त्वं द्रव्यं काङ्क्षति[144] गुर्विणी ।

येन येन हि मासेन यद्यत्कांक्षति[145] गुर्विणी ॥१९१॥

न प्राप्नोति यदा[146] तत्र शक्यरूपं[147] तदा शृणु ।

स[148] स भागः शिशोस्तस्य गर्भस्थस्य प्रपीड्यते ॥१९२॥

In the chapter entitled *Māhendravāruṇa* (*of the Kṛṣṇātreya tantra*), different types of *sattvās* (psychic disposition) are described. The foetus inside the womb possess one such *sattva* (mental faculty) and in accordance with the characteristic features of this *sattva* the enciente desires for different types of things. If the pregnant woman does not get the things which she desires in different months, then the respective organ (which has relationship with the thing desired) of the child gets afflicted.

अग्निवेशात्

'पञ्चमे मासि गर्भस्य मांसशोणितोपचयो[149] भवन्त्यन्येभ्यो मासेभ्यः तस्मात्तदा गर्भिणी कार्श्यमापद्यते विशेषेण। षष्ठे मासि गर्भस्य बलवर्णोपचयो भवत्यधिकमन्येभ्यो मासेभ्यः, तस्मात्तदा गर्भिणी बलवर्णहानिमापद्यते विशेषेण। सप्तमे मासि गर्भः सर्वैर्भावैराप्याय्यते, तस्मात्तदा गर्भिणी सर्वाकारैः क्लान्ततमा भवतीति ॥१६३॥

[चरक : शारीर४:२१-२३]

According to Agniveśa

In comparison to other months, during the fifth month of pregnancy, the foetus will have more of flesh and blood. Therefore, the pregnant woman becomes excessively emaciated during this period. During the sixth month, the foetus gets more of strength and complexion in comparison to other months. Therefore, at that time there will be excessive diminution of the strength and complexion of the pregnant woman. During the seventh month, the foetus gets nourished from all the aspects. Therefore, at that time, the pregnant woman becomes extremely exhausted in all forms.

'अगण्यमष्टमं मासं प्रवदन्ति मुनीश्वराः ।
तस्मान्न गणना कार्या गर्भस्यात्र[150] कदाचन ॥१६४॥

The great sages instruct against counting the eighth month. Therefore, this month of pregnancy should never be counted.

यदि काङ्क्षास्याद्गौरश्यामं लोहिताक्षं दीर्घबाहुं[151] पुत्रं जनयितुम्,[152] तदा लोहित-

कुक्कुटरसेन रक्तशाल्योदनमुपहितं भोजयेत्[153] । "दौहृदिनी सा तथैव[154] पुत्रं[155] जनयति । यदिचेदिच्छास्या कृष्णं वहलकेशं शुक्लदन्तं विस्तीर्णवक्षं जनयितुम्, सा कृष्णतिल-तैलेन कृष्णकुक्कुटरसेन भोजयेत्, दौहृदिनी कृष्णवस्त्रपरीधाना सा तु तथैव जनयति । एवं यद्रूपाणां[156] जनपदानां सदृशं सुतमिच्छेत् तेषां वेशभूषणाहारोपचारा-निप्सितान् सेवमाना दौहृदिनी तादृशं पुत्रं जनयति । यद्येवमिच्छा स्यात् विशालनेत्रहृदयं लोमशं पुत्रं जनयितुं, तदा माषसूपौदनेन तिलतैलौदनमिश्रं रसौदनं दापयेत्[157] ॥१६५॥"

If the parents desire to have a son having white or bluish black complexion, red eyes and long arms, then the mother should take red variety of *śāli* rice mixed with the meat soup of red cock. If during the bicardiac stage, the pregnant woman desires of such things then she will give birth to a child having the above mentioned characteristic features. If they have the desire to procreate a child having black colour, thick hair, white teeth and wide chest, then the mother should take food mixed with the oil of the black variety of *tila* (sesamum seed) or mixed with the meat soup of black cock. If during the bicardiac stage the woman wants to wear black cloth, then she will give birth to a child having the above mentioned characteristic features.

Similarly, the parents may like to have children resembling the inhabitants of different other countries. To achieve that purpose, the pregnant woman, during her bicardiac state, should wear the dress and ornaments, take the food and follow the regimens liked by those people.

If they desire to have a child having big eyes and heart and a hairy child, then the pregnant woman should eat rice mixed with the soup of *māṣa* or rice mixed with til oil or rice mixed with meat soup.

अथ सुश्रुतः

राजसंदर्शने यस्या[158] गर्भे श्रद्धा च जायते ।
अर्थवन्तं महाभागं कुमारं सा प्रसूयते ॥१६६॥

According to Suśruta

If a pregnant woman longs to see the king, then she will deliver a child endowed with great wealth and fortunes.

दुकूलपट्टकौशेयभूषणादिषु दौहृदात् ।
अलङ्कारैषिणं[159] पुत्रं ललितं सा प्रसूयते ॥१६७॥

[सुश्रुत : शारीर३:२२-२३]

If during the bicardiac state, the pregnant woman longs to have silken *paṭṭa* or wollen cloth or ornaments, then she will deliver a child who will also like to wear ornaments and to lead a luxurious (*lalita*) life.

देवताप्रतिमायां तु प्रसूते पार्षदोपमम् ।

[सुश्रुत : शारीर३:२४]

दर्शने व्यालजातीनां हिंसाशीलं प्रसूयते[160] ॥१६८॥

[सुश्रुत : शारीर३:२४]

आश्रमे संयतात्मानं धर्मशीलं[161] प्रसूयते ।

[सुश्रुत : शारीर३:२४]

गवां[162] मांसेन बलिनं सर्वक्लेशसहं सुतम्[163] ॥१६९॥

शारीर३:२५]

[164]वाराहमांसे स्वप्नालुं शूरं [165]च जनयेत्सुतम् ।
[166]मार्गाद्विक्रान्तजङ्घालं सदा वनचरं सुतम् ।
सृमराद्विघ्नमनसं [167]नित्यभीतं च तैत्तिरात् ॥२००॥

[सुश्रुत : शारीर३:२६-२७]

If she longs for the idol of the gods, then she will deliver a child who will have the characteristics of the members of the royal court. If she longs to see wild animals then she will deliver a child who will be addicted to violence. If she longs to see a disciplined saint in a hermitage then she will deliver a religious child. If she longs for beef, then she will deliver a child who will be very strong and be able to face hardships. If she longs for pork then she will deliver a child who will be sleepy (indolent) but brave. If she longs for the meat of deer, then she will deliver a child who will walk very fast, who will have strong calf muscles and who will be a forest dweller. If she longs to take the meat of *sṛmara* (a type of deer) then she will deliver a child having an anxious mind. If she longs to take the meat of *tittiri* bird then she will deliver a child who will be eternally fearful.

आत्रेयात्

पूप-पायस-पक्कान्न-दौहृदात्सुभगं सुतम् ।
प्रसूते मत्स्यकांक्षातः शुक्राढ्यं [168]श्लेष्मलं सुतम् ॥२०१॥

According to Ātreya

If the pregnant woman during her bicardiac state longs for *pūpa* (pastry), *pāyasa* (milk preparation) and *pakvānna* (fried food), then she will deliver a child who will be endowed with good fortunes. If she longs for fish during the bicardiac state, then she will deliver a child who will have excess of semen and *kapha*.

प्रजागरं दिवास्वापं कठिनासनसेविनम्[169] ।

विषमाः सर्वशश्चेष्टाः क्रोधेर्ष्या शोचनं भयम् ॥२०२॥

श्रमोपवासावत्यन्नं क्षुत्तृष्णासम्प्रधारणम् ।

अतिव्यवायं व्यायामं भारं प्रावरणं गुरुम् ॥२०३॥

संक्षोभितान्नं पानं च [170]श्रद्धावेगविधारणम् ।

तीक्ष्णोष्णं गुरुविष्टम्भि गर्भिणी परिवर्जयेत् ।

एभिर्वा च्यवते गर्भः शुष्येत् कुक्षौ म्रियेत वा ॥२०४॥

The pregnant woman should avoid the following :

1. Remaining awake at night;
2. Sleep during day time;
3. Sitting in a hard seat;
4. All the irregular postures of the body;
5. Anger, envy, worry, fear, exhaustion, fasting and intake of food in large quantity;
6. Suppression of the urges for food (hunger) and drink (thirst);
7. Excessive sexual intercourse;
8. Exercise and covering the body with heavy cloth;
9. Irritating food and drinks;
10. Suppression of the urge for liking a thing; and
11. Things which are sharp, hot, heavy and *viṣṭambhi* (wind forming in the colon).

If the pregnant woman resorts to the above mentioned things, then they may cause abortion, emaciation of the foetus or its death.

अग्निवेशात्

मद्यपानात्पिपासालुं निःसत्त्वं जनयेत्सुतम् ।
व्यवायनित्यान्निर्ह्रीका स्वल्पायुर्वा भवेत्ततः ।।२०५।।

स्वप्ननित्याल्पवाग्बुद्धि तन्द्रिणं लभते सुतम् ।
रात्रौ जागरणप्राया जागरूकं कृशाबलम् ।।२०६।।

शोकनित्या विरूपं तु कृशमल्पबलायुषम् ।
अमर्षणा[171]दौषधानां क्रुद्धं चण्डमसूयकम् ।।२०७।।

अभि[172]त्वात्बहुलाद्वीर्यं तेन मन्यीपतापिनम् ।
[173]वह्वायासाद्द्रोहशीलं भवेदात्मक्रियालसम् ।।२०८।।

उन्मत्तं जनयेन्नारी नग्नानावृतचारिणी ।
गर्भिणी कलहप्राया सूतेऽपस्मारिणं सुतम् ।।२०९।।

[174]बहुविप्लुतचित्तं तु [175]शीतपर्युषिताशिनी ।
गोधामांसाशनप्राया शर्कराश्मरिरोगिणम् ।।२१०।।

छागाशिनी द्विमूर्धानं माषप्राया श्वसिज्जनम् ।
स्वादुनित्या कफव्याधिं स्थूलं मूकं प्रमेहिणम् ।।२११।।

अम्लनित्यास्त्रपित्ताक्षिकुष्ठवीसर्परोगिणम् ।
वलीपलितखालित्यं प्रचुरं [176]लवणाशिनी ।।२१२।।

कटुनित्याबलं मंदं शुक्रप्रजनमैथुनम् ।

तिक्तनित्यानिलात्मानं रूक्षं स्वल्पबलं सुतम् ॥२१३॥

कषायसेविनी कृत्स्नम् अ्रसृगानाहरोगिणम् ।

सिन्धु-शालूक[177]-पिंडालु-सेवनात्स्फोट[178]युक्त्वचः ॥२१४॥

येषां येषां तु रोगाणां हेतुः सेवेत गुर्विणी ।

भृशं तद्व्याधिभूयिष्ठमपत्यं जनयेद्ध्रुवम् ॥२१५॥

According to Agniveśa

The diet and regimen of the mother during pregnancy determine the characteristic features of the child as follows :

Diet and regimen of the mother during pregnancy	*Characteristic features of the child*
(1)	(2)
1. Intake of alcoholic drinks.	The child would become constantly thirsty and without any energy.
2. Habitual cohabitation.	The child will be shameless and it will have a short span of life.
3. Excessive sleep.	The child will have less power of speech; less of intellect and more of drowsiness.
4. Habitually remaining awake at night.	The child will also remain awake and it will be thin and weak.
5. Constant grief.	The child will be disfigured and weak. It will have a short span of life.
6. Jealousy.	The child will be of wrathful disposition, ferocious and envious.

(1)	(2)
7. Ego.	The child will have more of strength and will inflict miseries upon others.
8. Becoming tired in excess.	The child will be quarrelsome and lazy in performing its own duties.
9. Moving naked without any cloth on the body.	The child will be insane.
10. Constantly quarrelsome disposition.	The child will be epileptic.
11. Intake of cold and stale food.	The child will have excessively instability of mind.
12. Constantly taking of the meat of Iguana.	The child will suffer from *śarkarā* (gravels) and *aśmari* (stone) in the urinary tract.
13. Intake of the meat of the goat.	The child will have two heads.
14. Habitually taking of *māṣa*.	The child will be asthmatic.
15. Habitually taking of sweet things.	The child will suffer from diseases caused by *kapha*; it will be fatty, dumb and diabetic.
16. Habitually intake of sour things.	The child will suffer from *raktapitta* (a disease characterised by bleeding from different parts of the body), eye diseases, *kuṣṭha* (obstinate skin diseases, including leprosy) and *visarpa* (erysipelas).

(1)	(2)
17. Intake of salt in excess.	The child will suffer from premature wrinkling of the skin, premature greying of hair and baldness.
18. Habitual intake of pungent things.	The child will be weak. It will have less of semen, less eye sight and less power of sexual intercourse.
19. Habitual intake of bitter things.	The child will suffer from diseases of *vāyu*. It will have dry skin and there will be less of strength.
20. Intake of astringent things.	The child will suffer from diseases of blood and constipation.
21. Intake of *sindhu*, *śālūka* and *piṇḍālu*.	There will be eruptions in the skin of the child.

If the pregnant woman takes diet and regimen which are responsible for the manifestation of various diseases, then the child will certainly be afflicted with those diseases.

सुश्रुतः

यस्या दक्षिणभागस्य स्तने प्राक् क्षीरदर्शनम्[179] ।
दक्षिणाक्षिमहत्त्वं[180] च सक्थ्युत्कर्षति दक्षिणम् ॥२१६॥
अभिध्यायति बाहुल्यात्तुमान्नामेति दोहदम्[181] ।
स्वप्नेषु चोपलभते नलकुङ्[182]नलमम्बुजम्[183] ॥२१७॥

तथाम्रादीनि चान्यानि पुन्नामान्येवमादिकम् ।
प्रसन्नमुखवर्णं च सा प्रसूते ध्रुवं सुतम् ॥२१८॥

एतद्विपर्यये ब्रूयाज्जनयिस्यति कन्यकाम् ।

According to Suśruta

The following are the characteristic features of a pregnant woman who will deliver a male child :

1. The appearance of lactation first in the right breast;
2. Enlargement of the size of the right eye;
3. Prominence of the right thigh;
4. Thinking of a male child in excess during the bicardiac stage of the pregnancy;
5. Appearance of the flowers of *nala, kuṁnalu*, lotus and mango in dreams; and
6. Appearance of happiness in the face and freshness in the complexion.

The characteristic features which are opposite to ones stated above indicate that the pregnant woman will deliver female child.

पार्श्वद्वयोन्नतं यस्याः पुरस्तान्निम्नतोदरं ॥२१९॥

प्राग्लक्षणेन शून्यं च जनयेत्सा नपुंसकम्[184] ।'

If both the sides of the abdomen are bulging and if there is depression in the centre of the abdomen and if the signs and symptoms described above are absent, then she will deliver a eunuch.

मूत्रं[185] च मातृकं रक्तमांससेदोगुदादिकम् ॥२२०॥

पैतृकं तु स्थितं शुक्रं धमन्यस्थिकचादिकम् ।

Urine, blood, flesh, fat, rectum including anus etc., are derived from the mother. Semen, vessels, bones, hair etc., in the foetus are derived from the father.

यदा धमति वायुस्तु देहस्तेनास्य वर्धते ॥२२१॥

Because of the blowing of the *vāyu* there is growth in the body of the foetus.

शिरोग्रीवापाणिपादपार्श्वपृष्ठोदरं ह्युरः[186] ।

अष्टावङ्गानि चैतानि पार्थिवानि विदुर्बुधाः ॥२२२॥

Head, neck, hands, feet, sides of the chest, back, abdomen, front part of the chest—these are the eight *aṅgas* (important divisions) of the body. According to wise people, these *aṅgas* are dominated by *pṛthvī mahābhūta*.

नासाचिबुकमोष्ठौ च श्रवणाङ्गुष्ठकाङ्गुलिः ।

[187] पार्ष्णिगुल्फप्रभृतयः प्रत्यङ्गानीति सर्वशः ॥२२३॥

Nose, chin, lip, ear, fingers and toes, ankle, wrist etc., are called *pratyaṅgas* (minor parts of the body).

शाखाश्चतस्रो मध्यं च षष्ठं शिर इति स्मृतम् ।

षडङ्गं प्रोच्यते ह्यस्य प्रविस्तारोऽघुनोच्यते ॥२२४॥

The body is called *ṣaḍaṅga* (composed of six important parts). These are the four limbs, (two upper limbs and two lower limbs), trunk (including the chest and the abdomen) and head (including neck). Now, their details will be described.

[188] नाभिवृक्कयकृत्क्लोमप्लीह्नोरन्त्राशयादिषु ।

कोष्ठ इत्यभिधीयन्ते ऋषयः सौनकादयः ॥२२५॥

According to sages, namely Saunaka etc., *nābhi* (umbilicus) *vṛkka* (kidney), *yakṛt* (liver), *kloman* (pancreas ?), *plihā* (spleen), *antra* (intestine), *āśaya* (visceras) etc., taken together are called *koṣṭha.*

रक्तमेदः प्रसादेन वृक्कः[189] संजायते ध्रुवम् ।
वृषणौ तु प्रसादेन मेदो मांसकफास्रजम् ॥२२६॥
कफशोणितयोश्चापि प्रसादो हृदयं स्मृतम् ।
तदाश्रयाश्चतुर्विंशधमनी रसवाहिनी[190] ॥२२७॥
तस्याधो वामतः प्लीहा दक्षिणे क्लोममुच्यते ।
[191]'सुषिरं स्यावधोवक्त्रं यकृत्प्लीहान्तरस्थितम् ।'
[192]'तत्रैव यकृतं विद्याद्धृदयं[193] चेतनं स्मृतम्' ॥२२८॥

Vṛkka (kidney) is certainly produced from the essence of the blood and the fat. The testicles are produced from the essence of the fat, muscle tissue, *kapha* and blood. *Hṛdaya* (heart) is produced of the essence of *kapha* and *śoṇita.* To this heart are attached 24 vessels which carry *rasa* (plasma). Below the heart towards the left side, *plihā* is located. Below this heart towards the right side *kloman* is located. Heart is having empty space inside it. It is curved downwards and it is located between the liver and the spleen. The *yakṛt* (liver) is located there. The heart is also called *cetanā* (seat of consciousness).

[194]'रत्नाकरात्

प्रसन्नाभ्यां कफासृग्भ्यां हृदयं पंकजाकृतिः ।
सुषिरं स्यादधोवक्त्रं[195] यकृत्प्लीहांतर[196]स्थितम्[197] ॥२२९॥

एतच्च चेतनास्थानं तदस्मिंस्तमसावृते ।
निमीलति स्वपित्यात्मा जाग्रत्यस्मिन्विकसत्यपि ॥२३०॥

According to Ratnākara

Hṛdaya is the product of the essence of *kapha* and *asṛk*. It is lotus like in shape. It has empty space inside and it faces downwards. It is located between the *yakṛt* (liver) and *plihan* (spleen). It is the location of consciousness. It gets closed when it becomes covered by *tamas* and when the person (*ātmā* = lit. Soul) sleeps. When the person gets awakened, it opens (blossoms). [reference *śloka* no. 228].

द्विधा[198] स्वप्नसुषुप्तिभ्यां[199] स्वापो बाह्येन्द्रियाणि चेत् ।
लीयन्ते[200] हृदि जाग्रन्ति चित्तं[201] स्वप्नस्तदुच्यते ।
मनश्चेल्लीयते प्राणे सुषुप्तिः स्यात्तदात्मनः[202] ॥२३१॥

Svāpa (sleep) is of two types viz., *svapna* (light sleep) and *suṣupti* (deep sleep). When the external senses get submerged in the heart while the *citta* (mind) is still awake (active), it is called the state of *svapna*. If the mind gets submerged in the *prāṇa* (elan vital), then it is called the state of *suṣupti*.

सर्वाङ्गसुन्दरात्

समानवायुः प्रध्मातादक्ताद्देहोष्मपाचितात् ।
किञ्चिदुच्छ्रितरूपस्तु जायते क्लोमसंज्ञितः ।
तत्तुल्यहेतुजे प्लीहयकृती भिषजां मते ॥२३२॥

[सर्वाङ्गसुन्दरी टीकाः अष्टाङ्गहृदय : शारीर ३:१२]

According to Sarvāṅga sundara

Rakta, impelled by *samāna vāyu*, undergoes *pāka* (metabolic transformation) and becomes slightly swollen which is called *kloman.* According to physicians, *plihan* (spleen) and *yakṛt* (liver) are also produced in the same manner.

पाराशरात्

प्राणिनां तु यकृत्प्लीह्नौ शोणितात्प्रभवौ मतौ ।
शोणितप्रभवफेनः तस्माज्जातो हि फुप्फुसः ।।२३३।।
यस्तु शोणितजः किट्टस्तस्मात्क्लोमं च जायते ।
मेदःशोणितसम्भूतं कोष्ठे अन्त्रं[203] प्रजायते ।।२३४।।
सार्ध-त्रिव्याम-मात्राणि पुरुषाणां हि तानि च ।
स्त्रीणां त्रिव्याममात्राणि अन्त्राणि मुनयो विदुः ।।२३५।।
[204]व्यामो वाह्वोः सकरयोः तिर्यगन्तरं इत्यर्थः[205] ।।२३६।।

According to Pārāśara

Yakṛt (liver) and *plihan* (spleen) in the human beings are produced from out of blood. The foam that comes out of the blood produces *phupphusa* (lungs). *Kloman* is made of the *kiṭṭa* (waste product or excreta) of the blood. The intestine in the *koṣṭha* (gastro-intestinal tract) is made of the fat and the blood. In males the size of the intestine is 3 1/2 *vyāma* (one *vyāma* = 182.88 cm.). In females the size of the intestine is 3 *vyāmas.* When the arms and hands are kept laterally extended in both the sides, then the distance from the tip of the finger of the one hand to the other is called *vyāma.*

अथ सुश्रुतः

उदरे पच्यमानानां[206] धातूनां द्रुमसारवत् ।
कफशोणितमांसानां साराज्जिह्वा प्रजायते ।।२३७।।

[सुश्रुत : शारीर४:२७-२८]

According to Suśruta

Like the heart-wood of a tree, tongue is the product of the essence of the *kapha*, *śoṇita* and *māṁsa dhātus*, metabolised in the stomach.

हरिश्चन्द्रात्

उदानवायोराधारः फुफ्फुसः प्रोच्यते बुधैः ।

207 208
रक्तवाहि शिरामूलं तथा प्रोक्तं महर्षिणा ॥२३८॥

According to Hariścandra

Phuphusa (lungs) is the substratum of *udāna vāyu*. According to the great sages, this is the *mūla* (source of origin) of the channels of circulation of blood.

यकृद्रंजकपित्तस्य स्थानं रक्तस्य संश्रयः ।

जलवाहिशिरामूलं तृष्णाच्छादनकं तिलम् ॥२३९॥

Yakṛt (liver) is the location of *rañjaka* type of *pitta* and it is the substratum of the blood.

Tila (?) is the source of origin of the channels of circulation of water in the body and it regulates thirst.

209
ज्ञेयो पुष्टिकरौ वृक्कौ मुष्कौ पुंभावसंभवौ ।

श्लेष्माशयः स्यादुरसि तस्मादामाशयस्त्वधः ॥२४०॥

Both the *vṛkkas* (kidneys) help in the nourishment of the body. Both the *muṣkas* (testicles) are responsible for the manifestation of the masculine features in the body. The *śleṣmāśaya* (viscera for the storage of *kapha*) is located in the chest. Below that is located the *āmāśaya* (the stomach where the food is stored before digestion).

210
'ऊर्ध्वमग्न्याशयो नाभेर्वामभागे व्यवस्थितः ।'

तस्योपरि तिलं[211] ज्ञेयं तदधः पवनाशयः ॥२४१॥

मलाशयस्त्वधस्तस्माद्बस्तिर्मूत्राशयः स्मृतः ।

जीवरक्ताश्रयमुरो[212] ज्ञेयाः सप्ताशयास्त्वमी ॥२४२॥

पुरुषेभ्योऽधिकाश्चान्ये नारीणामाशयास्त्रयः ।

धारा गर्भाशयः प्रोक्तः स्तनौ स्तन्याशयौ मतौ ।

'धात्वाशयान्तरस्था या मर्यादा सा कला विदुः[213] ॥२४३॥

Above the stomach and towards the left side of the umbilicus, *agnyāśaya* (?) is located. *Tila* (?) is located above the *agnyāśaya*. *Pavanāśaya* (colon ?) is located below the *tila*. *Malāśaya* (rectum) and *basti* (urinary bladder) which latter is the *mūtrāśaya* (organ for the storage of urine) are located below the *pavanāśaya*. *Uras* (chest) is the *āśaya* (organ for storage) of *jīva rakta* (blood which is responsible for life). These are the seven *āśayas* (organs for storage) in *males*. In females there are three more *āśayas*. These are the *dhārā* (uterus) which is *garbhāśaya* (bed of the foetus) and the two breasts which are the *stanyāśayas* (organs for the storage of breast milk).

The limiting membrane between the *dhātus* (tissue elements or contained material) and the *āśaya* (organ for storage) is called *kalā*.

वृद्धवाहडः

'धात्वाशयान्तरे तस्य यः क्लेदस्त्वधितिष्ठति ।

देहोष्मणा विपक्वो यः सा कलेत्यभिधीयते[214] ॥२४४॥'

According to Vṛddha vāhaḍa

The *kleda* (sticky material) which is located between the *dhātus* and the *āśayas* undergoes *pāka* (metabolic transformation) by the *dehoṣmā* (a group of enzymes of the body) and this is called *kalā*.

सप्तकला भवन्ति

प्रथमा मांसधरा, यस्या मांसे सिरास्नायुधमनीस्रोतसां प्रतानानि[215] भवन्ति ।।२४५।।

[सुश्रुत : शारीर४:८]

Seven varieties of Kalā

The first variety is called *māṁsa dharā kalā* because of which there are branches of channels like *sirās* (veins), *snāyus* (ligaments or nerves) and *dhamanis* (arteries) in the muscles.

यथा विसमृणालानि विवर्धन्ते समन्ततः ।

भूमौ पङ्कोदकस्थानि तथा मांसे सिरादयः ।।२४६।।

[सुश्रुत : शारीर४:६]

As stalks and stems of lotus grow in different directions with their base in the ground which is made of mud and water, similarly, vessels etc., pervade the muscles.

मेदसः स्नेहमादाय सिरास्नायुत्वमाप्नुयात् ।

सिराणां तु मृदुः[216] पाकः स्नायूनां च ततः[217] खरः ।।२४७।।

[सुश्रुत : शारीर४:२९-३०]

Sirās (vessels) and *snāyus* (ligaments and nerves) are formed out of the unctuous fraction of the *medas* (fat). *Sirās* are produced as a result of mild *pāka* (cooking) and *snāyus* are produced by *khara pāka* (lit. over cooking).

द्वितीया[218] रक्तधरा । ननु रसानन्तरं रक्तं ततो मांसं श्रूयते । अत्र कथं प्रागेव न

रक्तधरा उक्ता ? तत्रोच्यते रसाद्रक्तं [219] ततो मांसादि क्रमोऽयं पोषणे न तु धारणे । [220]

धारणार्थे कलानिर्दिष्टा, रक्तधराकलामांसाभ्यन्तरे तिष्ठति [221] ॥२४८॥

The second variety is called *rakta dharā kalā*. The question that may arise here is: as to why *rakta dharā kalā* has not been described before the description of *māṁsa dharā kalā*? It would have been appropriate because *rakta dhātu* precedes the *māṁsa dhātu* in the order of enumeration. This is not correct in the present context. The order of enumeration of *rasa*, *rakta* and *māṁsa* relates to the order of nourishment (*poṣaṇa*) of these *dhātus*. This order does not hold good in the matter of *dhāraṇa* (sustaining the body). *Kalās* are meant for the sustenance of the body. The *rakta dharā kalā* is located inside the muscles. Therefore, it is described after the description of *māṁsa dharā kalā*.

तत्र सुश्रुतः

वृक्षाद्यथाभिप्रहतात् [222] क्षीरिणः क्षीरमावहेत् ।
मांसादेवं क्षतात् क्षिप्रं शोणितं संप्रसिच्यते [223] ॥२४९॥

[सुश्रुत : शारीर४:११]

According to Suśruta

When a milky tree is injured or cut, the milky latex comes out of it. Similarly, when there is an injury or a cut in the muscle, blood comes out of it instantaneously.

तृतीया मेदोधरा, मेदो हि सर्वभूतानामुदरस्थमण्वस्थिषु च, महत्सु च मज्जा भवति ।

अल्पास्थिषु तनु मेदः अस्थ्नामन्तर्भवति ॥२५०॥

[सुश्रुत : शारीर४:१२]

The third variety is called *medodharā kalā.* In all living beings *medas* is located in the abdomen and small bones. The bigger bones carry *majjā* (marrow) inside it. Inside the small bones, soft type of *medas* (fat) is located.

तथा च

'स्थूलास्थिषु विशेषेण मज्जा त्वभ्यन्तरे भवेत्[224] ।

अथेतरेषु[225] सर्वेषु[226] सरक्तं मेद उच्यते ।

शुद्धमांसस्य[227] यः स्नेहः सा वसा परिकीर्तिता ध्रुवम् ॥२५१॥

[सुश्रुत : शारीर४:१३]

Majjā is specially located inside the big bones. Inside all the remaining bones, *medas,* which is red, is located.

The fatty substance of the pure form of muscle tissue is called *vasā.*

चतुर्थी श्लेष्मधरा, सा सर्वसन्धिषु संस्थिता ॥२५२॥

'स्नेहाभ्यक्ते यथा ह्यक्षे[228] चक्रं साधु प्रवर्तते ।

सन्धयः साधु वर्तन्ते संश्लिष्टाः श्लेष्मणा तथा ॥२५३॥

[सुश्रुत : शारीर४:१५]

The fourth variety is called *śleṣma dharā kalā.* It is located in all joints. A wheel moves properly if its axle is greased well. Similarly, the joints work effectively when the surfaces of the bones are well oleated with *śleṣmā* or *kapha.*

पञ्चमी पुरीषधरा । स उंदुकस्थं मलं विभजति । उंदुकः कोऽर्थः? पोटक[229] इत्यर्थः ॥२५४॥

The fifth variety is called *puriṣa dharā kalā.* It is located in the *unduka* (caecum). It helps in the separation of stool from the food particles. *Unduka* is also called *poṭaka*.

चरके[230]

यकृत्समन्तात् कोष्ठं च तथा नाभि[231] समाश्रिता ।

उन्दुकस्थं विभजते मलं मलधरा कला ॥२५५॥

[सुश्रुत : शारीर४:१७]

According to Caraka

The *mala dharā kalā*, located in the *unduka* is spread from the *yakṛt* (liver) through the *koṣṭha* (relevant portion of the gastro-intestinal tract) around the umbilicus. It is this *kalā* which separates the feces from the food particles.

'षष्ठी पित्तधरा नाम या कला परिकीर्तिता ।

पक्वामाशयमध्यस्था ग्रहणी सा प्रकीर्तिता[232] ॥२५६॥

[सुश्रुत : उत्तरतन्त्र४०:१६९]

The sixth variety is called *pitta dharā kalā*. It is located between the *pakvāśaya* (intestines) and *āmāśaya* (stomach). It is generally known as *grahaṇi*.

सप्तमी शुक्रधरा नाम,[233] सा प्राणिनां सर्वत्रव्यापिनी ।

[सुश्रुत : शारीर४:२०]

The seventh variety is called *śukra dharā kalā*. It pervades the entire body of the living beings.

स्त्रीणां दशकला ज्ञेया गर्भस्य स्तनयोस्तथा ॥२५७॥

Females have ten *kalās*. The additional three varieties of *kalās* are located in the uterus and the two breasts.

वसिष्ठः

[234] यवद्वयप्रमाणा च त्वक्संभूतिर्भवेदिह ।

क्षीरे संतानिका यद्वद्रम्भावल्कलवत्क्रमात् ॥२५८॥

Skin

According to Vasiṣṭha

The thickness of the skin is equal to the thickness of the two barley grains. It is like the *santānikā* (scum or cream) of the milk. As a banana tree is covered with its several layers of bark one after another, similarly the body is covered with several layers of skin one over the other.

[235] प्रथमाऽवभासिनी नाम, लसीकावारिधारिणी पद्मकंटकसिध्माऽधिष्ठानम्,

व्रीहेरष्टादशभागप्रमाणा । द्वितीया लोहितधरानाम[236] ज्ञेया, तिलकालकाधिष्ठाना,

व्रीहेः षोडशभागप्रमाणा ॥२५९॥

The first layer of the skin is called *avabhāsinī*. It carries *lasikā* (lymph) and *vāri* (water). Diseases like *padma kaṇṭaka* and *sidhma* are located in this layer. In thickness it is 1/18 th of a *brīhi*.

The second layer of the skin is called *lohita dharā*. Diseases like *tila kālaka* are located in this layer. In size it is 1/16th of a *brīhi*.

श्वेता तृतीया संख्याता स्थानं चर्मदलस्य[237] सा ।

ताम्रा चतुर्थी विज्ञेया किलासश्वित्रभूमिका ॥२६०॥

The third layer of the skin is called *śvetā*. The disease *carma dala* is located in this layer.

The fourth layer is called *tāmrā*. Diseases like *kilāsa* and *śvitra* are located in this layer.

पञ्चमी वेदिनी नाम, सा कुष्ठदद्रुगजचर्माधिष्ठाना, पंचभागप्रमाणा । षष्ठी [238]लोहितानीया, गलगण्डमालाबल्मीकश्लीपदाद्यधिष्ठाना, [239]ब्रीहिप्रमाणा । सप्तमी स्थूला मांसधरा सा, विद्रधीभगन्दरार्शो[ऽ]धिष्ठाना, ब्रीहिद्वयप्रमाणा ॥२६१॥

The fifth layer is called *vedinī*. Diseases like *kuṣṭha*, *dadru* and *gaja carma* are located in this layer. In size it is 1/5th of a *brīhi*.

The sixth layer is called *lohita*. Diseases like *gala gaṇḍa*, *gaṇḍa mālā*, *balmīka* and *ślīpada* etc. are located in this layer. In size it is like a *brīhi*.

The seventh layer which is very thick is called *māṁsa dharā*. Diseases like *vidradhi* (abscess), *bhagandara* (fistula-in-ano) and *arśas* (piles) are located in this layer. In size it is like two *brīhis* taken together.

अङ्गुष्ठोदरमाना च त्वचा उदरकण्ठयोः ॥२६२॥

The skin in *udara* (abdomen) and *kaṇṭha* (neck) is of the size of the thickness of *aṅguṣṭha* (thumb).

[240]‘श्रवणनयनगुदेन्द्रियवदनघ्राणोर्ध्वतालुदशरंध्राः समाख्याता वह्निर्मार्गानुसारिणः ।’
स्त्रीणां त्रयोदशः तथा । स्तनयोश्चासृक्स्रवश्च अधः ॥२६३॥

Randhra

There are ten *randhras* (external openings) in the body of males, namely, two ears, two eyes, anus, genital tract, mouth, two nostrils and *ūrdhva tālu* (opening in the anterior frontanalle).

Females have thirteen openings. The three additional openings are, the two openings of the breasts and the genital tract through which the menstrual blood flows.

[अस्थि]

'षष्ठित्रिशतमस्थीनि भाषन्ते वेदवादिनः ।

शल्यतन्त्रेषु त्रिण्येव शतानीति विदुर्बुधाः[241] ॥२६४॥

Bones

According to *veda vādis* (those who believe in the *vedas*) there are three hundred and sixty bones. According to surgical texts the number of bones is only three hundred.

तानि पञ्चविधानि; तद्यथाः

कपालरुचके चैव तरुणो वलयस्तथा ।

नलकश्चेति नामानि तेषां भेदा ह्यनेकशः ॥२६५॥

तत्र जानुनितम्बांसगलतालुशंखशिरःसु कपालानि । दशनास्तु रुचकाः । घ्राणकर्ण-

ग्रीवाक्षिकोशेषु तरुणानि । [242]'पादपृष्ठोदरोरःसु वलयानि । शेषाणि नलक-

[243]संज्ञकानि ॥२६६॥

These are of five varieties viz., *kapāla* (flat bones), *rucaka* (peg like bones), *taruṇa* (tender and thin bones), *valaya* (ring like bones) and *nalaka* (tube like elongated bones). These bones are of different types. *Kapāla* variety of bones are located in the *jānu* (knee joint), *nitaṁba* (hips), *aṁsa* (scapular region), *gala* (neck), *tālu* (palate), *śaṁkha* (temporal region) and *śiras* (head). *Rucaka* variety of bones are the teeth. *Taruṇa* variety of bones are located in the sockets of nose, ears, throat and eyes. *Valaya* variety of bones are located in the feet, back, abdomen and chest. All the remaining bones are of *nalaka* variety.

तत्र भोजः

हस्तपादाङ्गुलितले कूर्चे च मणिबन्धयोः ।

बाहुजङ्घाद्वये वापि जानीयान्नलकानि तु ॥२६७॥

According to Bhoja

Nalaka bones are located in hands, legs, fingers, toes, metaphalangeal and metatarsal regions, wrist and ankle joints, arms and thighs.

'सन्धयश्च द्विविधाश्चेष्टावन्तः, स्थिराश्च ये[244] ।

शाखासु हन्वोः कट्यां च चेष्टावन्तस्तु[245] सन्धयः ।

शेषास्तु सन्धयः सर्वे विज्ञेया स्यु स्थिरा बुधैः ॥२६८॥

[सुश्रुत : शारीर५:२४-२५]

Joints

Joints are of two varieties viz., *ceṣṭāvanta* (mobile) and *sthira* (immobile). The first variety of joints are located in the limbs, mandibles and hips. All the remaining joints belong to the latter variety.

[सन्धि]

संख्याताः सन्धयः सर्वैर्दशाधिकशतद्वयम् ।

अस्थ्नां[246] तु सन्धयो ह्येते केवलाः परिकीर्तिताः ॥२६९॥

पेशीस्नायुसिराणां च सन्धेः संख्या[247] न विद्यते ।

[सुश्रुत : शारीर५:२८]

According to all scholars, joints are two hundred and ten in number. This pertains to the number of joints of bones only. There are other joints of muscles, ligaments and vessels which are innumerable.

[248] ते चाष्टधा भवन्तीहि प्रोक्ता शल्यार्थपारगैः ॥२७०॥

तद्यथा

उदूखला मण्डलाश्च सामुद्गा लूनसेविनी[249] ।
शंखावर्त्ता प्रतरा च कोरा वायसतुण्डिका ॥२७१॥
कक्षावक्षोरुदन्तेषु ज्ञेया सन्धिरुदूखला ।
कण्ठहृन्नयनक्लोमनाडीष्वपि च मण्डला ।
नितंबांसे गुदे पीठे सामुद्गा चरणेषु च ॥२७२॥

समुद्गाः संपुटास्तदाकृतिर्भवाः सामुद्गाः ॥२७३॥

शिरः कटीकपालेषु भवेत्सा लूनसेविनी[250] ।
श्रोत्रे श्रृङ्गाटके चैव शंखावर्त्ता मता बुधैः ।
प्रातराश्च बुधैर्ज्ञेया ग्रीवायां पृष्ठवंशयोः ॥२७४॥

प्रतरो भल्लकः, तदाकृतयः प्रातराः ॥२७५॥

[251] 'मणिबन्धे गुल्फयोश्च कोराख्या जानुकूर्परे ॥२७६॥

कोरो नाम कर्णस्तदाकृतयः, कोरः कलिका तदाकृतयो वा ॥२७७॥

हन्वोरुभयतश्चैव मता वायसतुण्डिका ।"[252]
शिरास्नाय्वस्थिपर्वाणि सन्धयश्च शरीरिणाम् ।
पेशीभिः संवृतान्यत्र बलवन्ति भवन्त्यतः ॥२७८॥

[सुश्रुत : शारीर ५:३८]

The joints according to experts in surgery are of eight varieties, as follows :

1. *Udūkhala* (Ball & socket joint) : These are located in the axilla (shoulder), chest, thighs (hips) and teeth;

2. *Maṇḍala* : These are located in throat, cardiac region, eyes and *kloma nāḍi* (trachea);

3. *Sāmudga* : These are located in hip, shoulder, anal region and legs. They are called *sāmudga* because they are like *sampuṭa* (two vessels kept face to face and sealed);

4. *Lūna sevini* : These are located in the head and hips;

5. *Śaṅkhāvarta* : These are located in the ears and *śṛṅgāṭaka* (sphenoidal region);

6. *Prstara* : These are present in the neck and the vertebral column. *Pratara* means *bhallaka* (spear). The joints having that shape are called *prātara*;

7. *Kora* : These joints are present in the wrist, ankle, knee and elbow. The term *kora* means ear or a bud. Joints of the shape of an ear or a bud are called *kora*; and

8. *Vāyasa tuṇḍikā:* These are present in the mandibular region and both the thighs.

The vessels, ligaments, bones, phalanges and joints in living beings are covered (attached) with muscles. Therefore, they are endowed with strength.

[पेशी, कण्डरा]

'सा पेश्यः समाख्याताः[253] याश्च शतं बुधैः। स्त्रीणां तु विंशत्याधिकाः। कण्डराश्चैव

षोडशः[254] ॥२७६॥'

Muscles and Tendons

Muscles are one hundred in number. Females have twenty more muscles.

Tendons are sixteen in number.

[मांसरज्जु]

रत्नाकरः

'पार्श्वयोः पृष्ठवंशस्य चतस्रो मांसरज्जवः ।' 255

Māṁsa rajjus

According to Ratnākara

In both the sides of the vertebral column there are four *māṁsa rajjus* (muscles which serve the purpose of ligaments).

[नाडी]

द्वात्रिंशत्सहस्त्राणि नाड्यो देहे व्यवस्थिताः ॥२८०॥

सार्धं त्रिलक्षं शंसन्ति केचित्स्वेदवहा इति ।

स्थूलमूलाः सुसूक्ष्माग्राः पत्रशाखाप्रतानवत् 256

शाखोपशाखया तद्वत्तेषां संख्या न विद्यते ॥२८१॥

Nāḍi

In the body there are thirty two thousand *nāḍis* (vessels). According to some scholars, the *nāḍis* carrying sweat are three and half lakhs in number. They are thick at the root and very thin at their ends. They spread by ramification like branches, sub-branches and leaves of a tree. Therefore, it is not possible to enumerate them.

[शिरा]

वैद्यके

नाभेरधः प्रसृत्य यो दशयान्त्यधस्तादूर्ध्वं कृतानुसृतयो दश तद्वदेव ।

द्वे द्वे शिरे प्रवितते प्रसृते च तिर्यक्, युक्ताश्चतुर्भिरिति विंशतिरत्र काये ॥२८२॥

[257] आसां च सूक्ष्मप्रसृतिशुषिराणि शतानि सप्तसु तानि यैरसकृदन्नरसं वहद्भिः ।

आप्याय्यते वपुरिदं [358] हि नृणाममीषां, अम्भःस्रवद्भिरिव सिन्धुशतैः समुद्रः ॥२८३॥

Śirā

According to Medical texts

Ten *śirās* move from the umbilicus downwards. Ten *śirās* move from the umbilicus upwards. Two *śirās* in each side move from the umbilicus sidewards. Thus, in the body there are twenty four *śirās*. They have seven hundred subtle branches. With the help of these vessels, the end product of the food is carried to different parts of the body, for providing nourishment to human beings. It is on the analogy of water flowing through hundreds of rivers towards the sea.

आपादतः प्रभृति गात्रमशेषमेषामामस्तकादपि च नाभिभुवस्तलेन ।

एतन्मृदङ्गमिव चर्ममयेन काये, [259] नद्धं नृणामिति शिराशतसप्तकेन ॥२८४॥

The entire body beginning from the sole of the feet to the topmost part of the head is nourished by these vessels originating from the umbilicus. As a drum, the body is covered with the skin and vibration is caused through these seven hundred vessels in the human beings.

[स्नायु, कण्डरा]

स्नायुश्चतुर्विधा [260] विद्यात्तास्तु सर्वा निबोध मे ।

प्रतानवत्यो वृत्ताश्च पृथ्व्यश्च शुषिरास्तथा ।

प्रतानवत्यः शाखासु सर्वसन्धिषु [261] चाप्यथ ॥२८५॥

[सुश्रुत : शारीर५:३०-३१]

Snāyu and Kaṇḍarā

Snāyu (ligament) is of four varieties viz., *pratānavati* (having branches), *vṛttā* (round), *pṛthu* (thick) and *śuṣirā* (having porosity). The first variety of ligaments are present in all the joints of the limbs.

तेषु ये वर्त्तुला स्थूलाः कण्डरास्ते प्रकीर्तिताः ।
'आमपक्वाशयान्तेषु बस्तौ च शुषिराः खलु ।
पार्श्वोरसि तथा पृष्ठे पृथुलाश्च शिरस्यथ ॥२८६॥
[सुश्रुत : शारीर५:३२]

From amongst these ligaments, those which are round and thick are called *kaṇḍarā* (tendons). The *śuṣira* type of ligaments are present inside the *āmāśaya*, *pakvāśaya* and *basti* (urinary bladder). The *pṛthula* type of ligaments are present in the sides of the chest, in the chest, in the back and in the head.

'महाभारसहाः[262] स्थूलाः ॥२८७॥

The *sthūla* (thick) variety of ligaments which are called tendons are capable of tolerating very heavy weight.

[धमनी]

गर्गः

धातूनां बन्धनकराः दोषधातुवहाः[263] स्थिराः ।
धमन्ते[264] पवनं देहे धमन्य इति कीर्तिताः ॥२८८॥

Dhamanī

According to Garga

Dhamanis (arteries) keep the tissue elements adhered to each other. They carry the *doṣas* and *dhātus* (nutrition for the tissue elements). They remain stable (*sthira*). They cause *dhamana* (blow or carry by pulsation) of air in the body because of which they are called *dhamani*.

महाभारसहाः स्थूलाः कण्डराः कंडनक्षमाः ।

स्नायुबन्धनयोग्या च आपादतलमस्तकाः ॥२८९॥

The *kaṇḍarās* (tendons) are capable of carrying heavy weight. They are thick and they can not be torn. *Snāyus* (ligaments) help in binding the joints all over the body—right from the feet upto the head.

तासां प्रभंजनवहाः दशनाड्यो भवन्ति हि ।

दशपित्तवहास्तद्वद्भवन्ति श्लेष्मवाहिकाः ॥२९०॥

265

दशरक्तवहा ज्ञेया यकृत्प्लीह्नोर्द्वयं द्वयम् ।

Ten *nāḍis* carry *vāyu*. Ten other *nāḍis* similarly, carry *pitta*, ten others carry *kapha* and ten of these *nāḍiṣ* carry *rakta*. In the liver and the spleen there are two *nādis* in each one of them.

स्वशिरासु यदा दोषः कुपितः संप्रवर्त्तते ॥२९१॥

कुर्वन्ति विविधान्रोगान्निरामान्सामजांस्तथा ।

When *doṣas* get aggravated in their own *nāḍis* (channels) then they cause different types of *sāma* and *nirāma* diseases.

तत्रारुणा वातवहाः नीला पित्तवहास्तथा ।

गौरा कफाद्रक्तवहारुणानोष्णा न शीतलाः ।

The vessels carrying *vāyu* are *aruṇa* (reddish) in colour. Those carrying *pitta* are blue in colour. Those vessels carrying *kapha* are white in colour. Vessels carrying *rakta* are *aruṇa* (reddish) in colour and they are neither hot nor cold to touch.

[सेवनी]

सेवन्यः पञ्चशिरसि द्वे जिह्वालिङ्गयोर्मते ॥२६३॥

गुदर्लिंगान्तरे चैका भारद्वाजोऽब्रवीद्ध्रुवम् ।

Sevani

According to *Bharadvāja*, there are five *sevanīs* (sutures) in the head, two sutures in tongue and the penis and one between the anus and the penis.

[मर्म]

सप्तोत्तरं मर्मशतं नृणां देहे व्यवस्थितम् ॥२६४॥

मांसमर्मशिरामर्मस्नायुमर्मो[266]ऽस्थिमर्मकम् ।

सन्धिमर्म तथैतेषां संख्येदानीं प्रचक्ष्यते[267] ॥२६५॥

Marma

In the body of human beings there are one hundred seven *marmas* (vital spots). These are of five varieties viz., *māṁsa marmas* (vital spots in the muscles), *śirā marmas* (vital spots having the vessels), *snāyu marmas* (vital spots having ligaments and nerves), *asthi marma* (vital spots in the bones) and *sandhi marmas* (vital spots in the joints).

Now the number of *marmas* will be described.

तत्रैकादश मांसे तु शिरासु त्रिशताधिकम् ।

सप्ताधिका विंशतिस्तु स्नायुर्मर्म[268]विदो विदुः ॥२६६॥

अष्टावास्थिषु मर्माणि संधिमर्माणि विंशतिः ।

सप्ताधिकशतं चैव भवत्येवंविधं पुनः[269] ॥२६७॥

The number of various types of *marmas* is as follows :

1. *Māṁsa marma*	...	11
2. *Śirā marma*	...	41
3. *Snāyu marma*		27
4. *Asthi marma*		8
5. *Sandhi marma*		20
Total		107

सद्यः प्राणहराणि स्युः कालान्तरहराणि च ।
विशल्यघ्नानि वैकल्यकराणि रुक्कराणि च ॥२९८॥

These *marmas* are also divided into the following categories:

1. *Sadya prāṇa hara* (which cause instantaneous death);
2. *Kālāntara prāṇa hara* (which cause death after some time);
3. *Viśalyaghna* (which cause death when the foreign body is taken out);
4. *Vaikalya kara* (which cause deformity); and
5. *Rukkara* (which cause pain).

'शृङ्गाटकान्यधिपतिः शङ्खौ कण्ठसिरागुदम् ।
हृदयं बस्तिनाभ्यौ च घ्नन्ति सद्यो हतानि तु ॥२९९॥'

[सुश्रुत : शारीर६:९]

'चत्वारि शृङ्गाटकानि कण्ठशिराष्टौ मातृका ॥३००॥'

270

ग्रीवायाः उभयपार्श्वयोः याश्च शिराः ताः अष्टौ शिराममर्णि चतुरंगुलानि सद्योमारकाणि,' एकोनविंशति सद्योघ्नानि ॥३०१॥'

Sadya prāṇa hara

Śṛṅgāṭaka, adhipati, two *śaṅkhas, kaṇṭha sirā, guda* (anus), *hṛdaya* (heart), *basti* (urinary bladder) and *nābhi* (umbilicus) belong to this category. Any injury to these places cause instantaneous death.

Śṛṅgāṭakas are four in number. *Kaṇṭha śirās* are eight in number. These *śirās* or vessels, are also called *mātṛkā*. These are located in both the sides of the neck—four in each side. They belong to the category of *śirā marma*. These are four *aṅgulas* in size. Any injury to these *marmas* causes instantaneous death. Thus, in total, there are nineteen *marmas* belonging to *sadya prāṇa hara* category.

271

'अथ कालान्तरप्राणहराणि त्रयस्त्रिंशत् ।

वक्षोमर्माणि सीमन्ततलक्षिप्रेन्द्रबस्तयः ॥३०२॥

कटिकतरुणे सन्धिः पार्श्वयोर्बृहती च या ।

नितम्बाविति चैतानि कालान्तरहराणि तु ॥३०३॥

[सुश्रुत : शारीर६:१०-११]

Kālāntara prāṇa hara

These are thirty three in number. These are called *vakṣa marma, simanta, tala, kṣipra, indra basti, kaṭika taruṇa, sandhi and bṛhati,* which are located in the sides and both the *nitambas*. Any injury to these *marmas* cause death of the patient after some time.

'त्रीणि विशल्यघ्नानि ॥३०४॥'

[सुश्रुत : शारीर६:८]

'उत्क्षेपौ स्थपनी चैव विशल्यघ्नानि निर्दिशेत् ।

Viśalyaghna

These are three in number. They are two *utkṣepa* and *sthapanī*. Any injury to these *marmas* causes the death of the patient only when the foreign body is taken out.

चतुश्चत्वारिंशत् वैकल्यकराणि ॥३०५॥

[सुश्रुत : शारीर६:८]

लोहिताक्षाणि जानूर्वीकूर्चविटपकूर्पराः ।
कुकुन्दरे कक्षधरे विधुरे सकृकाटिके ॥३०६॥
अंसांसफलकापाङ्गा नीले मन्ये फणौ तथा ।
वैकल्यकरणान्याहुरावर्तौ द्वौ तथैव च ॥३०७॥

[सुश्रुत : शारीर६:११-१३]

Vaikalya kara

These are 44 in number. These are called *lohitākṣa* (4), *āṇi* (4), *jānu* (2), *urvi* (4), *kūrca* (4), *viṭapa* (2), *kūrpara* (2), two *kukundaras*, two *kakṣadharas*, two *vidhuras*, two *kṛkāṭikas*, *aṁsa* (2), *aṁsa phalaka* (2), *apāṅga* (2), two *nilas*, two *manyās*, two *phaṇas* and two *āvarttas*.

अष्टौ रुजाकराणि ॥३०८॥

[सुश्रुत : शारीर६:८]

गुल्फौ द्वौ मणिबन्धौ द्वौ द्वे द्वे कूर्चशिरांसि च ।
रुजाकराणि जानीयादष्टावेतानि बुद्धिमान् ॥३०९॥

[सुश्रुत : शारीर६:१४]

Rukkara

These are eight in number. They are called two *gulphas*, two *maṇi bandhas*, two *kūrcas* and two *kūrca śirās*. Any injury to these *marmas* causes pain.

'सद्यःप्राणहराणि स्युर्भूयिष्ठाग्नि गुणानि वै ।
क्षीणे ह्यग्निगुणे यस्मात्प्राणो यात्यविलम्बितः ॥३१०॥
सौम्याग्निगुणयुक्तानि कालान्तरहराणि च ।
वायव्यगुणकान्याहुर्विशल्यघ्नानि यानि च ॥३११॥
यावच्छल्यः मुखे रुद्धो वायुस्तिष्ठति देहिनाम् ।
तावत्संतिष्ठते प्राणौ म्रियते मारुते गते ॥३१२॥[273]

The *sadya prāṇa hara mārmas* are dominated by the attributes of *agni mahābhūta*. When these attributes of *agni guṇa* get reduced as a result of injury, the person dies instantaneously. *Kālāntara prāṇa hara marmas* are dominated by the attributes of *saumya* (*jala*) and *agni mahābhūtas*. The *viśalyaghna marmas* are dominated by the attributes of *vāyu mahābhūta*. Till the opening of the injury is blocked by the foreign body, *vāyu* remains obstructed inside the body and the patient survives. But when this foreign body is removed, the patient dies because of the elimination of *vāyu*.

वसिष्ठः

[274]'पाकात्पतितशल्योऽपि म्रियते नात्र संशयः ।
वैकल्यकरणान्याहुर्यानि सौम्यगुणानि च ॥३१३॥
सोमस्थिरत्वात्सौम्याच्च कुर्यात्प्राणावलम्बनम् ।
वाय्वग्निगुणयुक्तानि रुक्कराणि भवन्ति हि ॥३१४॥

According to Vasiṣṭha

If the foreign body in *viśalyaghna marmas* fall down after

suppuration, even then, the person dies and there is no doubt about it. The *vaikalya kara marmas* are dominated by the attributes of *jala mahābhūta. Jala mahābhūta* is stable and cooling. Therefore, any injury to these *marmas* does not result in death. The *rukkara marmas* are dominated by the attributes of *vāyu* and *agni mahābhūtas*.

सद्यःप्राणहराणि स्युः शल्याद्वासप्तरात्रतः ।

पक्षान्मासाद्द्विमासाद्वा हन्ति कालान्तरस्त्वतः ॥३१५॥

वैकल्यरुक्कराणिस्युर्घ्नन्ति चाधिकताडनात् ।'[375]

Injury to the *sadya prāṇa hara marmas* results in death within seven nights. Injury to the *kālāntara prāṇa hara marmas* results in death within a fortnight, or a month, or two months. If there is excessive injury in *vaikalya kara* and *rukkara marmas*, then this also results in the death of the patient.

'सोममारुततेजांसि रजःसत्त्वतमांसि च ॥३१६॥

मर्मसु प्रायशः पुंसां भूतात्मा चावतिष्ठते ।

मर्मस्वभिहतास्तस्मान्न जीवन्ति शरीरिणः ॥३१७॥'

[सुश्रुत : शारीर६:३५-३६]

In the *marmas* (vital spots) of human beings generally, the *bhūtātmā* (individual soul) is located along with *jala, vāyu, agni rajas, satvta* and *tamas*. Therefore, injury to these *marmas* of a person does cause death of the living beings.

देहप्रसुप्तिर्गुरुता हृण्मोहः शीतकामिता ।

स्वेदो मूर्च्छा वमिः श्वासो मर्मविद्धस्य लक्षणम् ॥३१८॥

Numbness of the body, heaviness, unconsciousness, desire for cold things, sweating, fainting, vomiting and dysponea—these are the signs and symptoms of a person whose vital spots have been injured.

प्राणघाती न[276] जीवेच्च क्वचिद्वैद्यगुणेन[377] चेत् ।
असमग्राभिघाताच्च सोऽपि वैकल्यमश्नुते ॥३१९॥

A person whose vital spots are injured, normally does not live. But at times, his life in saved because of the excellence of the physician. If the vital spot is partially injured, then instead of death, there will be deformity of the person.

मर्माभिघातः स्वल्पोऽपि प्रायशो बाधते भृशम् ।
तस्मात्क्षारविषाग्न्यादीन् यत्नान्मर्मसु वर्जयेत् ।
भल्लातकादितैलेन वह्निसाध्यं सुसाधयेत् ॥३२०॥

Even a little injury to the vital spot causes excessive pain in the patient. Therefore, these vital spots should be carefully avoided while administering alkalies, poisons and cauterization therapies. If a disease in a vital spot needs cauterization for cure, then this should be performed by the help of the oil of *bhallātaka* etc.

खरनादः

विक्षिप्यते भृशं दीनः शून्यो भ्रमति वेपते ।
हृदयं दह्यतेऽत्यर्थं नैकस्थानेऽवतिष्ठते[278] ॥३२१॥
मर्मोपविद्धान्मरणमेतैर्लिंगैरवाप्नुयात् ।

According to Kharanāda

A person, whose vital spots are injured, succumbs to death, and before that, the following signs and symptoms are manifested in him :

1. He throws his limbs here and there very frequently;
2. There is frustration, emptiness, giddiness and shivering in him;
3. There is excess of burning sensation in his heart; and
4. Such a person will not be able to stay in one place.

मर्मविद्धोऽपि च [279]नरस्तोदभेदादिपीडितः ॥३२२॥

अतिप्रस्रुतरक्तश्च सद्यस्त्यजति जीवितम् ।

स्नायुमांसातिविद्धानां सलक्षणचिकित्सितम् ॥३२३॥

सद्योव्रणचिकित्सायां कथयिष्यामि तत्त्वतः ।

When a vital spot of the body is injured, then the person suffers from different types of pains like *toda* (as if a pointed weapon is inserted into the body) and *bheda* (as if the portion of the body has been incised). There will be excessive bleeding, and thereafter, the person dies instantaneously. If there is injury to the *snāyu marma* and *māṁsa marma* then the signs and symptoms which are manifested and their treatment will be described elaborately in the Chapter dealing with the treatment of fresh wounds (of *Kharanāda saṁhitā*).

मध्ये पादतलस्याहुरभितो [280]मध्यमाङ्गुलिम् ॥३२४॥

[281]तलहृन्नामरुजया तत्र विद्धस्य पञ्चता ।

अङ्गुष्ठाङ्गुलिमध्यस्थं क्षिप्रमाक्षेपमरणम् ॥३२५॥

तस्योर्ध्वं द्व्यङ्गुले [282]कूर्चः पादभ्रमणकम्पकृत् ।

गुल्फसन्धेरधः [283]कूर्चशिरः [284]शोफरुजाकरम् ॥३२६॥

जङ्घाचरणयोः सन्धौ [285]गुल्फो रुक्स्तम्भमान्द्यकृत् ।

जङ्घान्तरे त्विन्द्रबस्तिर्मारयत्यसृजः [286]क्षयात् ॥३२७॥

जङ्घोर्वोः सङ्गमे जानुः खञ्जता तत्र जीवतः ।

जानुनस्त्र्यङ्गुलादूर्ध्व[287]माण्यूरुस्तम्भशोफकृत् ॥३२८॥

[उर्व्यूरुमध्ये तद्भेदात्सक्थिशोषोऽस्रसङ्क्षयात्]

288
ऊरुमूले लोहिताख्यं हन्ति पक्षमसृक्क्षयात् ।

मुष्कवङ्क्षणयोर्मध्ये विटपं षण्ढताकरम् ॥३२९॥

[अष्टाङ्गहृदय : शारीर४:२८]

289
कक्षाक्षमध्ये कक्षाधृक् कुणित्वं तत्र जायते ।

[अष्टाङ्गहृदय : शारीर४:६]

290 291
मूत्राशयो धनुर्वक्रो बस्तिरल्पास्रमांसगः ॥३३०॥

[अष्टाङ्गहृदयः शारीर४:१०]

292
'उध्वधोऽस्रकफापूर्ण कोष्ठो नश्येत्तयोः क्रमात् ।'

[अष्टाङ्गहृदय : शारीर४:१४]

In the centre of the sole of the feet on the middle toe, the *tala hṛdaya marma* is located. If this *marma* is injured then the patient dies after suffering from pain. Between the great toe and the second toe, the *marma* called "*kṣipra*" is located. Any injury to this vital spot leads to death after *ākṣepa* (clonic and tonic contractions). Two *aṅgulas* above this vital spot is located the *marma* called "*kūrca*". Any injury to this vital spot will cause shaking movement (shivering) of the leg. Below the ankle joint the *marma* called "*kūrca śiras*" is located. Injury to this vital spot causes swelling and pain. In the joint between the calf and the leg, the *marma* called "*gulpha*" is located. Injury to this vital spot causes pain, rigidity and sluggishness. In the middle of the calf region the *marma* called "*indra basti*" is located. Any injury to this vital spot results in death because of excessive bleeding. Between the calf region and the thigh is located the *marma* called "*jānu*". Any injury to this vital spot causes *khañjatā* (limping movement). Three *aṅgulas* above the knee joint in the thigh is located the *marma* called '*āṇi*'. Any injury to this vital spot causes *urustambha* (rigidity of thighs) and swelling. The *marma* called "*urvī*" is located in the centre of the thighs. Injury to this vital spot results in the emaciation of the thighs because of the loss of blood. The *lohitāks(khy)a marma* is located at the root of the thighs. Injury to this vital spot causes hemiplegia as a result of the loss of blood. Between the testicles and the pelvic bone the *marma* called "*viṭapa*" is located. Injury to this vital spot causes sterility. Between the axilla and the clavicle the *marma* called *kakṣādhṛk* is located. Injury to this vital spot results in *kuṇitva* (inability to move the upper limb). *Basti* is curved like a bow and it is the reservoir of urine. It has less amount of blood and muscle tissue. If there is injury above this vital spot then the death occurs as a result of the *koṣtha* (abdominal cavity) being filled up with blood. If there is injury below this vital spot then death occurs as a result of the *koṣṭha* being filled up with *kapha*.

पृष्ठवंशोरसोर्मध्ये तयोरेव च पार्श्वयोः ॥३३१॥

[अष्टाङ्गहृदय : शारीर४:१६]

293 'ऋतेऽश्मरी [व्रणा] द्विद्धस्तत्राप्युभयतश्च यः ।'

294 'मूत्रस्राव्येकतो भिन्ने व्रणो रोहेच्च यत्नतः ॥३३२॥

[अष्टाङ्गहृदय : शारीर४:११-१२]

If there is injury in both the sides of this urinary bladder and between the vertibral column and the chest (except the ulcer caused by the surgical operation for taking out the stone in the urinary bladder) then urine comes out from the ulcer and it will heal with great difficulty.

स्तनरोहितमूलाख्ये द्वयङ्गुले स्तनयोर्वदेत् ।

[अष्टाङ्गहृदय : शारीर४:१४]

295 'अर्धोऽसकूटयोर्विद्यादपालापाख्यमर्मणी ॥३३३॥'

तयोः कोष्ठेऽसृजा पूर्णे नश्येद्यातेन[296] पूयताम् ।

The *marma* called *stana rohita* is located at the distance of two *aṅgulas* from the nipples in the breast. *Apālāpa marma* is located below the shoulder joint. If there is injury to the two vital spots, the chest cavity becomes filled up with blood and death occurs because of suppuration.

पार्श्वयोः पृष्ठवंशस्य श्रोणी कर्णौ प्रतिष्ठितौ ॥३३४॥

वंशाश्रिते स्फिजोरूर्ध्वं कटीकतरुणे स्मृते ।

तत्र रक्तक्षयात्पाण्डुर्हीनरूपो[297] विनश्यति ॥३३५॥

In the sides of the vertibral columns two *marmas* called *śroṇi karṇa* are located. Adjacent to the vertibral column and above the buttocks, there are two *marmas* called *kaṭika taruṇa*. Injury to this vital spot leads to loss of blood, anemia, loss of complexion and death.

पृष्ठवंशं[298] ह्युभयतो यौ सन्धी कटिपार्श्वयोः ।

जघनस्य[299] बहिर्भागे मर्मणी तौ कुकुन्दरौ[300] ।

चेष्टाहानिरधःकाये[301] स्पर्शाज्ञानं च तद्व्यधात्[302] ॥३३६॥

[अष्टाङ्गहृदय : शारीर४:१६-२०]

Two *kukundara marmas* are located in both the sides of the vertibral column near the lumber region. They are outside the *jaghana* (thighs). If there is injury to these vital spots, then there will be loss of activity as well as sensation in the lower limbs.

नितम्बावप्येवम् ॥३३७॥

Two *nitamba marmas* have the above mentioned characteristics.

[303] स्तनमूलार्जवे भागे पृष्ठवंशाश्रये [304] सिरे ।

[305] बृहत्यौ, तत्र विद्धस्य मरणं रक्तसङ्क्षयात् ॥३३८॥

Just at the back of the *stana mūla marma*, resting on the vertibral column there are two *sirās* (vessels) which are called *bṛhati*. If there is injury to this vital spot, then there will be death because of excessive bleeding.

बाहुमूलाभिसम्बद्धे पृष्ठवंशस्य पार्श्वयोः ।

अंसयोः फलके [306] बाहुस्वापशोषौ तयोर्व्यधात् ॥३३९॥

[अष्टाङ्गहृदय : शारीर४:२३-२५]

By the sides of the vertibral column, there are two *marmas* called *aṁsa phalaka*. These are connected to the root of the arms. Injury to these vital spots leads to numbness and wasting of the arms.

[307] एवं वंशौ ॥३४०॥

Two *vaṁśa marmas* have also got the above mentioned characteristics.

[308] कण्ठनाडीमुभयतः सिराः हनुसमाश्रिताः ।

पृथक्चतस्रस्ताः सद्यो घ्नन्त्यसून्[309]मातृकाह्वया ।

In both the sides of *kaṇṭha nāḍi* (trachea), there are four separate vessels. These vessels are connected to the mandibles. These are called *mātṛkā*. Injury to these vital spots cause instantaneous death.

कृकाटिके शिरोग्रीवासन्धौ, तत्र चलं [310] शिरः ॥३४१॥

[अष्टाङ्गहृदय : शारीर४:२८-२९]

There are two *marmas* called *kṛkāṭikā* in the joint between the head and the neck. If there is any injury to these two vital spots then there will be shaking of the head.

अनुकर्णं ललाटान्ते शङ्खौ सद्यो विनाशनौ ।
केशान्ते शङ्खयोरूर्ध्वमुत्क्षेपौ, स्थपनी पुनः ।
भ्रुवोर्मध्ये त्रयोऽप्यत्र शल्ये जीवेदनुद्धृते ॥३४२॥

[अष्टाङ्गहृदय : शारीर४:३५-३६]

At the end of the region of forehead and near the ears, there are two *śmarmas* called *śaṁkha*. Injury to these vital spots leads to instantaneous death.

At the end of the hairline and above the *śaṁkha marmas*, two other *marmas* called *utkṣepa* are located. Another *marma* called *sthapani* is located between the two eye-brows. If there is injury to these three vital spots and if the foreign body is removed then the patient succumbs to death.

कपाले सन्धयः पञ्च सीमन्तास्तिर्यगूर्ध्वगाः ।
भ्रमोन्मादमनोनाशैस्तेषु विद्धेषु नश्यति ॥३४३॥

[अष्टाङ्गहृदय : शारीर४:३५-३६]

There are five joints in the skull and these five *marmas* are called *simanta*. Some of suturing joints move obliquely and some upwards. If there is injury to these vital spots, the patient suffers from giddiness, insanity and mental afflictions and ultimately succumbs to death.

रोमावर्ताप्येवम् ॥३४४॥

Two *romāvarta marmas* have also got the above-mentioned characteristics.

वृद्धवाग्भटात्

'स्तनचूचुकयोरूर्ध्वं[311] स्तनरोहितसंज्ञकम्[312] ॥३४५॥'

॥इति मर्मकथनम्॥

According to Vṛddha Vāgbhaṭa

The *marma* called *stana rohita* is located above the nipples of the breasts.

Thus, ends the description of *marmas* or vital spots.

'पञ्चाभिभूतास्त्वथ पञ्चकृत्वः पञ्चेन्द्रियं पञ्चसु भावयन्ति ।
पञ्चेन्द्रियं पञ्चसु भावयित्वा पञ्चत्वमायान्ति विनाशकाले ॥३४६॥

[सुश्रुत : शारीर९:११]

Description of the Process of Death

The *dhamanis* (arteries) which are made up of five *mahābhūtas*, effect an intimate contact between the five sensory faculties and the five sensory organs for fivc timos. Thereafter, these five sensory faculties establish contact with the five *mahābhūtas* at the time of the death or *pañcatva* (disintegration of five *mahābhūtas*) of the individual.

स्वस्थस्य[313] रक्षणं कुर्यादस्वस्थस्य[314] तु बुद्धिमान् ।
[315]क्षपयेद्बृंहयेद्वापि पारंपर्योपदेशतः ॥३४७॥

[सुश्रुत : सूत्र१५:४०]

Health and Ill-health

The wise physician should make efforts for the maintenance of the positive health of a healthy person. When, however, the body is afflicted with diseases, then the physician should reduce the increased *doṣas* etc., and increase the reduced *dhātus* etc., on the basis of medical instruction followed traditionally.

वैलक्षण्याच्छरीराणामस्थायित्वात्तथैव च ।

दोषधातुमलानां[316] तु परिमाणं न विद्यते ॥३४८॥

[सुश्रुत : सूत्र १५:३७]

Quantity of Doṣas etc.

It is very difficult to ascertain the quantity of *doṣas, dhātus* and *malas* in the body because there is considerable variation in the bodies of different individuals and also because the quantity of *doṣas* etc., is very unstable.

'दोषादीनां च समतां[317] ह्यनुमानेन लक्षयेत्[318] ।

अन्नं प्रार्थयते नित्यं लघ्वन्नं खादते सुखम् ॥३४६॥

भुक्तं सम्यक् प्रपचति वर्णवान्बलवान्भवेत् ।

प्रसृष्टा वातविण्मूत्रशुक्रादीनां तथैव च ।

पञ्चेन्द्रियार्थोपपन्नं सम्यक्स्वप्नं प्रयच्छति[319] ॥३५६॥

Equilibrium of Doṣas etc.

The equilibrium of *doṣas* etc., is determined by inference. The following are the characteristic features of a person who has equilibrium of *doṣas* etc., in his body:

1. There is regular desire for food;
2. He feels comfortable when he takes light food;
3. There is proper digestion of the ingested food;
4. The person is endowed with excellent complexion and strength;

5. There is proper elimination of flatus, stool and urine and ejaculation of semen;

6. The five senses are able to perceive their objects properly; and

7. There is good sleep.

सुश्रुतः

समदोषः समाग्निश्च समधातुमलक्रियः ।

प्रसन्नात्मेन्द्रियमनाः स्वस्थ इत्यभिधीयते ॥३५१॥

[सुश्रुत : सूत्र१५:४१]

According to Suśruta

A person who has equilibrium of *doṣas*, *agnis*, *dhātus*, *malas* and other activities of the body, who has happiness of *ātman* (individual soul), *indriya* (senses) and *manas* (mind) is called *svastha* (or a healthy person).

320

कथं शरीरे धातूनां वैषम्यं न भवेदिह ।

समानां चानुबन्धः स्यादित्यर्थं क्रियते क्रिया ॥३५२॥

[चरक सूत्र१६:३५]

Objective of Therapeutics

The objectives of therapeutics are to prevent any change in the equilibrium of *dhātus* and to maintain the continuity of the *dhātus* which are in a state of equilibrium.

या ह्युदीर्णं शमयति नान्यं व्याधिं करोति च ।

सा क्रिया, न तु या व्याधिं हरत्यन्यमुदीरयेत् ॥३५३॥

[सुश्रुत : सूत्र३५:२३]

Therapeutics

The measure which alleviates the aggravated conditions of *doṣas* in the body without producing any other disease is called a therapy. The measure which cures one disease but simultaneously produces another should not be called a therapy.

'शीते शीतप्रतीकारमुष्णे चोष्णनिवारणम् ।
कृत्वा कुर्यात् क्रियां प्राप्तां क्रियाकालं न हापयेत् ॥३५४॥

Line of Treatment in General

Remedial measures should be adopted for cold during the winter season and for hot during the summer. One should not ignore the time when there is indication for the administration of the therapy.

अप्राप्ते वा क्रियाकाले प्राप्ते वा न कृता क्रिया ।
क्रियाहीनाऽतिरिक्ता वा साध्येष्वपि न सिद्‌ध्यति ॥३५५॥

[सुश्रुत : सूत्र३५:२१-२२]

Timely Administration

If therapies are administered before the appropriate time, if these are not administered during the appropriate time and if there is either less or excess of these therapies, then even the curable diseases do not get cured.

क्रियायास्तु गुणालाभे क्रियामन्यां प्रयोजयेत् ।
पूर्वस्यां शान्तवेगायां न क्रियासंकरो हितः ॥३५६॥

[सुश्रुत : सूत्र३५:४८]

Change of Therapy

When the physician fails to get the results by administering one type of therapy, then another type of therapy should be administered only after all the effects of the previous therapy are over. *Kriyā saṁkara* (mixture of therapies) is not useful.

क्रियाभिस्तुल्यरूपाभिः क्रियासाङ्कर्यमुच्यते ।

पूर्वस्यां शान्तवेगायां तस्मिन्नन्यां प्रयोजयेत् ।।३५७।।

भिन्नरूपतया तास्तु[321] न च कुर्वन्ति दूषणम् ।

गुणालाभे तु कर्त्तव्याः विश्राम्यान्तरिताः क्रियाः ।।३५८।।

सैव सैवाऽन्यथा[322] तस्मात्पूर्ववत्संकराद्भयम् ।

When several therapies of the same category are simultaneously administered this is called *kriyā saṁkara.* When the effects of the earlier therapy are over only then an other therapy should be administered. Since these two therapies are different in nature they do not produce any harmful effect. If the desired effect is not achieved, then after giving a pause, the other therapy should be started. Since these two therapies are different, there is the danger of *kriyā saṁkara* as described before.

षड्भिः केचिदहोरात्रात्केचित्सप्तभिरेव च ।।३५९।।

इच्छन्ति मुनयः प्रायो रसस्य परिवर्तनम् ।

परिवृत्या रसस्यैव शान्तवेगा क्रियाभवेत् ।।३६०।।

According to sages, *rasa* (chyle or plasma) gets converted into successive *dhātus* after an interval of six or seven days. The effect of a particular therapy becomes over by the time when this transformation of *rasa* takes place.

उत्पद्यते हि साऽवस्था देशकालबलं प्रति ।

यस्यां कार्यमकार्यं स्यात्कर्मकार्यं च वर्जितम् ।

एवं सम्यक्परिज्ञाय कुर्यात्प्रशमनीं क्रियाम् ।।३६१।।

Depending upon the nature of the locality and time, such situations may arise in which a therapy which is indicated does not prove effective and a therapy which is normally contra-indicated may become useful. Therefore, after proper and careful examination therapies should be administered.

इति श्री महाराजाधिराजटोडरमल्लविरचिते टोडरानंदे आयुर्वेदसौख्ये शारीरकथनं नाम चतुर्थोहर्षः ।[323]

Thus, ends the fourth Chapter of *Āyurveda saukhyaṁ* in *Ṭaḍarānanda* composed by the great king *Ṭoḍaramalla* which deals with various anatomical and physiological topics.

NOTES AND REFERENCES

1. 'यदन्नं देहधात्वोजोबलवर्णादिपोषकम् ।
तत्राग्निर्हेतुराहारान्न ह्यपक्वाद्रसादयः । इति आकरे पाठः
[चरक: चिकित्सा १५:५]

2. 'तत् सूर्यमण्डलम्' इति आकरे पाठः ।

3. 'प्रदीपवच्चापि नृणां तस्य' इति आकरे पाठः ।

4. [ ] पाठोऽयं मूलपुस्तकेषु नोपलभ्यते ।

5. 'जरायुमध्ये——काचकोशस्थदीपवत्' पाठोऽयं आयुर्वेदीयक्रियाशारीरमध्ये नोपलभ्यते ।

6. 'तिष्ठन् तेजो युक्तो गभस्तिभिः' इति आकरे पाठः ।

7. 'पल्लवानि' इति आकरे पाठः ।

8. 'सूर्यकान्तो मणिर्यथा' इति आकरे पाठः ।

9. 'वामपार्श्वाश्रितं नाभेः किंचित्सूर्यस्य मण्डलम् ।
तन्मध्ये मण्डलं सौम्यं तन्मध्येऽग्निर्व्यवस्थितः ।

जरायुमात्रप्रच्छन्नः काचकोशस्थदीपवत् ।' इति अष्टाङ्गहृदयस्य शारीर-स्थाने तृतीयोऽध्याये प्रक्षिप्तपाठः ।

10. 'तत्र' इति आकरे पाठः ।

11. 'अत्रोच्यते' इति आकरे पाठः ।

12. 'आग्नेयत्वात्——क्रियतेऽन्तरग्निरिति' पाठोऽयं द्वितीयषष्ठपुस्कयोः नोपलभ्यते ।

13. 'क्रोधशोकश्रमक्लान्तः' इति सर्वपुस्तकेषु पाठः ।

14. 'पक्वाशयजीवनम्' इति प्रथमपुस्तके पाठः ।

15. 'ह्याहारः' इति आकरे पाठः ।

16. 'गुणान् स्वानभिवर्धयेत्' इति आकरे पाठः ।

17. 'परिबृंहयेत्' इति आकरे पाठः ।

18. 'शेषान्' इति प्रथमपुस्तके पाठः ।
'समस्तोषधि' इति षष्ठपुस्तके पाठः ।

19. अन्नं पाकक्रमादिभिः इति आकरे पाठः ।

20. सुश्रुते पाठोऽयं भिन्नरूपेणोपलभ्यते
यथाः—
तत्र 'रस' गतौ धातुः, अहरहर्गच्छतीत्यतो रसः ।
स खलु त्रीणि त्रीणिकलासहस्राणि पञ्चदश च कला एकैकस्मिन् धातावतिष्ठते; एवं मासेन रसः शुक्रं स्त्रीणां चार्तवं भवति ।
भवति चात्र—
अष्टादशसहस्राणि सङ्ख्या ह्यस्मिन् समुच्चये ।
कलानां नवतिः प्रोक्ता स्वतन्त्रपरतन्त्रयोः ॥
स शब्दार्चिर्जलसन्तानवदणुना विशेषेणानुधावत्येवं शरीरं केवलम् ।
[सुश्रुत : सूत्र १४:१३-१६]

21. द्रष्टव्यम्—सुश्रुत : सूत्र १४:१७ ।

22. 'श्रेष्ठं कर्म क्रमात्स्मृतम् इति आकरे पाठः ।

23. पाठोऽयं उपलब्धायां चरकसंहितायां नोऽपलभ्यतें । डल्हणे तु निम्नवत् पाठः ।

स्थूलसूक्ष्ममलैः सर्व्वे भिद्यन्ते धातवस्त्रिधा ।

स्वः स्थूलोंऽशः परं सूक्ष्मो विण्मलं याति तन्मलः ।

अन्नात् पच्यमानात् विण्मूत्रं मलः सारो रसः । रसादग्निपक्वात् मलः कफः, स्थूलो भागो रसः, अणुभागो रक्तम् । रक्तादग्निपक्वात् मलः पित्तम्, स्थुलभागः शोणितम्, अणुभागस्तु मांसमिति । ततोऽपि आत्मपावकपच्यमानान्मलः श्रोत्रनासाकर्णाक्षप्रजननादिस्रोतोमलः, स्थूलो भागो मांसम्, सूक्ष्मो मेदः । ततोऽपि निजवह्निपच्यमानान्मलः स्वेदः, स्थूलांशो मेद एव, सूक्ष्मभागोऽस्थि । ततोऽपि पच्यमानात् मलः केशलोमश्मश्रूणि, स्थूलऽस्थि, सूक्ष्मस्तु मज्जा । ततोऽपि मज्ज्ञः पावकपच्यमानान्मलो नयनपुरीषत्वचां स्नेहः, स्थूलो भागो मज्जा, सूक्ष्मः शुक्रम् । ततः पुनः पच्यमानादत्र मलः नोत्पद्यते सहस्रधाध्मातसुवर्णवत्, स्थूलो भागः शुक्रमेव ।

[डल्हण : सुश्रुत : सूत्र१४:१०]

अष्टाङ्गसंग्रहे तु निम्नवत् पाठः—

तत्राहाररसो व्यानविक्षिप्तो यथास्वं सप्तसु धात्वग्निषु क्रमात्पच्यमानः स्वात्मभावप्रच्युतिसमनन्तरमेव प्राप्तरक्तादिधातुसंज्ञकः कालवदस्खलितबलप्रमाणो देहमूर्जयित्वा धातून् धातुमलांश्च पुष्णाति । अथान्नकिट्टमच्छं मूत्रं घनं शकृत् । रसस्य सारो रक्तं; मलः कफो लसीका च । रक्तस्य सारो मांसं कण्डराः सिराश्च; मलं पित्तम् । मांसस्य सारो मेदस्त्वचौ वसा च; किट्टं कर्णाक्षिनासिकास्यरोमकूपप्रजननमलाः । मेदसः सारोऽस्थिस्नायुसंधयः; किट्टं स्वेदः । अस्थ्नः सारो मज्जा; किट्टं केशलोमानि नखाः । मज्ज्ञस्तु सारः शुक्रं; मलोऽक्षिविट्त्वचां स्नेहः । शुक्रस्य सारमोजः । अत्यन्तशुद्धतया चास्मिन् मलाभावः । अन्ये पुनरत एव तस्य नेच्छन्ति पाकम् । आकरे पुनः शुक्रस्य सारं गर्भमेवामनन्ति ॥

[अष्टाङ्गसंग्रह : शारीरः६]

24. 'सन्ति' इति द्वितीयपुस्तके पाठः ।

25. स्वाग्निभिः पच्यमानेषु मलः षट्सु रसादिषु । न शुक्रे पच्यमानेऽपि हेमनीवाक्षये मलः । इति आकरे पाठः ।

[डल्हण : सुश्रुत : सूत्र १४-१०]

26. (क) कफः पित्तं मलाः खेषु प्रस्वेदो नखरोम च । स्नेहोऽक्षित्वग्विशामोजो धातूनां क्रमशो मलाः । इति आकरे पाठः ।

(ख) कफः पित्तं मलः खेषु स्वेदः स्यान्नखरोम च। नेत्रविट्त्वक्षु च स्नेहो धातूनां क्रमशो मलाः। इति सुश्रुते पाठः।

[सुश्रुत : सूत्र४६:५२९]

27. 'सत्कथं' इति पञ्चमपुस्तके पाठः।
28. 'तत्रास्मत्सम्मतम्' इति पञ्चमपुस्तके पाठः।
29. 'पुंभावसंभवाविति' इति पञ्चमपुस्तके पाठः।
30. 'आकृष्टाण्डकोशस्य पुंसः स्मश्रुपातात्, स्मश्रुकाणामण्ड एवं। संभव-शब्दोऽत्रपोषणेति जैजट'।। इतिपञ्चमपुस्तके पाठः।
31. 'केचिदत्रापिशुक्रतेजोष्मणाकृत्वायुवानपिडिका' इति पंचमपुस्तके पाठः।
32. 'न तु मलात्' इति पञ्चमपुस्तके पाठः।
33. द्रष्टव्यम्—डल्हण : सुश्रुत : सूत्र४६:५४९-५५०।
34. 'धर्मशास्त्रात्' इति पञ्चमपुस्तके पाठः।
35. 'सार्द्धाः स्वेदायनैसह' इति पञ्चमपुस्तके पाठः।
36. ततो हीनास्तु ते ये च हीनकूर्चा मता बुधैः इति पञ्चमपुस्तके पाठः।
37. स्त्रियो मसात्स्रवत्यस्मात्तस्मान्न खलति स्त्रियाः। इति द्वितीयपुस्तके पाठः।
38. 'हिसदृशात्' इति पञ्चमपुस्तके पाठः।
39. 'देहे प्रजायते' इति आदर्शपुस्तकेषु पाठः।
40. 'तत्कथं' इति आदर्शपुस्तकेषु पाठः।
41. रसाद्रक्तात्सितं मासं तत्कथं जायते नृणाम्। मांसात् स्निग्धं च शुक्लं च कथं मेदः प्रजायते। तस्माद्दृढं चातिखरं कथमस्थि प्रजायते। तस्माच्चातिमृदुर्मज्जा कथं भवति देहिनाम्। (प)ययोश्च परिणामेन बहिः शुक्रं प्रवर्त्तते। कथं सर्वगतं शुक्रं प्रवदन्ति मुनीश्वराः। पाठोऽयं समस्तादर्शपुस्तकेषु उपलभ्यते।
42. 'अथास्थिमध्ये मज्ज्ञश्च' इति आदर्शपुस्तकेषु पाठः।
43. 'भवति देहिनः' इति आदर्शपुस्तकेषु पाठः।
44. 'तच्च निःसरते कथम्' इति आदर्शपुस्तकेषु पाठः।

45. एवमुक्तस्तु शिष्येण गुरुः प्राहेदमुत्तरम् । तेजो रसानां सर्वेषां मनुजानां यदुच्यते । पित्तोष्मणः स रागेण रसो रक्तत्वमृच्छति ।

[चरक : चिकित्सा १५:२७-२८]

46. 'रंजितास्तेजसा ह्यापः' इति पंचमपुस्तके पाठः ।

47. 'तत्र' इति पञ्चमपुस्तके पाठः ।

48. 'रक्तार्त्तवयोरभेदं' इति डल्हणे पाठः ।

49. 'रसादेवस्त्रियारक्तं———स्वभावभेदं दर्शयन्नाह' पाठोऽयं पञ्चमपुस्तके नोपलभ्यते ।

50. 'ऋतुकालजरक्तमेव' इति डल्हणे पाठः ।

51. द्रष्टव्यम्—सुश्रुत : सूत्र१४:८ (डल्हण) ।

52. '———आर्त्तवशोणितं त्वाग्नेयमित्यन्ये पठन्ति । आर्त्तवञ्च तत् शोणितञ्चेति आर्त्तवशोणितम् । तु शब्दोऽत्रावधारणे । इति तु आकरे पाठः ।

53. 'अनुष्णं' इति पञ्चमपुस्तके पाठः ।

54. 'गर्भाशये——बुधे' पाठोऽयं षष्ठपुस्तके अधिकं भवति ।

55. पाठोऽयमशुद्धं प्रतिभाति ।

56. 'तदा' इति प्रथमपुस्तके पाठः ।

57. 'सुश्रुते तु पाठोऽयं पद्यवद्धं नोपलभ्यते आकरे तु "एवं मासेन रसः शुक्रं स्त्रीणां आर्त्तवं भवति ।"

[सुश्रुत : सूत्र१४:१४]

58. 'वृद्धवाग्भटः' इति षष्ठपुस्तके पाठः ।

59. अत्र आर्त्तवशब्दोऽयं शुक्रे वर्त्तते न तु रजसि । रजो हि रसाद्रक्तवत् सप्तमेऽहनि जायते । अथ यद्ययमार्त्तवशब्दः शुक्रे न वर्त्तते तदा अत्र शुक्रोत्पत्त्यधिकारे स्त्रीणां शुक्रस्यानुक्तत्वात् षड्धातुत्वं स्यात् । तस्मात् आर्त्तवशब्दः शुक्रे वर्त्तते, अन्ये तु पुनरत्रार्त्तवशब्दं रजस्येव वर्त्तयन्ति, चकारेण स्त्रीशुक्रं समुच्चिन्वन्तीति, शुक्रेऽपि गर्भजननशक्तिद्योतनार्थम् ।' इति डल्हणे पाठः ।

[डल्हणः सुश्रुत : सूत्र१४:१५]

60. मासेनोपचितं काले धमनीभ्यां तदार्त्तवम् ।

ईषत् कृष्णं विवर्णं च वायुर्योनिमुखं नयेत् ।
तद्वर्षाद्द्वादशात् काले वर्तमानमसृक् पुनः । इति सुश्रुते पाठः ।
[सुश्रुत : शारीर३:१०-११]

61. 'दृश्यते' इति आकरे पाठः ।

62. 'विद्यते' इति प्रथमपञ्चमपुस्तकयोः पाठः ।

63. द्रष्टव्यम्—जीवच्छरीरे रक्तदर्शनात्, मृतशरीरे चादर्शनात् ।
[डल्हण : सुश्रुत : सूत्र१४:८]

64. 'तालभागक्रमस्थानि' इति द्वितीयषष्ठपुस्तकयोः पाठः ।

65. द्रष्टव्यम्—चरक : चिकित्सा१५:२२-३५ ।

66. 'चापि' इति पञ्चमपुस्तके पाठः ।

67. द्रष्टव्यम्—चरक : चिकित्सा२:४:३६ ।
आयुर्वेदीयक्रियाशारीर पृष्ठ ५७५ ।

68. यथा पयसि सर्पिस्तु गूढश्चेक्षौ रसो यथा ।
शरीरेषु तथा शुक्रं नृणां विद्याद्भिषग्वरः, । इति सुश्रुते पाठः ।
[सुश्रुत : शारीर४:२१]

69. 'स्रोत्रस्तथा' इति द्वितीयपुस्तके पाठः ।

70. 'मार्द्रवं' इति षष्ठपुस्तके पाठः ।

71. 'वातात्मकोऽपि' इति प्रथमपुस्तके पाठः ।

72. 'सर्गत्वं' इति षष्ठपुस्तके पाठः ।

73. 'यदा' इति षष्ठपुस्तके पाठः ।

74. 'पञ्चात्मसंयुक्ता' इति द्वितीयषष्ठपुस्तकयोः पाठः ।

75. 'आत्मप्रकृतिभिर्युतः' इति प्रथमपुस्तके पाठः ।

76. [] पाठोऽयं आदर्शपुस्तकेषु नोपलभ्यते ।

77. 'कार्तवीर्यो' इति आदर्शपुस्तकेषु पाठः ।

78. 79. []पाठोऽयं आकरात् गृहीतः मूलादर्शपुस्तिकासु नोपलभ्यते ।

80. द्रष्टव्यम्—सुश्रुत : शारीर२:२६ ।
अष्टाङ्गहृदय : शारीर१:२६ ।

81. चरके तु पाठोऽयं श्लोकबद्धं नोपलभ्यते। गद्ये तु अथाप्येतौ स्त्रीपुंसौ स्नेहस्वेदाभ्यामुपपाद्य, वमनविरेचनाभ्यां संशोध्य, क्रमेण प्रकृतिमापादयेत्। संशुद्धौ चास्थापनानुवासनाभ्यामुपाचरेत्; उपाचरेच्च मधुरौषधसंस्कृताभ्यां घृतक्षीराभ्यां पुरुषं, स्त्रियं तु तैलमाषाभ्याम्।

[चरक : शारीर८:४]

82. 'प्रसूयेतायुक्ते' इति पञ्चमपुस्तके पाठः।

83. 'तस्यास्त्रिदिनमारभ्य' इति द्वितीयषष्ठपुस्तकयोः पाठः।

84. 'सर्वदाचारवर्जिता' इति द्वितीयपुस्तके पाठः।
'सदाचारवर्जिता' इति षष्ठपुस्तके पाठः।

85. 'प्रवर्त्तमाने रक्ते च यदि गच्छति मूढधीः।' इति प्रथमपुस्तके पाठः।

86. 'प्रजायेत व्यंगोमत्तोऽल्पजीवनः' इति प्रथमपुस्तके पाठः।

87. 'गर्भको' इति षष्ठपुस्तके पाठः।

88. द्रष्टव्यम्—सुश्रुत : शारीर२:३३-३४।

89. 'यत्तु' इति आकरे पाठः।

90. 'यच्चद्भिर्न्नविरंज्यते' इति प्रथमद्वितीयषष्ठपुस्तकेषु पाठः।

91. द्रष्टव्यम्—चरक : चिकित्सा३०:२२५-२२६।

92. 'गूढार्त्तवा स्त्रीत्येके तेषां मते यथा' इति द्वितीयपुस्तके पाठः।
'अद्रिष्टार्त्तवा केषांमते तद्यथा' इति पञ्चमपुस्तके पाठः।

93. द्रष्टव्यम्—चरक : शारीर८:५-७।
चरक : शारीर८:१४।
चरक : शारीर२:२५।
सुश्रुत : शारीर२:४६।

94. 'ततः शुक्लवाससौ स्रग्विणौ सुमनसावन्योन्यमभिकामौ संवसेयातां स्नानात् प्रभृति युग्मेष्वहःसु पुत्रकामौ, अयुग्मेषु दुहितृकामौ। न च न्युब्जां पार्श्वगतां वा संसेवेत' इति तु आकरे पाठः।

95. सुश्रुते तु पद्यात्मकोऽयं पाठः नोपलभ्यते।
आकरपाठस्तु—
ततोऽपराह्णे पुमान् मासं ब्रह्मचारी सर्पिः स्निग्धः सर्पिःक्षीराभ्यां शाल्योदनं भुक्त्वा मासं ब्रह्मचारिणीं तैलस्निग्धां तैलमाषोत्तराहारां नारीमुपेयाद्रात्रौ

सामभिरभिविश्वास्य; विकल्प्यैवं चतुर्थ्यां षष्ठ्यामष्टम्यां दशम्यां द्वादश्यां चोपेयादिति पुत्रकामः ।

अतः परं पञ्चम्यां सप्तम्यां नवम्यामेकादश्यां च स्त्रीकामः; त्रयोदशीप्रभृतयो निन्द्याः ।

[सुश्रुत : शारीर२:२८,३०]

96. द्रष्टव्यम्—चरक : शारीर८:५ ।
अष्टाङ्गहृदय : शारीर१:२७ ।

97. क. 'रजः प्रात्तारिसंभवेत्' इति षष्ठपुस्तके पाठः ।
ख. पाठोऽयं अशुद्धं प्रतिभाति; शुद्धस्तु बहुतर एव ।

98. 'तत्र या गच्छेद्ध्रुवं' इति प्रथमपञ्चमपुस्तकयोः पाठः ।

99. 'युग्मेषु———पुत्रं प्रसूयते' पाठोऽयं प्रथमपंचमपुस्तकयोः नोपलभ्यते ।

100. 'तत्र या गच्छेद्ध्रुवं' इति द्वितीयपुस्तके पाठः ।

101. 'तत्रवैश्वानसः' इति षष्ठपुस्तके पाठः ।

102. 'बहुलपक्षेतु' इति षष्ठपुस्तके पाठः ।

103. 'मस्तुलुंगोधिकायते' इति षष्ठपुस्तके पाठः ।

104. 'योगशारीरे' इति पञ्चमषष्ठपुस्तकयोः पाठः ।

105. 'त्वेहि शिमी' इति प्रथमपुस्तके पाठः ।

106. 'सिमीवालि' इति षष्ठपुस्तके पाठः ।

107. द्रष्टव्यम्—चरक : शारीर८:८ ।
अष्टाङ्गहृदय : शारीर१:३ ।

108. द्रष्टव्यम्—चरक : शारीर२:१२ ।

109. 'प्रविलीयते' इति आकरे पाठः ।

110. शुक्रसंयोगात्तथादिष्टस्य' इति द्वितीयपुस्तके पाठः ।

111. 'ततो———षंढो जायते' पाठोऽयं षष्ठपुस्तके उपलभ्यते ।

112. 'सुजायतेत्वाक्षिप्तवेगायाः' इति पञ्चमपुस्तके पाठः ।

113. 'प्रतिष्ठिता' इति आकरे पाठः ।

114. 'गर्भशय्यां' इति आकरे पाठः ।

115. "गर्भस्तु मातुः पृष्ठाभिरेकोर्द्ध शिराः संकुचाङ्गान्यास्ते कुक्षौ गर्भाशयस्य।" पाठोऽयं आदर्शपुस्तकेषु उपलभ्यते, तत्तु सम्यक् न प्रतिभाति।

116. 'वामपार्श्वे' इति द्वितीयपुस्तके पाठः।

117. 'सद्योगृहीतगर्भाया लिङ्गानि' इति सुश्रुते पाठः।

118. 'आश्लेषगन्धाविकृतिः भवेत्कृष्णमुखौ स्तनौ' इति द्वितीयपुस्तके पाठः।

119. द्रष्टव्यम् —सुश्रुत : शारीर३:१३-१५।
चरक : शारीर२:२३।
अष्टाङ्गहृदय : शारीर१:३५-३६।

120. 'केदारं' इति द्वितीयपुस्तके पाठः।

121. 'प्रदृश्यते' इति प्रथमपुस्तके पाठः।

122. 'तस्य' इति पञ्चमपुस्तके पाठः।

123. द्रष्टव्यम्—चरक : शारीर२:१२-१६।

124. 'यदा नार्यावुपेयातां वृषस्यन्त्यौ कथंचन।
मुञ्चतः शुक्रमन्योन्यमनस्थिस्तत्र जायते।' इति आकरे पाठः।

125. 'हीन्यधिकाङ्गावधिरावटुकुक्षौ' इति द्वितीयपुस्तके पाठः।

126. 'कुनपो' इति प्रथमपुस्तके पाठः।

127. 'उत्तुशिशखयः सत्वं रजः शितज्ञौतमोर्कशितभौमौ एतैतंरान्मनः स्वा प्रकृति प्रयछतिरसन्वरजशा मया। यस्यांशे भास्करस्तादृक् वलिनाशदृशा मूर्त्तिः बुद्धा चा जातिकुलदेशान्। इति सारावल्याम्।' इति पञ्चमपुस्तके अधिको पाठः।

128. द्रष्टव्यम्—सुश्रुत : शारीर३:१८।
चरक : शारीर४:६-११।
अष्टाङ्गहृदय : शारीर१:३७-५४।

129. 'यथा' इति द्वितीयपुस्तके पाठः।

130. 'भागाश्चतुर्थे' इति द्वितीयपुस्तके पाठः।

131. 'दोहृदं' इति द्वितीयपुस्तके पाठः।

132. 'समायाति'———कृष्णश्यामसमेचकः' पाठोऽयं प्रथमपञ्चमपुस्तकयोः नोपलभ्यते।

133. 'अष्टमे मासि भवत्योजस्तत्र जातो न जीवेत्।
निरोजत्वान्निरितिर्भागधेयत्वाच्च। तत्र मांसोदनं दापयेत्'। इति आदर्श-पुस्तकेषु पाठः।

134. 'अपि' इति द्वितीयपुस्तके पाठः।

135. द्रष्टव्यम्—नवमदशमैकादशद्वादशानामन्यतमस्मिञ्जायते। अतोऽन्यथा विकारी भवति।

[सुश्रुत : शारीर३:३०]

136. 'वशिष्ठः' इति पञ्चमपुस्तके पाठः।

137. क. 'ह्ये तद्विण्मूत्रोपद्रसेविनाम्' इति प्रथमपुस्तके पाठः।
ख. 'ह्ये तद्विण्मूत्रोपद्रघ्नसेविनाम्' इति पञ्चमपुस्तके पाठः।
ग. 'ह्ये तद्विण्मूत्रोपघ्नसेविनाम्' इति षष्ठपुस्तके पाठः।

138. 'तदाह्लक्षणम्' इति षष्ठपुस्तके पाठः।

139. 'कोलाम्लमधुरौषधैः' इति प्रथमपुस्तके पाठः।

140. 'विदाहेनाऽपि पच्यतेपि इति षष्ठपुस्तके पाठः।

141. 'चतुर्थे———गर्भः।' पाठोऽयं द्वितीयपुस्तके नोपलभ्यते।

142. 'गुर्विणी' इति आदर्शपुस्तिकाषु पाठः।

143. 'तदात्मकं' इति पञ्चमषष्ठपुस्तकयोः पाठः।

144. 'च श्रद्धां' इति प्रथमपुस्तके पाठः।

145. 'द्रव्यकांक्षति' इति षष्ठपुस्तके पाठः।

146. 'तदा' इति द्वितीयपुस्तके पाठः।

147. 'तत्त्ववशक्यरूपं' इति द्वितीयपुस्तके पाठः।

148. 'समं' इति षष्ठपुस्तके पाठः।

149. 'भवत्यधिकमन्येभ्यो' इति आकरे पाठः।

150. द्रष्टव्यम्—चरक : शारीर४:२४।

151. 'वीर्यबाहु'' इति द्वितीयपुस्तके पाठः।

152. 'सदा' इति प्रथमपुस्तके पाठः।

153. 'रक्तशल्योदनमुपदौह्रदंभोजयेत्' इति द्वितीयपुस्तके पाठः।

154. 'दोहृदिनी' इति षष्ठपुस्तके पाठः ।

155. 'स्यात्तथैव' इति द्वितीयपुस्तके पाठः ।

156. 'जगद्रूपाणां' इति प्रथमपुस्तके पाठः ।

157. द्रष्टव्यम्—चरक : शारीर८:९ ।

158. 'दौहृदं जायते स्त्रियाः' इति आकरे पाठः ।

159. 'अलङ्कारैषिणां' इति प्रथमद्वितीयषष्ठपुस्तकेषु पाठः ।

160. 'प्रजायते' इति प्रथमपुस्तके पाठः ।

161. 'धर्ममूलं' इति सर्वादर्शपुस्तकेषु पाठः ।

162. 'मांसे तु' इति आकरे पाठः ।

163. 'तथा' इति आकरे पाठः ।

164. 'वराहमांसात्' इति आकरे पाठः ।

165. 'संजनयेत् सुतम्' इति आकरे पाठः ।

166. 'मार्गविक्रान्तजंघालं' इति आदर्शपुस्तकेषु पाठः ।

167. 'नृत्यशीलं' इति आदर्शपुस्तकेषु पाठः ।

168. 'श्लेष्मकं' इति द्वितीयपुस्तके पाठः ।

169. 'कठिनोत्कटुकासनं' इति प्रथमपुस्तके पाठः ।

170. 'शुद्धावेगविधारणम्' इति षष्ठपुस्तके पाठः ।

171. 'अमर्षंदाक्षोषधानां' इति प्रथमपञ्चमपुस्तकयोः पाठः ।

172. 'अभिलषाकुलावीयं' इति षष्ठपुस्तके पाठः ।

173. 'वहुकायाद्रोहशीलं' इति द्वितीयपुस्तके पाठः ।

174. 'बहुविष्णुतचित्तं' इति द्वितीयपुस्तके पाठः ।

175. 'शीलपर्युषिताशिनी' इति प्रथमपुस्तके पाठः ।

176. द्रष्टव्यम्—चरक : शारीर८:२१ ।
सुश्रुत : शारीर३:२०-२९ ।

177. 'सूर' इति प्रथमपुस्तके पाठः ।

178. 'सेवनात्स्फोटमुक्त्वचः' इति द्वितीयपुस्तके पाठः ।

179. 'प्राक् दर्शनं भवेत्' इति द्वितीयपुस्तके पाठः ।

180. 'दक्षिणकुक्षिमहत्त्वं' इति तु आकरे पाठः ।

181. 'दौर्हृदम्' इति तु आकरे पाठः ।

182. 'नलकुण्डलमम्बुजम्' इति पञ्चमपुस्तके पाठः ।

183. 'पद्मोत्पलकुमुदाम्रातकादीनि' इति तु आकरे पाठः ।

184. द्रष्टव्यम्—सुश्रुत : शारीर३:३४ ।

185. 'मूत्रयं च समातृकं' इति द्वितीयपुस्तके पाठः ।

186. 'करः' इति द्वितीयपुस्तके पाठः ।

187. 'पार्ष्णीगुल्फप्रभृतयः' इति षष्ठपुस्तके पाठः ।

188. 'नाभिहृद्यकृत्' इति द्वितीयपुस्तके पाठः ।

189. 'वक्षः' इति द्वितीयषष्ठपुस्तकयोः पाठः ।

190. द्रष्टव्यम्—सुश्रुत : शारीर३:३३ ।
सुश्रुत : शारीर४:३१ ।
चरक : शारीर३:६-१३ ।

191. 'शुषिरं———स्थितां' पाठोऽयं द्वितीयपुस्तके नोपलभ्यते ।

192. 'तत्रैव———स्मृतम्' पाठोऽयं द्वितीयपुस्तके अधिको भवति ।

193. 'चेतना' इति षष्ठपुस्तके पाठः ।

194. 'शलाकरात्' इति षष्ठपुस्तके पाठः ।

195. 'वक्र' इति प्रथमपुस्तके पाठः ।

196. 'यकृत्क्रीडीतरस्थितम्' इति द्वितीयपुस्तके पाठः ।

197. 'रत्नाकरात्———स्थितम्' पाठोऽयं पञ्चमपुस्तके नोपलभ्यते ।

198. 'द्विधा' इति षष्ठपुस्तके पाठः ।

199. 'सुषुप्तिः स्यात्तदात्मनः' इति द्वितीयपुस्तके पाठः ।

200. 'लीयन्ते———स्यात्तदात्मनः' पाठोऽयं द्वितीयपुस्तके नोपलभ्यते ।

201. 'जागर्न्तिचित्तं' इति पञ्चमपुस्तके पाठः ।

202. द्रष्टव्यम्—सुश्रुत : शारीर४:३२-३७ ।

203. 'यन्त्रं' इति द्वितीयपुस्तके पाठः ।
'यन्त्रे' इति पञ्चमपुस्तके पाठः ।

204. 'व्यामो वाहोंससकरयोः तिर्यगनामितादधः' इति द्वितीयपुस्तके पाठः।

205. द्रष्टव्यम्—सुश्रुत : शारीर५:६।

206. 'पच्यमानानामाध्मानाद्रुक्मसारवत्' इति आकरे पाठः।

207. 'रक्तवाहि' इति षष्ठपुस्तके पाठः।

208. 'धरामूलं' इति प्रथमपुस्तके पाठः।

209. 'प्रोक्तौ पुष्टिकरौ तौ तु वृक्कौ पुंभावसम्भवौ' इति द्वितीयपुस्तके पाठः।

210. 'ऊर्ध्वमग्न्याशयोर्नाभेर्वामभागे व्यवस्थितः' इति आदर्शपुस्तकेषु पाठः।

211. 'मलं' इति षष्ठपुस्तके पाठः।

212. 'जीवरक्ताशयमुरो' इति षष्ठपुस्तके पाठः।

213. द्रष्टव्यम्—सुश्रुत : शारीर४:५–७।

214. द्रष्टव्यम्—अष्टाङ्गहृदय : शारीर३:६।

215. 'प्रताना' इति आकरे पाठः।

216. 'च' इति आदर्शपुस्तकेषु पाठः।

217. 'तथा' इति आदर्शपुस्तकेषु पाठः।

218. मांसस्याभ्यन्तरतः, तस्यां शोणितं विशेषतश्च सिरासु यकृत्प्लीह्नोश्च भवति। इति सुश्रुते पञ्चमपुस्तके च पाठः।

[सुश्रुत : शारीर४:१०]

219. द्रष्टव्यम्—सुश्रुत : शारीर४:८ डल्हणः।

220. 'रक्तधारणे' इति द्वितीयपुस्तके पाठः।

221. द्रष्टव्यम्—सुश्रुत : शारीर४:१०।

222. 'वृक्षाद्यथाप्रतिहतात्' इति आदर्शपुस्तकेषु पाठः।

223. 'समप्रवर्त्तते' इति आदर्शपुस्तकेषु पाठः।

224. त्वभ्यन्तराश्रितः इति आकरे पाठः।

225. 'अण्वन्तरेषु' इति आदर्शपुस्तकेषु पाठः।

226. 'सर्वेषु' तु आकरे पाठः।

227. 'शुद्धमांसभवः' इति द्वितीयपुस्तके पाठः।

228. 'वाक्षे' इति द्वितीयपुस्तके पाठः।

229. 'पोट' इति द्वितीयपुस्तके पाठः।

230. पाठोऽयं चरके नोपलभ्यते पाठोऽयं सुश्रुते उपलभ्यते।

231. 'अन्त्राणि' इति आकरे पाठः।

232. द्रष्टव्यम्—चरक : चिकित्सा१५:५६।

233. 'या सर्वप्राणिनां सर्वशरीरव्यापिनी' इति आकरे पाठः।

234. 'शुक्रासृग्रू ष्मणा चापि त्वक्संभूतिर्भवेदिह' इति प्रथमपुस्तके पाठः।

235. 'प्रथमा मांसधरा नाम' इति द्वितीयपुस्तके पाठः।

236. 'लोहिता नाम सा ज्ञेया' इति प्रथमपुस्तके पाठः।

237. 'च मण्डलस्य' इति द्वितीयपुस्तके पाठः।

238. 'रोहिणी' तु आकरे पाठः।

239. द्रष्टव्यम्—सुश्रुत : शारीर४:४।
चरक : शारीर७:४।

240. 'श्रवणनयन————वहिर्मार्गानुसारिणः' पाठोऽयं द्वितीयषष्ठपुस्तकयोः नोपलभ्यते।

241. द्रष्टव्यम्—सुश्रुत : शारीर५:१८।

242. 'पादपृष्ठोदरोरः— — —सञ्ज्ञकानि' पाठोऽयं द्वितीयपुस्तके नोपलभ्यते।

243. द्रष्टव्यम्—सुश्रुत : शारीर५:२०।

244. 'स्थिराश्च' इति आकरे पाठः।

245. 'चेष्टावन्तस्थिराश्च ये इति प्रथमपुस्तके पाठः।

246. 'सन्धयस्त्वेते' इति द्वितीयपुस्तके पाठः।

247. 'संख्या हि भिद्यते' इति द्वितीयपुस्तके पाठः।

248. 'भावा एवंविधास्तेहः' इति द्वितीयषष्ठपुस्तकयोः पाठः।

249. 'सामुद्गतुन्नसेवनी' इति आकरे पाठः।

250. 'सेवनी' इति आकरे पाठः।

251. 'मणिवन्धाङ्गुलीगुल्फे कोराख्या जानुकूर्परे' इति प्रथमपञ्चमपुस्तकयोः पाठः।

252. द्रष्टव्यम्—सुश्रुत : शारीर५:२७।
253. 'यः समानो नृणां' इति द्वितीयपुस्तके पाठः।
254. द्रष्टव्यम्—सुश्रुत : शारीर५:११।
255. द्रष्टव्यम्—सुश्रुत : शारीर५:१४।
256. 'यत्र शाखाप्रतानवत्' इति द्वितीयपुस्तके पाठः।
257. 'सूक्ष्मसुचिराणि' इति द्वितीयपुस्तके पाठः।
258. 'नृणामनीषामम्भ' इति प्रथमपुस्तके पाठः।
259. क. 'कायं नद्धं' इति षष्ठपुस्तके पाठः।
ख. 'काये नद्धं' इति प्रथमपुस्तके पाठः।
260. 'प्रोक्तात्तास्तु' इति आदर्शपुस्तकेषु पाठः।
261. 'चाप्यधः' इति षष्ठपुस्तके पाठः।
262. पाठोऽयं प्रथमपञ्चमपुस्तकयोः नोपलभ्यते।
263. 'शिरा' इति प्रथमपुस्तके पाठः।
264. 'धमन्ति' इति प्रथमपुस्तके पाठः।
265. 'रसरक्तवहा' इति पञ्चमपुस्तके पाठः।
266. 'स्नायुमर्मा समस्तकम्' इति द्वितीयपुस्तके पाठः।
267. 'प्रचक्षते' इति प्रथमपुस्तके पाठः।
268. 'न्यायैर्मर्मविदो विदुः' इति द्वितीयपुस्तके पाठः।
269. द्रष्टव्यम्—सुश्रुत : शारीर६:३-४।
270. 'ग्रीवायाः———सद्योमारकाणि' पाठोऽयं षष्ठपुस्तके अधिकं भवति।
271. द्रष्टव्यम्—सुश्रुत : शारीर६:६डल्हणः।
272. द्रष्टव्यम्—सुश्रुत : शारीर६:८।
273. द्रष्टव्यम्—सुश्रुत : शारीर६:१६।
274. क. 'पाकात्पतंतिशल्योऽपि' इति षष्ठपुस्तके पाठः।
ख. 'पाकात्पतितशल्यो वा जीवति' इति आकरे पाठः।
275. द्रष्टव्यम्—सुश्रुत : शारीर६:१६।

276. 'च' इति द्वितीयपुस्तके पाठः।

277. 'कश्चिद्वैद्य' इति प्रथमपञ्चमपुस्तकयोः पाठः।

278. 'श्वानेवतिष्ठते' इति द्वितीयपुस्तके पाठः।

279. 'नरः छेदभेदादि' इति प्रथमपुस्तके पाठः।

280. 'मध्यमांगुलिः' इति द्वितीयपुस्तके पाठः।

281. 'तलहृन्नाभि' इति द्वितीयपुस्तके पाठः।

282. 'कूर्मः' इति आदर्शपुस्तकेषु पाठः।

283. 'कूर्चः शिरः' इति आदर्शपुस्तकेषु पाठः।

284. 'संधिरुजाकरम्' इति आदर्शपुस्तकेषु पाठः।

285. क. 'गुल्फौ रुक्स्तभकौ यकृत्' इति द्वितीयपुस्तके पाठः।
ख. 'गुल्फौ नुक्स्तम्भकौन्यकृत्' इति प्रथमपुस्तके पाठः।

286. 'क्षणात्' इति द्वितीयपुस्तके पाठः।

287. 'जानुनस्त्र्यङ्गुलादूर्ध्वमन्योरूस्तंभशोफकृत्' इति प्रथमपुस्तके पाठः।

288. 'पक्षकफक्षयात्' इति प्रथमपुस्तके पाठः।

289. क. 'कक्षास्थि' इति द्वितीयपुस्तके पाठः।
ख. 'कक्षाक्षि' इति प्रथमपुस्तके पाठः।

290. 'मूत्राशये' इति आदर्शपुस्तकेषु पाठः।

291. 'वसुरत्वाशमाशनात्' इति आदर्शपुस्तकेषु पाठः।

292. 'ऊर्ध्वाधोसृक्ककफापूर्णे कोष्ठे यस्यैतयोः क्रमात्' इति द्वितीयपुस्तके पाठः।

293. 'ऋतेऽश्मरी द्विधा तस्य तत्राप्युभयतश्च यः' इति आदर्शपुस्तकेषु पाठः।

294. 'मूत्रस्रावे कृते नृणां व्रणा रोहन्ति यत्नतः' इति आदर्शपुस्तकेषु पाठः।

295. 'अधोंर्शकूटयोर्विद्यादपलापापमर्मणी' इति द्वितीयपुस्तके पाठः।

296. 'तस्यष्टेतेन' इति द्वितीयपुस्तके पाठः।

297, 'रिक्तरक्तक्षयात्पाण्डुर्हीनरूपो' इति द्वितीयपुस्तके पाठः।

298. 'पृष्ठवंशे' इति आदर्शपुस्तकेषु पाठः।

299. 'जंघस्य तु' इति द्वितीयपुस्तके पाठः।

300. 'कुकुंचनौ' इति प्रथमषष्ठपुस्तके पाठः ।

301. 'चेष्टाहानिरुजः' इति द्वितीयपुस्तके पाठः ।

302. 'रुद्धता' इति आदर्शपुस्तकेषु पाठः ।

303. 'स्वनकूलाजवे' इति द्वितीयपुस्तके पाठः ।

304. 'तथा' इति द्वितीयपुस्तके पाठः ।

305. 'बृहती' इति द्वितीयपुस्तके पाठः ।

306. 'चाहुः स्वापशोषौ' इति द्वितीयपुस्तके पाठः ।

307. 'चासौ' इति द्वितीयपुस्तके पाठः ।

308 'कंठनाडीमुभयतो शिराजिह्वां समाश्रिताः' इति आदर्शपुस्तकेषु पाठः ।

309. 'घ्नन्त्यसून्मातृकावधात्' इति आदर्शपुस्तकेषु पाठः ।

310. 'बलं शिराः' इति द्वितीयपुस्तके पाठः ।

311. 'स्तनचूचुकयोरूर्ध्वं' इति तु आकरे पाठः ।

312. द्रष्टव्यम्—सुश्रुत : शारीर६:२५ ।

313. 'समस्य' इति द्वितीयपुस्तके पाठः ।

314. 'कुर्यादसमस्य च बुद्धिमान्' इति द्वितीयपुस्तके पाठः ।

315. 'क्षपयेद्बृंहयेच्चापि दोषधातुमलान् भिषक्' इति आकरे पाठः ।

316. 'दोषधातुमलादीनां' इति आदर्शपुस्तकेषु पाठः ।

317. 'शमतां' इति प्रथमपुस्तके पाठः ।

318. 'दोषादीनां त्वसमतामनुमानेन लक्षयेत्' इति आकरे पाठः ।

[सुश्रुत : सूत्र१५:३९]

319. 'प्रपश्यति' इति षष्ठपुस्तके पाठः ।

320. 'भवेदिति' इति आकरे पाठः ।

321. 'तासु' इति द्वितीयपुस्तके पाठः ।

322. 'सैव यथा' इति द्वितीयपुस्तके पाठः ।

323. 'इति श्री टोडरानन्दे शारीरकथनम्' इति द्वितीयषष्ठपुस्तकयोः पाठः ।

CHAPTER 5

[1] 'श्रीदाममित्रं यमुनोपकूलात् वहन् परे मे स रतिं विदध्यात् ।

भांडीरकं नाम वनं नरेन्द्रे सर्वाश्रये टोडरमल्लसंज्ञे' ॥१॥

Lord Kṛṣṇa who is the friend of Śrīdāma and who was playing in the forest called Bhāṇḍīraka, may bestow affections upon the king called Toḍara malla, who is the protector of all.

[There appears to be some mistakes in this invocation].

आयुरादौ परीक्षेत पश्चात् कार्यं चिकित्सितम् ।

[2] आयुर्हीनमनुष्याय भेषजैः किं प्रयोजनम् ॥२॥

The physician should first of all examine the span of life of the patient, and only thereafter, initiate his treatment. If the span of life is over then where is the need for treatment ?

[दूतपरीक्षा][3]

धूमं दृष्ट्वा यथा वह्निः दूरादेवानुमीयते ।

तथैवान्ते परोक्षे च सिद्धिर्दूतेन लक्ष्यते ॥३॥

Examination of Dūta

As the fire of a distant place can be inferred from the smoke, similarly, the success or otherwise in the treatment of a patient can be ascertained both by inference and direct observation from the characteristic features of the *dūta* (messenger who comes to call the physician).

'दूतदर्शनसंभाषा वेषचेष्टितमेव[4] च ।

ऋक्षं वेला तिथिश्चैव निमित्तं शकुनोऽनिलः[5] ॥४॥

देशो वैद्यस्य वाग्देहमनसां च विचेष्टितम् ।

कथयन्त्यातुरगतं शुभं वा यदि वाऽशुभम्' ॥५॥

[सुश्रुत : सूत्र २९:३-४]

The success or failure of the treatment is determined on the basis of the following :

1. Appearance, talk, dress and movement of the messenger;
2. The *nakṣatra* (location of the star); *velā* (time of the day and night) and *tithi* (day of the fortnight) etc., when the physician is called;
3. *Nimitta* (auspicious or inauspicious events);
4. The characteristic features of birds, wind and the locality; and
5. The speech, movements of the body and mental action of the physician.

'स्वजातिर्वा[6] स्वगोत्रो वा दूतः कार्यकरः[7] शुभः ।'

[सुश्रुतः : सूत्र २६:२४]

If the messenger belongs to the same caste or the same clan as that of the patient, then there will be success in treatment and auspiciousness.

दूतं[8] नष्टं गतं [भ्रष्टं][9] वाक्यमित्यादि वर्जयेत् ॥६॥

The messenger who speaks hurriedly and whose sentence of speech is either not heard or who commits mistakes in speaking, should be avoided.

आत्रेयः

यः श्वेतवस्त्रावृत्तपूर्णपाणिः सम्पूर्णताम्बूलमुखः प्रशस्तः ।
द्विजः[10] तथा क्षत्रियकः सुशीलः प्रज्ञाधिकश्चाह्वयते सुखाय ॥७॥

According to Ātreya

If the messenger who has worn white cloth, whose hands are full (of presents), who has *tāmbūla* (betel leaf) in his mouth, who is skillful, who is a *dvija* (either *brāhmaṇa*, *kṣatriya* or *vaiśya*), who is of good conduct and who is intelligent calls the physician, then this results in happiness.

रजतमुकुलवस्त्रं[11] गन्धताम्बूलहस्तम्,[12] स्रजविकं च सरोजं पद्मकिंजल्कपुष्पम् ।
विनयवचनवादी पाठकः स्वच्छवेषो, भिषजमनसुतोषी रोगनाशाय दूतः[13] ॥८॥

If the messenger who has worn silver like white cloth, who has fragrant betel in the hand, who has worn garlands of water lilly and lotus, who is polite in speech, who is engaged in recitation, who has worn clean dress and who is pleasing to the mind of the physician comes to the physician, then the disease of the patient will be cured.

आगत्योदीच्यपूर्वमथ वरुणदिशामैशान्यासृत्य शान्तो[14] ।
दृष्ट्वा वैद्यं प्रहस्य प्रवदति निपुणं नातिनीचं न चोच्चम् ॥९॥
उत्तिष्ठेति प्रसादं कुरु वचनमिदं सौख्यवार्त्तां तनोति ।
प्राज्ञः स्वार्थं प्रकृष्टं सुखमगदकरं रोगिणां वैद्यलाभः[15] ॥१०॥

If the messenger who has come from the *udicya* (north), *varuṇa* (west) and *aiśānya*, (north-east), who is peaceful, who speaks to the physician with smiling face, who is skillful in talking, who speaks neither in a very low voice nor in a very loud voice, who requests the physician respectfully to grace the patient, who is intelligent and who is expert in accomplishing his own objectives, approaches the physician, then the patient will be free from his disease.

रक्तपित्तातिसारेषु प्रमेहेषु विशेषतः[16] ।
प्रशस्तो [17]जलरोधेषु दूतवैद्यसमागमः ॥११॥

[सुश्रुत : सूत्र २९:२२]

The meeting of the messenger and the physician near the dam of a water reservoir is good if the patient is suffering from *rakta-pitta* (a condition characterised by bleeding from different parts of the body), *atisāra* (diarrhoea), and *prameha* (obstinate urinary disorder including diabetes).

[18]'स्वग्पालि श्वेतवस्त्रो द्रविणयुतकर[19][क्षत्रियो] ब्राह्मणो वा ।
तांबूलाढ्यः सुशीलशुभवचनवदत्स्यात्प्रशस्तोऽत्र दूतः ॥१२॥

The messenger who has a garland in hand, who has worn white cloth, who has carried money in his hand, who is either *kṣatriya* or *brāhmaṇa* by caste, who has eaten *tāmbūla* (betel), who is of good conduct and who speaks politely is auspicious.

शस्ता योषिन्न दौत्ये न च जन [युगलं][20] नांगहीनो न रोगी ।
शोकार्त्तो वा रूदन्वानातप्तहतपतितमभृष्टशब्दान् ब्रुवाण:' ॥१३॥

A woman messenger is not conducive to auspiciousness. Two persons should not be sent together as messenger. A person who is *aṅga hīna* (short of any organ of the body), who is a patient, who is engulfed in grief, who is crying, and who speaks words like *ātapta*, *hata*, *patita* and *abhṛṣṭa*. is not useful as a messenger.

यक्ष्मिणां तु विसृष्टं[21] स्यात्तस्नेहानुपदर्शनम् ।
'गर्दभोष्ट्रथप्राप्ता: प्राप्ता वा स्युः परम्परा:' ॥१४॥

[सुश्रुत : सूत्र २९:६]

If the messenger has come with oil in hand, or on a vehicle of donkey or camel. or many of them come in line, to call the physician to attend to a patient suffering from tuberculosis, then the physician should not go there.

पाशदण्डायुधधरा: पाण्डुरेतरवाससः ।

[सुश्रुत : सूत्र २९:७]

न्यूनाधिकाङ्गा उद्विग्ना विकृता रौद्ररूपिण: ॥१५॥

[सुश्रुत : सूत्र २९:८]

छिन्दन्तस्तृणकाष्ठानि स्पृशन्तो नासिकां स्तनम्[22] ।
कपालोपलभस्मास्थितुषाङ्गारकराश्च ये ॥१६॥

[सुश्रुत : सूत्र २९:११]

फलं पक्वमसारं[23] च गृहीत्वाऽन्यच्च तादृशम्[24] ।

[सुश्रुत : सूत्र २९:१२]

तैलकर्दमदिग्धाङ्गा[25] रक्तस्रगनुलेपनाः ॥१७॥

[सुश्रुत : सूत्र २९:१२]

वैद्यं य[26] उपसर्पन्ति दूतास्ते चापि गर्हिताः ।

[सुश्रुत : सूत्र २९:१५]

If a messenger who has carried a noose, a staff or a sword, who has worn a cloth having colour other than grey, who has deformity, who is anxious, who is not in his self, who is ferocious, who bites grass and wood pieces, who is touching the nose and the breasts, who has *kapāla* (piece of broken earthen jar), *upala* (cow dung cake), *bhasma* (ash), *asthi* (bone), *tuṣā* (husk) and *aṅgāra* (charcoal) in hand, who has carried a ripe but immature fruit or similar other things in his hand, who has smeared his body with oil and mud and who has worn a garland smeared with blood, comes to the physician, then it is very inauspicious.

दूतमुखोत्थितवर्णान् द्विगुणी कृत्य त्रिभिर्हरेद्भागम् ॥१८॥

शून्येनोर्वऋते वा मृत्युं जीवनमादिशेद्वैद्यः ।

The alphabets in the statement of the messenger should be multiplied by two and the resultant number should be divided by three. If the residue of this division is zero, then the patient will die, otherwise, the patient will survive.

'वैद्यस्य दैवे पैत्र्ये वा कार्ये चोत्पातदर्शने ॥१९॥

मध्याह्ने चार्धरात्रे[27] वा सन्ध्ययोः कृत्तिकासु च ।

आर्द्राश्लेषामघामूलपूर्वासु भरणीषु च ॥२०॥

चतुर्थ्यां[28] च नवम्यां[29] च षष्ठ्यां संधिदिनेषु च ।'

[सुश्रुत्र : सूत्र २९:१७-१९]

रज्जुसंमार्जनीशूर्पहस्तो दूतो न शस्यते ॥२१॥

If the messenger comes to the physician when the latter is engaged in offering prayer to the gods or manes or when there is turbulance or during midday, midnight, dawn and dusk, or when in the sky there are stars like *kṛttikā*, *ārdrā*, *aśleṣā*, *maghā*, *mūlā* and *bharaṇi* or during *caturthī* (fourth day of the fortnight), *navami* (ninth day of the fortnight) and *ṣaṣṭhi* (sixth day of the fortnight) or during *sandhi dina* when a person is supposed to offer prayer to the gods and the manes or if he comes with *sammārjani* (rope used for *yajña*) and *sūrpa* (winnowing-basket) then it is very inauspicious.

ग्रन्थान्तरात्

30

'सतात्यश्लेषारौद्रपूर्वासु शुक्रे रोगोत्पत्तिर्जायते यस्य पुंसः ।

तद्भैषज्यं व्यावृता निःप्रयत्नं स्याल्लब्धाब्दे लब्धजन्मापि वैद्यः ॥२२॥

According to another medical text if a disease occurs in a man when the planet *Śukra* is in conjunction with constellations like *Aśleṣā* and *Raudra* then administration of therapies is prohibited. A physician who could cure such discases is extremely rare.

31

उरगशतभिषाद्रस्वातिनक्षत्रपूर्वा कृमिवहनविशाखापापवारेणयुक्ताः ।'

तिथिषु नवमी षष्ठी द्वादशी वा चतुर्थी भवति हरिहरोक्तो रोगिणां मृत्युकालः ॥२३॥

If a disease occurs in a constellation like *Uraga*, *Śatabhiṣā*, *Ārdrā*, *Svāti*, *Kṛmi*, *Dahana*, and *Viśakhā* coupled with *pāpavāra* (bad days) or in *tithi* like *navami*, *ṣaṣṭhi*, *dvādaśī* and *caturthī* then this certainly results in the death of the patient according to Harihara.

काष्ठस्य शुष्कवृक्षस्य स्थाने शुष्कजलाशये ।

शाखामृगमयूराणां संपाते तित्तिरादिषु ॥२४॥

समागतो यक्ष्मिणं वै ध्रुवं दूतस्तु दारुणः ।

If a messenger of a patient suffering from tuberculosis meets the physician near the wood of a dry tree or near a dry pond or when there is fall of *śākhā mṛga*, *mayūra*, *tittira* etc., then it is certainly inauspicious.

रूक्षस्थाने प्रदोषे वा कृशो रूक्षः क्षुधातुरः ॥२५॥

गर्हितो वातरोगेषु दूतो वैद्यमुपागतः ।

If the messenger of a patient suffering from *vāta roga* meets the physician in a dry place or during dusk and if he is emaciated, dry and hungry then it is inauspicious.

'स्विन्नाभितप्ता मध्याह्ने ज्वलनस्य समीपतः ॥२६॥

32

गर्हिताः पित्तरोगेषु कफोत्थेषु सुखप्रदाः ।'

If a messenger of a patient suffering from *pitta roga* meets the physician, when the former is sweating or afflicted with heat, during mid-day or near a fire, then it is inauspicious. On the other hand, it is auspicious if the patient is suffering from *kapha roga*.

जलाशयाः सोदकाश्च प्रमेहेषु विगर्हिता ॥२७॥

If the messenger meets the physician near a pond or along with water, then this is bad, if the patient is suffering from *prameha*.

आश्रितस्तु प्रनाडीषु गृहे वारिपथेषु च ।

अतीसारे प्रमेहे वा दूतः कार्यविनाशकः ॥२८॥

If the messenger meets the physician in a house having water channels or near a water channel, then it is inauspicious if the patient is suffering from *atisāra* or *prameha*.

शुक्रमूत्रगृहे शस्तो वमने रेचने तथा ।

If the patient is suffering from vomiting or diarrhoea then the meeting of his messenger with the physician in a house having semen and urine is inauspicious.

शाकुन्तिकाः शौकरिकाः प्रोन्मत्ताश्चातिनिन्दिताः ॥२६॥

Messenger who has birds or pigs and who are mad, are extremely despisable.

रोगिणां कालचक्रेण ज्ञात्वायुर्निश्चयं वदेत् ।
भेषजं येन साफल्यं जायते सिद्धिः दुर्लभम् ॥३०॥

A physician should ascertain the span of life of the patient with the help of a *kāla cakra* and then determine the success or otherwise of his treatment.

तद्यथा

ऋतुर्दहर नयन (३) करौ (२) बुद्धि (४) मुनि (७)
33
रस (६) वेंदो (४) ग्नि (३) चन्द्र (१) दिक् (१०) दुर्गा (६) ॥३१॥

बिन्यस्याधो विलिखेदादीन् हान्ताँस्तथा वर्णान् ।
दूतातुरयोर्नामनोर्वसुभिः संशोधितासु संख्यासु
जीवत्यधिके रोगी म्रियते हीने समे वापि ॥३२॥

As per the details given below the physician should write the number and the *devanāgari* alphabets. In the houses of alphabets the names of the messenger and the patient should be spotted. The corresponding number according to the alphabets of these names in the houses below should be added. This number should be divided by nine. If the residue exceeds the total number of alphabets of the names of the patient and the messenger, then the patient survives. If the residue is equal to or less than this number, then the patient dies.

[34]

१	३	२	४	७	६	४	३	१	१०	९
अ	आ	इ	ई	उ	ऊ	ए	ऐ	ओ	औ	अं
क	ख	ग	घ	ङ	च	छ	ज	झ	ञ	ट
ठ	ड	ढ	ण	त	थ	द	ध	न	प	फ
ब	भ	म	य	र	ल	व	श	ष	स	ह

आदौ जीवगृहं भूत्वा पश्चाच्छून्यगृहं[35] यदि ।

दूतस्तत्र मृतं विद्धि यस्य प्रश्नः कृतो भवेत् ॥३३॥

If the question of the messenger begins from *jiva gṛha* and ends in the house of zero then the patient about whom the question has been put will die.

पूर्वं शून्यालये भूत्वा यातो जीवालये यदि ।

दूतो वदति चेत्तत्र मृतावस्थोऽपि जीवति[36] ॥३४॥

If the question begins from the house of zero and ends in *jiva gṛha*, then even a moribund patient survives.

'जीवेनाधिष्ठिता पूर्णा रिक्ता[37] तेन विवर्जिता ।

पूर्णायां गच्छतः सिद्धिः रिक्तके[38] रिक्तता भवेत् ॥३५॥

॥इति दूतलक्षणं[39] शुभाशुभम् ॥

The whole (even) numbers are the life givers, the odd numbers are the indicators of death. If the question goes to the even number then the patient survives. If the question goes to an odd number then there will be the death of the patient.

Thus, ends the characteristic features of the auspicious and inauspicious messengers.

40 नक्षत्रवारैस्तिथिभिः समस्तैः कार्यं न किंचिच्छकुने विरुद्धे ।

दोषोऽपि तेषां शकुनेऽनुकूले सदैव सिद्ध्यन्ति समीहितार्थः ॥३६॥

One should not initiate any action on a *nakṣatra* (star), *vāra* (week days) and *tithi* (days of the *pakṣa* or fortnight) which are inauspicious because such actions have harmful effects. If action is initiated when these are auspicious then the objectives of such action are always accomplished.

राजा गजो द्विजमयूरकखंजरीटः चाषः शकुन्तः रजकः सितवस्त्रयुक्तः ।

पुत्रान्विता च युवती गणिका च कन्या श्रेयः सुखाय यशसे परिदर्शयन्ति ॥३७॥

सर्वत्रेति शेषः ।

If one sees the king, elephant, *dvija* (a person of *brāhmaṇa*, *kṣatriya* and *vaiśya* caste), peacock, *khañjarīṭa*, *cāṣa*, *śakunta*, washerman with white cloth, young lady with a male child, prostitute or virgin girl, then these auspicious things invariably lead to happiness and fame.

41 'मांसोदकुम्भच्छत्रं च वाजिवारणगोवृषाः ।'

फलमामं सवत्सा गौ मोदकाः स्वस्तिकं दधि ॥३८॥

42 'हिरण्याक्षतपात्रं च रत्नानि सुमनांसि च ।'

43 'अप्रशान्तोऽनलो मीनः प्रस्थाने श्रेष्ठ उच्यते' ॥३९॥

During the time of journey to the patient's house the best auspicious things are meat, jar full of water, umbrella, horse, elephant, cow, bull, unripe fruit, cow with a calf, *modaka* (a type of sweet meat), *svastika* (an auspicious *yantra* used in sacred rituals), curd, gold, vessel full of unbroken rice, gems, flowers, flame of fire which is not subdued and fish,

श्रादाय रिक्तं कलशं जलार्थी यदि व्रजेत्कोऽपि सहाध्वगेन ।

पूर्णं समादाय निवर्ततेऽन्यो भवेत्कृतार्थो भिषजस्तथैव ॥४०॥

If the physician, during his journey, comes across a person carrying empty jar and going to fetch water with his associate or if he sees a person who is returning with a jar full of water then he succeeds in accomplishing his objectives.

हंसा रवं स्यात् यदि वामतो न क्षितेक्षितिर्दक्षिणपादघातैः ।

कंडूयते दक्षिणमङ्गभागं वैद्यं[44] तुरङ्गो जयमादधाति ।४१॥

If the sound of swans is heard from the left side, if the horse kicks the earth with his right leg [the meaning of this portion is not clear] and if the horse itches its right side, then the physician is sure to be successful.

कंडूयमानावितरेतरस्य स्कन्धं रदैः पश्यति गर्दभौ यः ।

वैद्यः प्रयाणे यदि वा प्रवेशे भवत्यसौ रोगविनाशहेतुः ॥४२॥

If a couple of donkeys itching each other's neck with the help of their teeth is seen by the physician on his journey or during the entry to the patient's house, then the disease of the patient will be cured.

रौति प्रवेशे यदि दक्षिणेन स्यादक्षतातत्करणीयसिद्धिः ।

स्त्री लाभदाः स्युः सुरताधिरूढा धुन्वन्हि देहं न कदापि सिद्ध्यै ॥४३॥

When the physician is about to enter into the patient's house if he sees a crying woman in his right side, then this is auspicious. If the woman is passionate then it is auspicious and if she is shaking her body then it is not auspicious.

ब्रह्मदुन्दुभिजीमूतशंखवेणुरथस्वनाः ।

'सिंहगोगजहंसानां[45] नादश्चातीव शोभनः' ॥४४॥

The sounds of *brahma dundubhi*, *jīmūta*, *śaṁkha*, *veṇu*, *ratha*, *siṁha*, *go*, *gaja* and *haṁsa* are exceedingly auspicious.

दृष्टे शवे रोदनशब्दहीने महार्थसिद्धिः कथिता प्रयाणे ।

If, during the journey, one comes across a dead body being carried without any cry, then this indicates a great success.

मृदुः शीतोऽनुकूलश्च सुगन्धिश्चानिलः शुभः ॥४५॥

The wind, which is blowing slowly, which is cooling and which has pleasing fragrance, is auspicious.

46 'ग्रन्थ्यबुर्दादिरोगेषु छेदशब्दः सुपूजितः ।

If the sound of the word '*cheda*' (incise) is heard, then it is good for a person suffering from *granthi* (enlargement of glands), *arbuda* (tumour) etc.

विद्रध्युदरगुल्मेषु भेदशब्दः सुखावहः ।

If the sound of the word '*bheda*' (excise) is heard, then it is good for a person suffering from *vidradhi* (abscess), *udara* (ascitis) and *gulma* (phantom tumour).

रक्तपित्तातिसारेषु रुद्धशब्दः प्रशस्यते' ॥४६॥

[सुश्रुत : सूत्र २९:४२-४३]

If the sound of the word '*ruddha*' (obstruct) is heard, then it is good for a patient suffering from *rakta pitta* (a disease characterised by bleeding from different parts of the body) and *atisāra* (diarrhoea).

प्रस्थाने यायिनः श्रेष्ठा वाचश्च हृदयङ्गमाः ।

For a traveller, cordial speech just before the onset of the journey, is auspicious.

सर्पेषु यो धन्वननामधेयः प्रयाणकाले स तु वाममागे ॥४७॥

दृष्टः शुभः सिद्धिकृदुन्नताग्ररितष्ठत्यथोर्द्धं यदि राजलाभः ।

If a snake called '*dhanvana*' is seen in the left side while travelling, then it indicates the accomplishment of the objective. If the snake raises its head when it is seen then this endows the person with a kingdom.

'पुन्नामानः खगाः वामाः स्त्रीसंज्ञाः दक्षिणाः शुभाः' ॥४८॥

[सुश्रुत : सूत्र २६:३६]

Birds having names with masculine gender (in Sanskrit language) on left side and those having names with feminine gender on the right side are auspicious.

किमत्र बहुनोक्तेन संक्षेपेणाघुनोच्यते ।

A detailed description of such events is unnecessary. Therefore, now we shall give the description in brief.

47
दौर्मनस्यं च वैद्यस्य यात्रा काले न पूजितम् ॥

विपरीतमनः साक्षाद्विपरीतफलप्रदम् ॥४९॥

Anything that produces unhappiness in the mind of the physician during his journey is not useful. If the mind is unfavourable then this will also yield unfavourable results.

48
"अथ ग्रन्थान्तरात्

कन्या गो क्षीरयुक्ता दधि फलकुसुमं पावकं दीप्यमानं,

नागाश्वं भेरिशंखः द्विजवरगणिकाः पूर्णकुंभाः द्विजाश्च ॥५०॥

पद्मान्नं गीतनृत्यं नरपतिवृषभं श्वेतवस्त्रं च वीणा,

निर्जीवं मांसभारं गमनमभिमुखे सर्वकार्यार्थसिद्धिः ॥५१॥

According to Other Texts

During the journey, if a person comes across a virgin girl, milching cow, curd, fruit, flower, growing flame of fire, elephant, horse, *bheri* (a musical instrument), *śaṁkha* (conch shell), *brāhmaṇa*, prostitute, jar full of water, *dvija*, lotus, food, song, dance, king, bull, white cloth, *viṇā* (violin) and load of dead meat, then he is surely to accomplish his work.

तृणतुषफणिचर्मांगारकार्पासपंकैः,

लवणगुडसमुच्चक्लीवतैलौषधैश्च ॥५२॥

रिपुविडसितधान्यं व्याधिताभ्यंततैलं,

गमनमभितो मुंडो मत्तवातैर्न सिद्धिः" ॥५३॥

॥इति शुभाशुभशकुनलक्षणम्॥

During the journey, if a person comes across grass, husk, *phaṇi* (snake with a hood), skin, charcoal, cotton, mud, salt, jaggery, eunuch, oil, drugs, enemy, stool, black paddy, oil massage of a patient (?) and wild-wind, then he will not be able to accomplish his work.

Thus, ends the characteristics of good and bad omens.

फलाग्निजलवृष्टीनां पुष्पधूमाम्बुदा यथा ।

ख्यापयन्ति भविष्यत्वं तथारिष्टानि पञ्चताम् ॥५४॥

Prognostic signs

As the flower, smoke and cloud indicate the onset of fruit, fire and rain respectively, similarly *ariṣṭas* (signs of bad prognosis) indicate the shortly appearing death.

अग्निवेशः

अतिह्रस्वाति वा वृद्धिः प्रकृतेर्वा विपर्ययः ।

प्राणिनामायुषि क्षीणे तज्जीवं चलितं ध्रियम् ॥५५॥

According to Agniveśa

When the span of life is coming to an end, there will be less manifestation, excessive manifestation or irregular manifestation of the *prakṛti* (natural characteristic features) and the *śri* (graceful appearance) of the person will disappear.

49
यश्चेन्द्रियेष्विन्द्रियार्थे सधातुषु विपच्यते ।

तज्जलिङ्गमरिष्टाख्यं ज्ञेयं मृत्युपुरःसरम् ॥५६॥

If there is *dhātu pāka* (catabolic process in the tissue elements) in the sensory organs which are the receptors of the senses, then the signs and symptoms produced as a result of this are called *ariṣṭa.* The death occurs immediately after the manifestation of such signs and symptoms.

गोपुरः

'शीतोष्णफलपुष्पाणि वर्षं चोभयथा यथा ।'

कालेन च[50] प्रजायन्ते तथा मृत्युः शरीरिणाम्[51] ॥५७॥

According to Gopura

As cold, heat, fruit, flower and rain take place in appropriate time, similarly, death occurs in human beings in appropriate time.

अकालमृत्युनाशार्थं ज्ञेयं वैद्यप्रयोजनम् ।

धीमता तदनुष्ठेयं स्वास्थ्यं येनोपजायते[52] ॥५८॥

The role of a physician is to prevent untimely death. A wise man should observe all the medical instructions by which he can maintain positive health.

53
'विज्ञातं बहुशः सिद्धं विधिवच्चावचारितम् ।

न सिध्यत्यौषधं यस्य नास्ति तस्य चिकित्सितम् ॥५९॥

[अष्टाङ्गहृदयः शारीर ५:१२४-१२५]

When a medicine which is well known, which has successfully cured diseases of many patients and which has been administered following the proper procedure does not effect cure of the patient, then such persons cannot be treated i.e. they are sure to die.

करं संस्थापयेद्भूमौ[54] कुञ्चयेन्मध्यमाङ्गुलिम् ।

ध्रुवं[55] तस्य भवेन्मृत्युर्यद्युत्तिष्ठत्यनामिका ॥६०॥

The person should keep the palms of his hands flat on the ground and then extend backwards the middle fingers. If the index fingers get automatically extended then his death is certain.

नाभिस्थानगुदं यस्य कंपते तालुका मुहुः ।

छागगन्धि शरीरं च मानवो[56] न स जीवति ॥६१॥

If there is frequent trembling in the umbilical region, anus and the palate and if goat's smell emanates from the body of a person, then he will not survive.

हुंकारः शीतलो यस्य फूत्कारो वह्निसन्निभः ।

नासा च शीतला यस्य स जीवेत्प्रहरद्वयम् ॥६२॥

If the *huṁkāra* (producing the sound of *huṁ*) of a person is cold and if his *phūtkāra* (blowing of air through the mouth) is hot like fire and if his nose is cold then he lives for two *praharas* (six hours) only.

अरुन्धतीं ध्रुवं गंगां[57] विष्णोस्त्रीणि पदानि च ।

आयुर्हीनाः न पश्यन्ति चतुर्थं मातृमण्डलम् ॥६३॥

Persons, who have no span of life left cannot see the three steps of *Viṣṇu* viz; *Arundhatī*, *Dhruva* and the *Gaṅgā* of the sky as well as the *Mātṛ maṇḍala*.

अरुन्धती भवेज्जिह्वा ध्रुवो नासाग्रमेव च ।
भ्रुवोर्मध्ये विष्णुपदं नाभि स्यान्मातृमण्डलम्[58] ।'

[योगरत्नाकर : पृष्ठ १३]

देवमार्गं भवेद्गङ्गा विज्ञेया कुशलैः सदा ॥६४॥

तारका मातृमण्डलमित्येके ॥६५॥

Arundhatī is the tongue, *Dhruva* is the tip of nose, *Viṣṇu pada* is the mid-point between the two eye brows, *Mātṛ maṇḍala* is the umbilicus of *Viṣṇu*. The *Gaṅgā* in the sky is the path of the gods. According to some scholars the stars constitute *Mātṛ maṇḍala*.

नेत्राग्रस्थितया यस्य कराङ्गुल्यः[59] तु दृश्यते ।
नोदितः पूर्णिमाचन्द्रो दिनमेकं स जीवति ॥६६॥

If a person can see the tip of the finger placed just in front of his eyes and if he can not recognise the full-moon, then he will live only for one day.

यस्य प्रभातेन शिरोव्यथा स्यात् दीपैः परिवेषमवेक्षमाणः[60] ।
अवश्यतोऽसौ म्रियते मनुष्यो येनामृतं पीतमनेकधापि ॥६७॥

If a person seeing the lamps around him in the early morning gets headache he is certainly to die even if he has taken *amṛta* (ambrosia) for several times.

रक्तोर्ध्वदृष्टिरुष्णार्त्तः स्थूलौष्ठौ जांबवोपमौ ।
स्पर्शाज्ञत्वं[61] भवेद्यस्य द्विदिनं तस्य जीवितम्[62] ॥६८॥

If a person looks upwards being afflicted with heat, if his lips have become thick and black like a *jāmun* fruit and if he is unable to recognise the touch sensation, then he lives only for two days.

जिह्वा कृष्णा मुखं रक्तं हृच्छूलं च मनोभ्रमः ।
63
श्वासः क्षामस्वरो यस्य स जीवेद्दिवसत्रयम् ॥६९॥

If the tongue of a person has become black, if his face has become red, if he has pain in the heart, if he suffers from giddiness or delusion of mind, if he suffers from dyspnoea, and if his voice has become thin, then he lives only for three days.

नासाग्रं रसनाग्रं च चक्षुषैवोष्ठसंपुटम् ।
यो न पश्येत्पुरादृष्टं स चतुर्थेऽह्नि गच्छति ॥७०॥

If a person cannot see the tip of his nose, tip of his tongue and his lips through his eyes, even though he had seen them earlier, then he succumbs to death on the fourth day.

वायुना वीजितस्यापि सिक्तस्य पयसा मुहुः ।
देहे यस्य न रोमांचः पञ्चरात्रं स जीवति ॥७१॥

If a person does not get horripilation even if he is fanned after frequently and sprinkled with water, then he lives only for five nights.

स्नातमात्रस्य यस्यैते त्रयः शुष्यन्ति तत्क्षणात् ।
हृदयं हस्तपादौ च षड्रात्रं तस्य जीवितम् ॥७२॥

If immediately after taking bath, three places, viz., heart, palms and sole of the feet get dried immediately, then he lives only for six nights.

64
यस्य स्वदेशाच्चलितौ कर्णौ तु मृदुतां गतौ ।
भ्रुवोर्मध्यं न यः पश्येत्सप्तरात्रं स जीवति ॥७३॥

If the ears of a person have changed their place, if they become soft and if he is unable to see the point between the two eyebrows, then he lives only for seven nights.

शैत्यं न हन्यात्तपतोऽपि यस्य संतापकारी भवतीह सोमः ।

न वेत्ति यो वा तुहिनं न चोष्णं विनश्यते त्वष्टदिनेनासौ वै ॥७४॥

A person feels cold even if he is considerably heated, if cold produces heating sensation in the body and if he is not able to recognise the touch of ice or hot things, then he succumbs to death within eight days.

कर्णे[65] दण्डादिघातेन राजीनैव च दृश्यते[66] ।

अनिमित्तं च वाधिर्यं यस्य स ग्रहवासरात्[67] ॥७५॥

If a person gets striated spots in his ears when injured by a staff etc., and if he develops deafness without any perceptible reason, then he dies within nine days.

घृते तैले जले चापि दर्पणे यस्तु पश्यति ।

शिरोरहितमात्मानं दशरात्रं स जीवति ॥७६॥

If a person sees his body without his head through ghee, oil, water or a mirror, then he lives only for ten nights.

यस्य स्फुटन्ति नाङ्गुल्यः समाकृष्टेन वायसाः ।

दत्तं बलिं भक्षयन्ति स गच्छेत् रुद्रवासरात् ॥७७॥

If there is no cracking sound in the fingers of a person, if crows get attracted towards him and if they take the *bali* (food) given by the person, then he succumbs to death on the eleventh day.

शिरोविरहितं देहं परेषां यस्तु पश्यति ।

प्रतिलोमं[68] च वा पश्येत् सः गच्छेत् द्वादशोदिनैः ॥७८॥

If a person sees other persons without their heads, or sees in a reverse manner, then he dies on the twelfth day.

तारा दिवा दिक्षुरजो निपांत यो विद्युतं पश्यति च निरभ्रे ।

इन्द्रायुधं च स्वयमेव रात्रौ मासद्वयात्तस्य वदन्ति नाशम् ॥७९॥

A person who sees stars during day time, dust in different directions when they are actually clear, lightening when there is no cloud and rainbow during night, he succumbs to death within two months.

दीपे प्रणष्टे नहि वेत्ति गन्धं छायां निजां पश्यति मूर्धहीनाम् ।

घंटास्वनं यः शृणुतेऽन्तरालान्मासत्रयान्ते स विपद्यते ना ॥८०॥

If a person cannot get the smell of a lamp when it is extinguished, sees his own shadow without the head and if he can hear the sound of a bell beyond a great interval, then he succumbs to death within three months.

यस्य मस्तकमारुह्यासरटो बहुवर्णकः ।

दर्शयेद्बहुरूपं स चतुर्थे मासि नश्यति ॥८१॥

If *varaṭas* (a type of bee or wasp) having variagated colour, surrounds the head of a person and produce different types of movements, then such a person dies within four months.

खंजं पदं यस्य भवेत्कदाचित्पंकाकुले वा पथि पांसुले वा ।

स पञ्चमे मासि विहाय सर्वं प्रयाति याम्यं सदनं मनुष्यः ॥८२॥

If a person becomes lame by accidentally entering into a place having mud or on a road having ash, he dies within five months.

यस्य न स्फुरति ज्योतिः पीडिते नयनद्वये ।

मरणं तस्य निर्दिष्टं षष्ठे मासि विनिश्चितम् ॥८३॥

If a person does not see *jyoti* (vision of sparkling spots) by putting pressure on his eyes, he certainly dies within six months.

मध्याङ्गुलीनां त्रितयं च वक्रं रोगं विना शुष्यति यस्य कण्ठः ।

मुहुर्मुहुर्विस्मरणं च जाड्यं षड्भिः स मासैः प्रलयं प्रयाति ॥८४॥

If the three middle fingers of a person suddenly become curved, if his throat gets dried up without any disease, if his memory fails very frequently and if suddenly he becomes dumb, then he dies within six months.

वृद्धिर्वराङ्गस्य भवेदकस्मात्पीत्वा जलं यस्य न याति तृष्णा ।

भुक्त्वा भृशं नोधृतिरस्ति यस्य स सप्तमे मासि मृतिं लभेत ॥८५॥

If there is sudden increase in the size of the head of a person, if his thirst does not subside in spite of taking adequate quantity of water and if he does not get satisfied even after taking a lot of food, then he succumbs to death within seven months.

क्वचित्पश्यति वो दीप्तं सौवर्णं वृक्षकाननम् ।

विरूपाणि च भूतानि वसुमासं स जीवति ॥८६॥

If a person at times sees flame in a piece of gold, in a tree or in the forest and if he sees living beings in a distorted manner, then he lives only for eight months.

69

कृष्णमृत्पिण्डसंकाशं व्यभ्रेऽर्कं यः प्रपश्यति ।

चित्रं सूर्यं पश्यते वा नवमासं स जीवति ॥८७॥

If a person sees the sun like a black clod of earth when the sky is free from cloud and if he sees the sun in a distorted manner, then he lives only for nine months.

70 71

श्रवणौ पाणिपादौ च नासायुग्मस्तथा मुखम् ।

श्यावं स यस्य मेढ्रान्तं दशमासं स जीवति ॥८८॥

If the ears, hands, legs, both the nostrils, face and the tip of the penis of a person become *śyāva* (greyish blue) then he lives only for ten months.

पीतारक्तारुणाः नीलाः केशाः स्युः प्राणसंक्षये ।

प्रसाध्यमानाः जटिलाः रूक्षाः वाभ्यक्तसन्निभाः ॥८९॥

If the hair of a person becomes yellow, red, *aruṇa* (reddish) or blue in colour, if they appear to have been combed, if the hair becomes matted or dry and if the hair appears to be greased, then the person succumbs to death.

स्थूलांगोऽपि कृशं कृशोऽपि सहसा स्थूलत्वमालंबते ।

श्यामो वा कनकप्रभो यदि भवेद्गौरोऽपि कृष्णच्छविः ॥९०॥

शूरो भीरुरथापि धर्मनिपुणः शान्तो विकारी पुमान् ।

इत्येवं प्रकृतेस्तूशन्ति मुनयो दिङ्मासकैर्जीवनम्[72] ॥९१॥

If a fatty person suddenly becomes thin, if a thin person suddenly becomes fatty, if a black person suddenly becomes golden in colour, if a white person suddenly becomes black, if a brave person suddenly becomes coward, if a devilish person suddenly becomes peaceful and religious, then he lives, according to the sages, only for ten months.

प्रभवति पटुः हृष्टः[73] केशराभः कृशानुः ।

शशधरसमलेखा धारिणीनां[74] ललाटे ॥९२॥

भवति हि धमनीनां जालवान्भालदेशो ।

ह्यतिथिरिव स देही मासे चैकादशे स्यात् ॥९३॥

If the fire (aura or digestive power) inside a person becomes very sharp, well-nourished and saffron coloured, if in his forehead moon-like spots appear, and if there is a network of vessels in his forehead, then he is a guest in this world only for eleven months.

करांगुष्ठस्य मूलं तु समं यस्य न चेष्टते ।
स भवेद्वत्सरे पूर्णे क्षयरोगी न संशयः ॥६४॥

If the base of the thumb of a person does not move regularly, he undoubtedly suffers from tuberculosis within one year.

[75] संस्तब्धौ चारुणौ श्यामौ शीतौ मांसविवर्जितौ ।
स्विन्नाविव तथा पीतौ पादौ ज्ञेयौ गतायुषः ॥६५॥

If the legs of a person become numb, reddish or black in colour, cold, without flesh, as if boiled or yellow in colour, then he is to die soon.

[76] 'शरीरार्द्धे शरीरे वा मुखार्द्धेषु मुखेषु वा ।
हर्षो ग्लानिस्तथा स्नेहं रौक्षं वाऽपि गतायुषाम् ॥'६६॥

If there is happiness and sorrow and unctuousness and dryness simultaneously in half of the body, or the whole body, and in the half of the face or on the whole of the face, then he succumbs to death.

शुचिभिर्ज्ञातिभिर्मित्रैरुपभोगैश्च पुष्कलैः ।
[77] न प्रहृष्यति योऽकस्मात् सः गच्छेद्यममन्दिरम् ॥६७॥

If a person suddenly does not feel happy even when surrounded with relations and friends having purity of mind and when there is lot of wealth for enjoyment, then he succumbs to death.

'यस्य गोमयचूर्णाभं रजस्तीव्रमुदीर्यते ।
अङ्गेभ्यः शिरसो वापि यथा प्रेतस्तथैव सः[78] ॥६८॥'

If from the body or head of a person particles like the powder of a cow-dung cake fall in large quantity, he is as good as a dead person.

यस्य सन्धौ बाहुमूले प्रस्वेदाः लवणोपमाः ।
कणाः शुभ्राः प्रजायन्ते कुष्ठं तस्य भवेद्ध्रुवम् ॥९९॥

If in the joints and axillae of a person sweat appears in the form of salt in white particles, he certainly suffers from leprosy.

'यस्याधरोष्ठः पतति क्षिप्रं चोर्द्ध्वं तथोत्तरम् ।
79
उभौ वा लंबितौ यस्य सोऽपि सद्यो मरिष्यति ॥१००॥'

A person whose upper and lower lips suddenly become loose or get retracted upwards, or both the lips become elongated, he succumbs to death instantaneously.

अग्निवेशात्

नानापुष्पसमो गन्धो यस्य वाति दिवानिशम् ।
पुष्पितस्य वनस्येव नानाद्रुमलतावतः ॥१०१॥
तमाहुः पुष्पितं धीराः नरं मरणलक्षणैः ।

According to Agniveśa

If the fragrance of different types of flowers of a forest having different types of trees and creepers emanate from the body of a person day and night, he is called "*puṣpita*". This is a sign of imminent death.

मद्यानां मधुराणां च कुसुमानां प्रवाति च ॥१०२॥
विण्मूत्रकुणपानां च गन्धो यस्य शुभाशुभः ।
शरीरे जायतेऽसौ वै वर्षमेकं न जीवति ॥१०३॥

If the good and bad smells of sweet alcoholic drinks, flowers, stool, urine and dead body emanate from the body of a person, he does not survive for one year.

नदत्यनाहतं कांस्य यस्य वेश्मनि घट्टितम् ।
प्राग्रूपं मरणस्यैतद्विज्ञेयं नान्यथा ध्रुवम् ॥१०४॥

If a pot of bell metal resounds without having been beaten in the house of a person, then this certainly is the premonitory sign of his death.

आतुरस्य गृहे यस्य भिद्यन्ते वा पतन्ति वा ।
अतिमात्र [च [80] पात्राणि] दुर्लभं तस्य जीवनम् ॥१०५॥

If in the house of a patient, pots including utensils fall and break in excess, then his life is certainly coming to an end.

सुगन्धं चैति दुर्गन्धं दुर्गन्धं च सुगन्धताम् ।
यूकाः ललाटमायान्ति मृताः यूकाः पतन्ति च ॥१०६॥
ह्रीश्रियौ [81] नश्यतेऽकस्माद्धसतश्चापि दृश्यते ।
[82] दंतमांसं च केशेषु सीमन्तश्चोपजायते ॥१०७॥
'चुलेति चाक्षिपक्ष्माणि यथा प्रेतस्तथैव सः [83] ।'
'स्नातानुलिप्तं यं [84] चापि भजन्ते नीलमक्षिकाः ॥'१०८॥

[सुश्रुत : सूत्र ३०:१०]

If to a person good smell appears as bad smell and *vice versa*, if *yūkā* (lice) come to his forehead, if dead lice fall from his head, if he loses *hri* (humility) and *śri* (auspicious characteristics), if while laughing suddenly, his gum muscles are visible, if *simantas* (parting line of the hair) appear in the head, if there is matting of the eyelashes and if *nila makṣikā* (blue bee) moves around him after he has taken bath and applied unction, then he is as good as dead.

"घोणा[85] वा वक्त्रतो[86] याति वक्त्रुकामश्च मुह्यति ।

अकस्मादिन्द्रयोत्पत्तिर्यथाप्रेतस्तथैव सः ॥१०९॥"

If *ghoṇā* (foam ?) comes out of the mouth of a person, if he faints when he desires to speak and if his sense organs manifest their action all of a sudden, then he is as good as dead.

निर्मेघेऽह्नि वारिपूरितोमुखो मार्तण्डं पृष्ठीकृतः ।

फूत्कृत्यांबुनि[87] शक्रचापमनिशं दीर्घायुरालोकते ॥११०॥

यस्तं नैव विलोकते स मनुजः षण्मासमात्रावधो ।

Person who has a long span of life should take a mouthful of water and keeping his back towards the sun, blow the water in very thin streams on a day when it is not cloudy. He will invariably find rainbow. If a person cannot see such a rainbow then he will succumb to death within six months.

कोनाशस्य पुरीं प्रयाति[88] नयने न स्यान्मलं तस्य चेत् ॥१११॥

If a person does not get excreta in his eyes, then he succumbs to death.

द्रुमाऽश्वाऽश्वतरोष्ट्रादि - दुष्टवारणरोहणम्[89] ।

नृपाहितमजीर्णं च दूरतः परिवर्जयेत् ॥११२॥

The physician should keep himself at a great distance from a person who climbs a tree, who rides over untamed animals like horse, *aśvatara* (mule), camel and elephant, who works against the king and who constantly suffers from indigestion.

[90] "रसायनः जपो होमः धर्म्येच्छा विप्रपोषणः ।

वैद्यवाक्यकृतस्यापि प्राप्तमुत्कर्षमायुषः ॥११३॥

तथा ब्रह्मचिदानंदस्मरणेनाधुना समः ।"

For a long span of life, one should use rejuvenation therapy, perform *japa* (recitation of *mantras*), *homa* (offer oblation to fire), religious activities and charity to the *brāhmaṇas.* He should act on the advice of the physician and always keep *Brāhman* in his memory.

रात्रौ दाहो भवति यदि वा जायते जागरत्वं ॥११४॥

कण्ठे श्लेष्मा मुखविरसता कुंकुमाकारता[91] वा ।

यस्मिञ्जिह्वा भवति शिथिला स्थूलसूक्ष्मा च नाडी ॥११५॥

तद्धं वर्ज्यं स्मरणमधुना रामरामेति नाम ।

If a person gets burning sensation and sleeplessness at night, if his throat becomes full of phlegm, if he does not experience any taste in his mouth or gets the taste of saffron in the mouth, if his tongue becomes curved and loose, and if his pulse becomes either very thick or very thin, then the medicine for him is to recite the name of lord Rāma (i.e. he succumbs to death).

काष्ठेन विलिखेद्भूमिं छिनत्तिदशनैर्नखान् ॥११६॥

शिरोरुहान्नखैश्छिन्द्याद्यः स रोगं न मुञ्चति[92] ।

If person scribles over the ground with the help of a piece of wood, if he cuts his nail with the help of his teeth and if he cuts his hair by the help of his nail, then he does not recover from his disease.

इन्द्रियाणि बलं शक्तिराहारो मांसशोणितम् ॥११७॥

93
यस्याशु परिहीयन्ते स जहात्याशु जीवितम् ।

निवर्तते महाव्याधिः सहसाग्निबलक्षयः ॥११८॥

If a person suddenly loses his power of senses, strength, energy, food intake, muscles and blood, then he instantaneously succumbs to death after he is attacked by a serious disease as a result of the diminution of the power of digestion and strength.

दुर्बलो बहुभुंक्ते वा स्वल्पमूत्रपुरीषकः ।

स्वल्पं वा यस्तु संभुक्ते बहुमूत्रपुरीषकः ॥११९॥

नासिकां स्पृशते वापि स याति यममन्दिरम् ।

इति संक्षेपतः प्रोक्तं ग्रंथविस्तारभीतितः ॥१२०॥

चिकित्सायां प्रवक्ष्यन्तेऽरिष्टाः रोगभवाः पृथक् ।

If a weak person eats more food but passes out less of urine and stool or eats less of food but passes more of urine and stool and if he frequently touches his nose, then he succumbs to death.

In order to avoid detailed description, the *ariṣṭa lakṣaṇas* are described here only in brief. In the section on the treatment of diseases (of this text) bad prognostic signs and symptoms in respect of each disease will be described.

॥इति स्वस्थारिष्टरोगारिष्टानि ॥१२१॥

Thus, ends the description of *ariṣṭas* (signs and symptoms of imminent death) of a healthy person and a patient.

94 95
स्वप्नानथ प्रवक्ष्यामि शुभाय मरणाय च ।

अनुभूतः श्रुतो दृष्टः प्रार्थितश्चिन्तितोऽपि वा ॥

दीर्घोऽतिव्याकुलो व्यक्तो दिवसे वातदोषजः ॥१२२॥

मूत्राविष्टे मलाविष्टे पुरुषेषु तथैव च ॥

इत्येते निष्फलाः स्वप्नाः फलदाः ये त्वतोन्यथा १२३॥

Hereafter, different types of dreams which are auspicious and which indicate impending death will be described.

The following types of dreams are *niṣphalā* (fruitless):

1. Dreams which are based on things already experienced, heard, seen, requested and thought;
2. Dreams which are of long duration, which are disturbed and well manifested;
3. Dreams which occur in sleep during day time because of aggravation of *vāyu*; and
4. Dreams which occur as a result of fullness of bladder (by urine) and rectum (by stool).

Dreams caused by factors other than those described above are *phaladā* (fruitful).

शुभं पश्यति धर्मेण चाधर्मेणाशुभं ध्रुवम् ।

By virtuous acts, one gets auspicious dreams and by sinful acts, one gets inauspicious dreams.

मनोवहेषु स्रोतःसु रुद्धेष्वनिलादिना ॥१२४॥

पश्यन्ति दोषजं स्वप्नं यथास्वं तुल्यलक्षणम् [96] ।

When the *manovaha srotas* (channel of the mind) gets obstructed by *vāyu* etc., then a person gets dreams caused by different *doṣas*. Such dreams are similar to the characteristics of the *doṣas*.

नृत्यगीतरतिर्यानं पातप्लवनधावनम् ॥१२५॥

व्यायामोर्ध्वंगतीत्यादि [97] स्वप्ने पश्यन्ति वातिका ।

A person having aggravation of *vāyu* gets dreams of dances, songs, sex indulgence, movement on vehicles, fall, swimming, running and flying into the sky.

कलिप्रहारक्रोधोष्णकृष्णरक्ताम्लपीतकम् ॥१२६॥

तथातितैजसं द्रव्यं स्वप्ने पश्यन्ति पैत्तिकाः ।

A person having aggravation of *pitta* gets dreams of quarrels, beating, anger, heat, black, red and yellow colour, sour taste and dazzling objects.

निद्रामेव हि [98]आलस्य सलिलं स्वादु शीतलम् ॥१२७॥

तथा चातिगुरु द्रव्यं पश्यन्ति श्लैष्मिकाः नराः ।

A person having aggravation of *kapha* gets dreams of sleep, laziness, water, sweet taste, cold things and excessively heavy articles.

रात्रौ [99]यत् प्रथमे यामे सवंत्सरविपाकवान् ॥१२८॥

द्वितीये चाष्टभिर्मासैस्त्रिभिर्मासैस्तृतीयके ।

अरुणोदयवेलायां दशाहेन फलं लभेत् ॥१२९॥

A dream during the first *yāma* (3 hours) of the night produces results within one year. The dream during the second *yāma* produces results in eight months. The dream during the third *yāma* produces results in three months. The dream at the time of the sun rise produces results within 10 days.

स्वप्नेषु शुभ्राणि सुखप्रदानि सर्वाणि चैतानि विवर्जयित्वा ।

कार्पासभस्मास्थिकपालमूलं [100]कुर्यान्नराणां विपदं रुजं वा ॥

All white things, except cotton, ash, bone, skull and root in the dream provide happiness to the person. Cotton etc., in the dream indicate danger, or disease.

कृष्णानि सर्वाणि विनिन्दितानि आरोग्यसत्कीर्तिविनाशकानि ।
तत्राऽपि चैतानि विवर्जयित्वा गोवाजिराजद्विजहंसमत्स्यान् ॥१३०॥

All black things except, cow, stallion, bird, swan and fish in the dream are despicable and they take away health as well as fame of the person.

आत्रेयः

मुकुरकुसुमभृङ्गाः आतपत्रं ध्वजं वा,
दधिफलमथ वस्त्रं चान्नताम्बूलपूगम् ॥१३१॥
कमलकलशशंखं भूषणं काञ्चनं वा,
दिनकरशशितारामण्डलं शोभनाय ॥१३२॥

According to Ātreya

Appearance of buds, flowers, black bee, umbrella, flag, curd, fruit, cloth, food, betel, areca nut, lotus, jar, conch shell, ornaments, gold, sun, moon and stars in the dream is auspicious.

विकचकमलपुञ्जं[101] पूर्णपद्माकराम्भः,
प्रमुदितकरराजी[102] जीवितः श्रोत्रियश्च ॥१३३॥
तरति सलिलराशिं दुग्धमद्यास्रपानं
धनसुखविभवाप्तिं[103] रोगिणां रोगमुक्त्यै[104] ॥१३४॥

Appearance of lotus flowers, pond full of lotus and water, hands in a blessing posture, *brāhmin* who is alive, swimming in great sea, intake of milk, alcohol or blood, procurement of wealth, happiness and other riches by a patient in the dream indicates that a person will be cured of the disease.

देवः द्विजो वा पितरौ नृपो वा,
स्वप्नेषु वाक्यं ब्रुवते यथैव ॥
तथैव नान्यच्च भवेन्मनुष्यो,
यद्यस्य तत्स्याद्विपदं रुजं वा ॥१३५॥

If in a dream, gods, *brāhmins*, manes or kings appear and predict something, then this actually happens to the person. If they predict about any danger or disease, then such incidents do occur.

गोवाजिकुञ्जरनृपाः सुमनः प्रशस्ताः ।
स्वप्नेषु पश्यति नरः सरुजः सुखाय ॥१३६॥

If a person suffering from a disease dreams of cow, horse, elephant, king and flower, then these lead to his recovery.

स्वप्ने पयः पानमतिप्रशस्तं पानं सुरायाश्च घृतस्य चापि ।
तथा यवागूकृशरौदनं वा क्षैरेयिका भोजनकं सुखाय ॥१३७॥

Drinking of milk in dream is very auspicious. Drinking of alcohol, as well as, ghee and intake of gruel, *kṛśarā*, boiled rice, *kṣaireyikā* (a milk preparation) in dreams lead to happiness.

यो धान्यराशि तिलतण्डुलानां गोधूमसिद्धार्थयवादिकानाम् ।
सुपुष्पवल्लीं[105] फलितद्रुमं वा पश्येद्धनाप्तिः[106] गदनाशनार्थम् ।

If heap of paddy, *tila*, rice, wheat, mustard, barley etc., a creeper with beautiful flowers, a tree with fruits and procurement of wealth appear in the dream of a person, he gets cured of his diseases.

सुश्वेतवस्त्रां रमणीं सुरम्यां स्वप्ने समालिङ्गति सौख्यहेतुः ॥१३८॥

In a dream, if a person embraces an exceedingly beautiful lady wearing white cloth, then this results in happiness.

107
अहिं वा वृश्चिकं कीटं स्वप्ने यस्तु प्रपश्यति ।
प्रप्नोति धनराशिं च यदा भीतो न पश्यति ।

If snake, scorpion and insect appear in the dream of a person and if he does not get terrified by their sight, then he acquires wealth.

मांसं मत्स्यं स्रजः श्वेताः वासांसि च फलानि च ॥१३९॥

[सुश्रुत : सूत्र २९:७७]

पश्येद्रोगविनाशार्थं धनलाभार्थमेव च ।

Appearance of meat, fish, garland, white apparel and fruits in dreams results in the cure of the disease of the person. He also gets wealth.

108 109
उरगो वा जलौका वा मक्षिका वा[ऽ]पि संदशेत् ॥१४०॥

[सुश्रुत : सूत्र २९:८०]

110
स्वकरेण स्वकं वापि छेदयेद्यस्तु मस्तकः ।

रोगी रोगविनिर्मुक्तो धनप्राप्तिमवाप्नुयात् ॥१४१॥

If in dream one gets bitten by snake, leech or bee, or if one cuts his head by his own hand, then he gets cured of his disease and gets wealth.

भगछेदं] यदा नारी पश्येद्धवमवाप्नुयात् ।

सफले धनसंपत्तिर्दीप्ते रोगविनाशनम् ॥१४२॥

[111] "सुखं च पुष्पिते ज्ञेयं सम्पूर्णे वाञ्छितं फलम् ।

If a woman dreams of the incision of her *bhaga* (genital organ) then she gets her husband. If fruits appear in her dream then she gets wealth. If dazzling object appears in her dream then her disease gets cured. If she dreams of menstruation then she gets happiness. If she dreams of all these items then she gets the fruit she desires.

शून्यागारं लोकते यो मनुष्यः प्रसादं वा देवहीनं च पश्येत् ।।१४३।।"

पातः सद्यपुष्पितानां द्रुमाणां क्षौद्रं तैलं वाऽपि वैद्यसंगता ।।१४४।।

अतसी तैलपिण्याकलोहानि लवणं तिलान् ।

लभेत स्नाति वा पक्वमन्नं यश्चासवं पिबेत् ।।१४५।।

मुहुराघ्रायते यस्तु श्वापदैर्विकृताननैः ।

हसन्तमभिजल्पन्तं भीमं क्षपणकं मुहुः ।।१४६।।

[112] गतायुषस्तु जानीयात् ध्रुवंतत्त्वविदो विदुः ।

If a person dreams of an empty house, a temple without any statue of the gods, fall of a tree having fresh flowers, honey, oil, association with a physician, receiving *atasi*, oil cake, metals, salt and sesame seed, taking bath, boiled rice, drinking *āsava* type of wine, if in dream, animals with ferocious face smell him frequently and if he dreams of ferocious looking *kṣapaṇaka* (religious mendicant) who is laughing and talking, then he succumbs to death.

स्नेहं बहुविधं स्वप्ने चाण्डालै सह यः पिबेत् ।।१४७।।

स्वप्ने तु वाग्भटः प्राह प्रमेहेन विनश्यति ।

If a person dreams of drinking various types of *sneha* (ghee, oil etc.) in association with *cāṇḍālas* (outscast men), then according to Vāgbhaṭa, he dies of *prameha* (obstinate urinary disorders including diabetes).

शाल्मलिं कोविदारं च पारिभद्रादिकं तथा[113] ।।१४८।।
पुष्पाढ्यं यस्तु संरोहेत्तस्य मृत्युरदूरतः[114] ।

If in dream, a person climbs trees like *śālmali*, *kovidāra* and *pāribhadra* which are full of flowers, then his death is not far off.

कुष्ठेन हन्यते स्वप्ने पद्मैर्वर्तिन पश्यति[115] ।।१४९।।

If a person dreams of being fanned by lotus, then he dies of of *kuṣṭha* (obstinate skin diseases including leprosy).

प्रमेहे चातिसारे च तोयपानेन नश्यति[116] ।

If a person dreams of taking water, then he dies of *prameha* (obstinate urinary disorders including diabetes) or *atisāra* (diarrhoea).

गुल्मेषु स्थावरोत्पत्तिः कोष्ठे मूर्ध्निशिरोरुजि ।।१५०।।

If a person dreams of growth of trees in his abdomen then he dies of *gulma* (phantom tumour). If a person dreams of growth of trees in his head, then he dies of diseases of head (headache).

शष्कुलीभक्षणं छर्द्यां मधु श्वासपिपासयोः ।

If a person dreams of eating *śaṣkuli*, then he dies of vomiting. If he dreams of taking honey, he succumbs to death as a result of *śvāsa* (asthma) and *pipāsā* (morbid thirst).

हरिद्राभक्षणं पाण्डौ रक्तपित्तेऽस्रभक्षणम् ।।१५१।।

चक्षुरोगी न जीवेत सूर्येन्दुग्रंहणेक्षणात् ।

If a person dreams of eating *haridrā* (turmeric), then he dies of *pāṇḍu* (anemia). If he dreams of taking blood, then he dies of *rakta pitta* (a disease characterised by bleeding from different parts of the body).

If a person suffering from eye diseases dreams of seeing the solar or lunar eclipse, then he succumbs to death.

ओदनं पिशितोपेतं यो वमेद्दक्षिणामुखं ॥१५२॥

प्रभञ्जनाच्च मरणं पित्तात् द्राक्षाम्लतस्तथा ।

If, in dreams, a person facing towards the South, vomits rice mixed with meat, then he dies of *vāta roga*. If he dreams of vomiting *drākṣā* (grape fruit) and other sour things, then he dies of *pitta roga*.

117
प्राप्नोति च कफान्नूनं छर्दिर्वामनदर्शनात् ॥१५३॥

If a person dreams of vomiting or a *vāmana* (dwarf person), then he dies of *kapha roga*.

॥इति रुद्रागमात् ॥१५४॥

The above-mentioned characteristic features of dreams are taken from *Rudrāgama*.

हेमप्रसादमारुह्य यो वा गायति नृत्यति ।

गुहां तमःप्रवेशो वा तमःकूपेऽथमज्जनम् ॥१५५॥

118
श्वभ्रे वाथ श्मशाने वा प्रवेशो वारिसंकटे ।

हिरण्यायसयोर्लाभः भेदनं पर्वतस्य वा ॥१५६॥

119
प्रपातः पाशचर्म्मणां ध्रुवं मरणमाप्नुयात् ।

If in dream, a person sings and dances by climbing a palace of gold, or enters into a cave or a dark place, sinks into a dark well, enters into cloud, crematorium or flood water, gets gold or iron and witnesses the cracking of mountain and fall of a noose or skin, then he succumbs to death.

120

रक्तवस्त्रां कृष्णवस्त्रां मुक्तकेशां महाभुजाम् ॥१५७॥

याम्यां रुदन्तीं गायन्तीं किक्किटन्तीं तथैव च ।

आक्रोशन्तीं च संक्रुद्धां समालिंगतीं चुंबतीं ॥१५८॥

आह्वयन्तिं तु यः पश्येद्यमलोकं स गच्छति ।

If a person dreams of a lady in red or black cloth, having her hair loose, having big hands, crying, singing, chewing her teeth, dragging, embracing, kissing and calling with wrath and anger at night, then he succumbs to death.

121

स्वप्नानेवंविधान्दृष्ट्वा प्रातरुत्थाय यत्नवान् ॥१५९॥

दद्यान्माषांस्तिलां लोहं हिरण्यं ब्राह्मणाय वै ।

जपेन्मृत्युंजयं मन्त्रं गायत्रीं त्रिपदां तथा ॥१६०॥

न चाचक्षीत कस्मैश्चिद्दृष्ट्वा स्वप्नमशोभनम् ।

122

देवतायतने चैव वसेद्रात्रित्रयं बुधः ॥१६१॥

If a person gets dreams in the above-mentioned manner, he should give *māṣa*, *tila*, or iron and gold to a *brāhmaṇa*. He should recite *Mṛtyuñjaya mantra* and *Gāyatri mantra*, the latter having three steps. One should never speak of his evil dreams to others. He should reside inside a temple for three nights.

विष्णुत्रयं त्रीणि च पुष्कराणि

वह्नित्रयं त्रीणि पदानि विष्णोः ।

रुद्रस्त्रिनेत्रस्त्रिपथा च गंगा

एतानि दुःस्वप्नविनाशनानि ॥१६२॥

॥इति शुभाशुभस्वप्नानि॥

Three forms of Lord Viṣṇu, three *puṣkaras* (sacred ponds), three forms of *vahni*, three steps of Lord Viṣṇu, Rudra having three eyes, the Gaṅgā having three channels—all these counteract the effects of bad dreams.

Thus, ends the description of the auspicious and inauspicious dreams.

इति श्रीमहाराजाधिराजटोडरमल्लविरचिते टोडरानन्दे आयुर्वेदसौख्ये शुभाशुभ-दूतपरीक्षा-कालचक्र-शुभाशुभ-शकुनलक्षणारिष्टलक्षण-पंचस्वर-शुभाशुभस्वप्नकथनं नाम पञ्चमो हर्षः ।

Thus, ends the fifth Chapter of *Āyurveda saukhyaṁ* in *Ṭoḍarānanda* composed by the great king Ṭoḍara malla which deals with the following topics :

1. Auspicious and inauspicious messenger;
2. *Kāla cakra*;
3. Auspicious and inauspicious *śakuna* (events);
4. Signs and symptoms indicating *ariṣṭa* (bad prognosis);
5. *Panca svara*; and
6. Auspicious and inauspicious **dreams.**

NOTES AND REFERENCES

1. 'श्री दाममित्रं———टोडरमल्ल संज्ञे' पाठोऽयं द्वितीयषष्ठपुस्तकयोः नोपलभ्यते। 'यमुनोयकूलात्' पाठस्य अर्थसंगतिः न सम्यगवगम्यते।
2. 'आयुर्हीना मनुष्याये' इति द्वितीयपुस्तके पाठः।
3. द्रष्टव्यम्—चरक : इन्द्रियस्थान १२:६-२५।

   अष्टाङ्गहृदय : शारीर ६-१६।

   सुश्रुत : सूत्र २९:३-२६।
4. 'वेषाश्चेष्टितमेव' इति आकरे पाठः।
5. 'शकुनोऽनलः' इति षष्ठपुस्तके पाठः।
6. 'स्वस्यां जातौ' इति आकरे पाठः।
7. 'स्मृतः' इति आकरे पाठः।
8. 'दूतः' इति द्वितीयपुस्तके पाठः।
9. 'भृष्टं' इति आदर्शपुस्तकेषु पाठः।
10. 'दीनां' इति द्वितीयपुस्तके पाठः।
11. 'रजतमुकुरवस्त्रं' इति प्रथमपुस्तके पाठः।
12. 'पूगताम्बूलहस्तम्' इति प्रथमपुस्तके पाठः।
13. 'हेतु' इति षष्ठपुस्तके पाठः।
14. 'आगत्योदीच्यपूर्वमथवरुणदिशामैशयाश्रित्यशान्तो' इति द्वितीय पुस्तके पाठः।
15. 'वैद्यलाभं' इति प्रथमपञ्चमपुस्तकयोः पाठः।
16. 'तथैव च' इति आकरे पाठः।
17. 'गलरोगेषु' इति आदर्शपुस्तकेषु पाठः।
18. 'स्वग्पील———ब्रूवाणः' इति पञ्चमपुस्तके अधिकः पाठः।
19. 'छत्रयो' इति पञ्चमपुस्तके पाठः।
20. 'जनजुगलं' इति पञ्चमपुस्तके पाठः।

21. 'विशिष्ट' इति द्वितीयपुस्तके पाठः।

22. 'स्तनौ' इति आदर्शपुस्तकेषु पाठः।

23. 'वा' इति आकरे पाठः।

24. 'तद्विधम्' इति आकरे पाठः।

25. 'तैलकर्दमलिप्तांशाः' इति षष्ठपुस्तके पाठः।

26. 'नुपसर्पन्ति' इति पञ्चमपुस्तके पाठः।

27. 'च' इति आदर्शपुस्तके पाठः।

28. 'वा' इति आकरे पाठः।

29. 'वा' इति आकरे पाठः।

30. 'सतात्यश्लेषारौद्रपूर्वांशु' इति पञ्चमपुस्तके पाठः।

31. द्रष्टव्यम्—सुश्रुत : सूत्र २९:१८-१९।

32. द्रष्टव्यम्—सुश्रुत : सूत्र २९:२०।

33. 'रसवेदाग्नि' इति प्रथमपुस्तके पाठः।

34.

६	३	२	४	७	६	४	३	१	१०	९	
अ	आ	इ	ई	उ	ऊ	ए	ऐ	ओ	औ	अं	
क	ख	ग	घ	ङ	च	छ	ज	झ	ञ	ट	इति षष्ठपुस्तके पाठः।
ठ	ड	ढ	ण	त	थ	द	ध	न	प	फ	
ब	भ	म	य	र	ल	श	ष	स	ह	क्ष	

35. 'पञ्चाछून्यगृहे' इति द्वितीयपुस्तके पाठः।

36. मात्रचतुर्गुण अक्षरदूनाभागज्वदीजै अक्षरनयना एकै शुन्ने मर्दविनाशदोर-
रहै तो तिरिषानास। पाठोऽयं षष्ठपुस्तके अधिकोपलभ्यते।

37. 'रिक्तां तेन' इति षष्ठपुस्तके पाठः।

38. 'सिद्धिरिक्तैः' इति द्वितीयपुस्तके पाठः।

39. "अत्रैव प्रसंगात् प्रश्नलग्नवशादपि रोगिणां शुभाशुभमाह।

राजचण्डेश्वरः—

रोगी किं भविता नीरुगितिप्रश्नाः भिषक् ।
चतुर्थमौषधं रोगं सप्तमो दशमो रजी ॥१॥
रोगी रोगस्तथा वैद्यो भेषज यो भवेद्बली ।
तद्बलान्निर्णयः कार्य रोगिणां रोगसंक्षये ॥२॥
तनौ पापे भिषग्दत्तैर्भेषजैरधिका (रुका) रुजः ।
शुभे मुहुर्त्ते भिषग्दत्तैर्भेषजैर्निरुगामया ॥३॥
एवं व्योम्नि शुभोरो स्ववुध्यैव निरामयः ।
स्वबुध्या दशमे पापैरोगवृद्धि वदेत्सुधीः ॥४॥
घूने पाप तदा रोगी दीर्घकालं सतिष्ठिति ।
शुभे च क्षीयते रोगः पथ्याद्यैरौषधैर्विना ॥५॥
भूर्ये शुभे च तत्संख्यैरौषधैनीरुगामयी ।
दत्तैरफोषधैः वापै दीर्घरोगी भवेन्नरः ॥६॥
लग्नात्स्थिरे चरे राशौ सपापो रोगशान्तये ।
सशुभस्तु कियत्कालाद्रोगशान्तिकरो मतः ॥७॥
द्विः स्वभावेष्टमे रोगी रोगाद्रोगान्तरं ब्रजेत् ।
बहुकाले स्थिरे चैंव रोगीणां रोगसंस्थितिः ॥८॥
लग्नाच्चतुर्थचन्द्राक्कौं शुभदृष्टौ निरामयौ ।
सप्ताहात् पापदृष्टौ च रोगवृद्धिकरौ मतौ ॥९॥
स्मरे व्यये धने क्रूरे लग्ने मृत्यौरिपौशशिन।
सद्यो मृत्युकरो योगः क्रूरे वा चंद्रपार्श्वगे ॥१०॥
लग्ने रविः स्मरे चन्द्र रोगिणां मरणः प्रदः ।
पापार्क्षप्रश्नलग्ने तु पापसंयुतवीक्षिते ॥११॥
तथैव चाष्टमे स्थाने रोगिणां मरणो वदेत् ।
युग्मपापगताः पापा रोगिणां बहुरोगदाः ॥१२॥

लग्नपंचाष्टसप्तस्थाः सौम्याः सौम्यनिरीक्षताः ।

त्रिषट्दशायचंद्रश्च वदन्ति रोगिणां शुभं ॥१३॥

उपर्युक्तः पाठः बहुप्रमादपूर्णः द्वितीय षष्ठपुस्तकयोः अधिकोपलभ्यते ।

40. 'सलग्नेः' इति प्रथमपुस्तके पाठः ।

41. 'मांसोदकुम्भातपत्रविप्रवारणगोवृषाः' इति सुश्रुते पाठः ।

[सुश्रुत : सूत्र २९:२७]

42. 'हिरण्याक्षतपात्रं वा रत्नानि सुमनो नृपः ।' इति सुश्रुते पाठः ।

[सुश्रुत : सूत्र २९:२९]

43. 'अप्रशान्तोऽनलो वाजी हंसश्चापः शिखी तथा ।' इति सुश्रुते पाठः ।

[सुश्रुत : सूत्र २९:२९]

44. 'वैद्यः' इति प्रथमपुस्तके पाठः ।

45. 'सिंहगोवृषनादाश्च ह्रे (हे) षितं गजबृंहितम् ।' इति सुश्रुते पाठः ।

[सुश्रुत : सूत्र २९:३०]

46. 'ग्रन्थ्यर्बुदादिषु सदा' इति आकरे पाठः ।

47. 'यात्रायां न प्रशस्यते' इति आकरे पाठः ।

48. 'अथ ग्रन्थान्तरात्— —मत्तबातैर्नसिद्धिः' पाठोऽयं षष्ठपुस्तके नोपलभ्यते ।

49. 'इन्द्रियेष्विन्द्रियार्थेषु' इति द्वितीयपुस्तके पाठः ।

50. 'काले भवत्यकाले च तथा मृत्युः शरीरिणाम्' इति प्रथमपुस्तके पाठः ।

51. द्रष्टव्यम्—अष्टाङ्गहृदय : शारीर ५:१ ।

52. 'स्वास्थ्यं येन भवेत् ध्रुवं' इति प्रथमपुस्तके पाठः ।

53. विज्ञाने' इति द्वितीयषष्ठपुस्तकयोः पाठः ।

54. 'संख्यापयेद्भूमौ' इति द्वितीयपुस्तके पाठः ।

55. 'याममध्ये' इति प्रथमपुस्तके पाठः ।

56. 'क्षणमेकं' इति प्रथमपुस्तके पाठः ।

57. 'चैव' इति आकरे पाठः ।

58. द्रष्टव्यम्—अष्टाङ्गहृदय : शारीर५:३३ ।

चरक : इन्द्रियस्थान ११:५ ।

सुश्रुत : सूत्र ३०:२० ।

59. 'कचांगुल्या' इति षष्ठपुस्तके पाठः ।

60. 'परीवेशमवीक्षमाणः' इति षष्ठपुस्तके पाठः ।

61. 'उर्द्धश्वासो' इति प्रथमपुस्तके पाठः ।

62. 'जीवनं' इति प्रथमपुस्तके पाठः ।

63. 'कुहरस्थः' इति प्रथमपुस्तके पाठः ।

64. 'स्वदेहाच्चलितौ' इति षष्ठपुस्तके पाठः ।

65. 'कशा' इति प्रथमपुस्तके पाठः ।

66. 'प्रदृश्यते' इति प्रथमपुस्तके पाठः ।

67. 'ग्रहवासरान्' इति प्रथमपुस्तके पाठः ।

68. 'प्रतिलोमे' इति प्रथमपुस्तके पाठः ।

69. 'व्यमेकं' इति षष्ठपुस्तके पाठः ।

70. 'श्रवणौ———स जीवति' पाठोऽयं द्वितीयषष्ठपुस्तकयोः नोपलभ्यते ।

71. 'नाशायायुस्तथा' इति प्रथमपुस्तके पाठः ।

72. 'दिङ्मासजीवेन्नरः' इति प्रथमपुस्तके पाठः ।

73. 'हृषूः' इति द्वितीयपुस्तके पाठः ।

74. 'धारणानां' इति प्रथमपुस्तके पाठः ।

75. 'संस्तब्धी' इति पञ्चमपुस्तके पाठः ।

76. 'शरीरेर्धे————गतायुषां' पाठोऽयं प्रथमपञ्चमपुस्तकयोः अधिकमुपलभ्यते ।

77. 'प्रहृष्येत्' इति प्रथमपुस्तके पाठः ।

78. द्रष्टव्यम्—चरक : इन्द्रियस्थान१२:३ ।

79. द्रष्टव्यम्—सुश्रुत : सूत्र ३१:५ ।

80. पाठोऽयं सम्यक् संगच्छते । आदर्शपुस्तिकासु च 'अतिमात्रममात्राणि' इति पाठः उपलभ्यते ।

81. 'नश्यते यस्य हसतश्चापि' इति प्रथमपञ्चमपुस्तकयोः पाठः।

82. 'दंतमांसेषु' इति षष्ठपुस्तके पाठः।

83. द्रष्टव्यम्—सुश्रुत : सूत्र३१:१०।

84. 'वापि' इति द्वितीयपुस्तके पाठः।

85. "घोणा———तथैव सः" पाठोऽयं षष्ठपुस्तके नोपलभ्यते। पाठस्यास्य अर्थसंगतिः न सम्यक् अवगच्छते।

86. 'वक्रतो चाति' इति पंचमपुस्तके पाठः।

87. 'फूत्कृत्याहनि' इति द्वितीयपुस्तके पाठः।

88. 'नयाति' इति षष्ठपुस्तके पाठः।

89. 'दुष्टवानररोहणम्' इति द्वितीयपुस्तके पाठः।

90. "रसायन————युषा समः" पाठोऽयं द्वितीयषष्ठपुस्तकयोः नोपलभ्यते।

91. 'कुंकुमाकारभावा' इति प्रथमपञ्चमपुस्तकयोः पाठः।

92. द्रष्टव्यम्—अष्टाङ्गहृदय : शारीर ५:११८।

93. 'यस्याश्रु' इति द्वितीयपुस्तके पाठः।

94. 'स्वप्नान् अतः प्रवक्ष्यामि' इति प्रथमपञ्चमपुस्तकयोः पाठः।

95. "सकले न च संप्राप्तिः दीप्ते रोगविनाशनं। सुखं च पुष्पिते ज्ञेयं संपूर्य वांछितं फलं। शून्यागारं लोकते यो मनुष्यः प्रासादं वादे वह्नीं च पश्यते। पातं सद्यः पुष्पितानां द्रुमाणां क्षौद्रं तैलं वापि वैद्यः संगता। अतसीतिलपिण्पाकलोहानि लवणं तिलान्। लभेता श्रीति वा पक्वमन्नं यश्चासवं पिवेत्। मुहुराघ्रायते यस्तु श्वापदै विकृताननैः। हसन्तमभिजल्पं तं भीमं क्षणकं मुहुः। गतायुषं तु जानीयात् ध्रुवं तत्त्वविदो विदुः। स्नेहं बहुविधं स्वप्ने चांडालैः सह यः पिवेत्। स्वप्ने तु वाग्भटः प्राह प्रमेहेन विनश्यति। शाल्मली कोविदारं च पारिभद्रादिकं समाः। पुष्पाढ्यं यस्तु संरोहेत्तस्य मृत्युर्विनिर्दिशेत्। कुष्ठे च हन्यते स्वप्ने पद्मं वर्तिन वक्षसि। प्रमेहे चाति-

सारे च तोयपानेन नश्यति । गुल्मेषु स्थावरोत्पत्तिः कोष्ठे मर्द्धिशिरोरुजि।
शक्कुली भक्षे मधुश्वास पिपासयोः........................।"
पाठोऽयं षष्ठपुस्तके अधिकोपलभ्यते ।

96. 'तस्य' इति द्वितीयपुस्तके पाठः ।
97. 'गमेत्यादि' इति द्वितीयपुस्तके पाठः ।
98. 'चालस्य' इति द्वितीयषष्ठपुस्तकयोः पाठः ।
99. 'यः मथमे' इति द्वितीयपुस्तके पाठः ।
100. 'कपालशूलं इति प्रथमपञ्चमपुस्तकयोः पाठः ।
101. 'विकचकमलकुंजैः' इति प्रथमपञ्चमपुस्तकयोः णठः ।
102. 'प्रमुदितगुरुराजी इति द्वितीयपुस्तके पाठः ।
103. 'धनसुखविभवाप्त्यै' इति द्वितीयपुस्तके पाठः ।
104. 'रोगमुक्तिः' इति प्रथमपञ्चमपुस्तकयोः पाठः ।
105. 'सुपुष्पछत्रीफलितद्रुमं' इति पञ्चमपुस्तके पाठः ।
106. 'पश्येद्धनप्तिं' इति प्रथमपुस्तके पाठः ।
107. 'विपश्यति' इति प्रथमपञ्चमपुस्तकयोः पाठः ।
108. 'भ्रमरो' इति प्रथमपुस्तके आकरे च पाठः ।
109. 'यं दशेत्' इति आकरे पाठः ।
110. 'समनुषः' इति प्रथमपञ्चमपुस्तकयोः पाठः ।
111. "सुखं———च पश्येत्" पाठोऽयं प्रथमपञ्चमपुस्तकयोः नोपलभ्यते ।
112. 'गतायुषं तं' इति प्रथमपञ्चमपुस्तकयोः पाठः ।
113. 'समाः' इति द्वितीयषष्ठपुस्तकयोः पाठः ।
114. 'मृत्युविनिर्दिशेत्' इतिषष्ठपुस्तके पाठः ।
115. 'वक्षसि' इति प्रथमपञ्चमपुस्तकयोः पाठः ।
116. 'पश्यति' इति द्वितीयपुस्तके पाठः ।
117. 'कफान्नूनं' इति द्वितीयपुस्तके पाठः ।

118. 'वापि' इति द्वितीयषष्ठपुस्तकयोः पाठः ।

119. 'पाशवर्मणां' इति द्वितीयषष्ठपुस्तकयोः पाठः ।

120. 'शुक्लकेशां' इति प्रथमपञ्चमपुस्तकयोः पाठः ।

121. 'सवासाजलमाविशेत्' इति द्वितीयपुस्तके पाठः ।

122. वसेद्द्वित्रिदिनं बुधः' इति द्वितीयपुस्तके पाठः ।

CHAPTER 6

1 “अचूचुरद्यो नवनीतपिंडं शिचिस्थितं विश्वहृदि स्थितोऽपि ।

पायान्नृपं टोडरमल्लसंज्ञं गोपांगनानेत्रचकोरचन्द्रः ॥१॥”

Lord Kṛṣṇa who ate by licking the bolus of butter kept in a *śiñcikā* (an implement of ropes hanged from the roof for safe keeping of household items) as if it was the cream of the thought in the heart of the people in the universe and who was looked anxiously by the cowherd women as if the *cakoras* were looking towards the moon, may bless and protect the king Ṭoḍara malla

[अथ नाडीज्ञानम्]

“सद्यः स्नातस्य भुक्तस्य तथा स्नेहावगाहिनः ।

क्षुत्तृष्णार्त्तस्य सुप्तस्य नाडी सम्यक् न बुध्यते ॥२॥

Description of Pulse Examination

The pulse of a person who has just taken bath or food, who has taken oil-bath, who is hungry and thirsty and who is sleeping cannot be examined accurately.

अङ्गुष्ठमूलभागे या धमनी जीवसाक्षिणी ।
[2] "तच्चेष्टया सुखं दुःखं ज्ञेयं कायस्य पंडितैः ।"

[योगरत्नाकर : नाड़ीपरीक्षा : ८-१०]

The artery at the base of the thumb is the witness of the life. By the movement of this artery, a wiseman can examine the pleasant and unpleasant events of the body.

दक्षिणे हस्तपादे च परीक्षेत् विधिवत् द्विजः ॥३॥

It should be examined by a physician in the right hand and right leg of the person according to the prescribed procedure.

चरकात्

'स्त्रीणां भिषग्वामहस्ते पादे वामे च यत्नतः ।
शास्त्रेण सम्प्रदायेन तथा स्वानुभवेन वै ॥४॥

[योगरत्नाकर : नाडी परीक्षा :११]

According to Caraka

In females, the artery of the left hand and the left leg should be examined. This examination should be conducted carefully according to the instructions in medical classics, according to the tradition and according to the experience of the physician.

[3] "एकाङ्गुलं परित्यज्याधरादगुंष्ठमूलतः ।

The physician should examine the pulse by leaving the space of one *aṅgula* (about half an inch) from the root of the thumb.

आद्यंगुले तु मरुतः स्थानं पित्तस्य मध्यमे ॥५॥

कफ[स्यान्ते][4] निजस्थाने गतिं स्वस्थासु वा शिराः ।"

Below the first (index) finger of the physician is the site of *vāyu*; below the middle finger is the site of *pitta* and below the last (ring) finger is the site of *kapha*. In a healthy person, the artery pulsates in the respective places with characteristic features of the concerned *doṣas*.

परीक्षेद्रत्नवच्चात्र[5] अभ्यासादेव जायते ॥६॥

The examination should be conducted with great care and like a gem. Proficiency in this examination is attained only by constant practice.

'अग्रे वातवहा नाडी मध्ये वहति पित्तला ।

अन्ते श्लेष्मविकारेण नाडी ज्ञेया सदा बुधैः ॥७॥

A wise physician should always know that the artery carrying *vāyu* pulsates below the first finger, the one carrying *pitta* pulsates below the middle finger and the one carrying *kapha* pulsates below the last (ring) finger.

सर्पजलौकादिगतिं वदन्ति विबुधाः प्रभंजनेन नाडीम् ।

Because of *vāyu*, the pulse moves like *sarpa* (snake), *jalaukā* (leech) etc.

पित्तेन काकलावकमण्डूकादिगतिं[6] विदुस्तथा चपलाम् ॥८॥

Because of *pitta*, the pulse moves like *kāka* (crow), *lāvaka* (sparrow), *maṇḍūka* (frog) etc. It is very fickle.

राजहंसमयूराणां पारावतकपोतयोः ।

कुक्कुटस्य गतिं धत्ते धमनी कफसङ्गिनी ॥९॥

Because of the association of *kapha*, the pulse moves like *rāja haṁsa*, *mayūra*, *pārāvata* (dove), *kapota* (pigeon) and *kukkuṭa* (cock).

मुहुः सर्पगतिं नाडी मुहुर्भेकगतिं तथा ।

वातपित्तसमुद्भूतां तां वदन्ति विचक्षणाः ॥१०॥

According to the experts in the subject, because of *vāyu* and *pitta* the pulse at times moves like a snake and at times like a frog.

सर्पहंसगतिं तद्वद्वातश्लेष्मवतीं वदेत् ।

Similarly, because of *vāyu* and *kapha*, the pulse moves like a snake and a swan.

हरिहंसगतिं धत्ते पित्तश्लेष्मान्विता धरा ॥११॥

Because of *pitta* and *kapha*, the pulse moves like a *hari* (frog) and a swan.

काष्ठकुट्टो यथा काष्ठं कुट्टते चातिवेगतः ।

स्थित्वा स्थित्वा तथा नाडी सन्निपाताद्भवेद्ध्रुवम् ॥१२॥

A *kāṣṭhakuṭṭa* (wood-pecker bird) strikes (pecks) the wood very frequently maintaining pauses. Similar is the movement of the pulse in *sannipāta* (simultaneous aggravation of all the three *doṣas*).

वृद्धहारीतः

स्पन्दते चैकमानेन त्रिंशद्वारं यदा धरा ।

स्वस्थानेन तदा नूनं रोगी जीवति नान्यथा ॥१३॥

According to Vṛddha Hārita

If the pulse pulsates in the same manner in its own place for at least thirty times, then the patient survives. Otherwise, he does not survive.

स्थित्वा स्थित्वा वहति या[8] सा ज्ञेया प्राणघातिनी ।

If the pulse pulsates after pauses, then this indicates impending death.

जिह्मं[9] जिह्मं शिथिलं शिथिलं व्याकुलं व्याकुलं वा ॥१४॥

स्थित्वा स्थित्वा वहति धमनी याति नाशं[10] च सूक्ष्मा ।

If the pulse pulsates in a curved manner, in a sluggish manner, in an irregular manner after pauses and if there is very thin pulsation, then the person succumbs to death.

पार्श्वे[11] स्कन्धे स्फुरति पुनरप्यङ्गुलीं संस्पृशेद्वा ।

भावैरेवं बहुविधतरैः सन्निपातादसाध्या[12] ॥१५॥

If the pulsation is felt (takes place?) in the sides of the shoulder and then in the fingers and if similar other features are observed then it should be determined as the pulse of *sannipāta.* A person having such type of pulse beat is incurable.

'पूर्वं[13] पित्तगतिं प्रभञ्जनगतिं श्लेष्माणमाविभ्रतीम् ।

स्वस्थानाद्‌गमनं मुहुर्विदधति चक्राधिरूढेव या ॥१६॥

भीष्मत्वं दधति कलापिगतिकां सूक्ष्मत्वमातन्वतीं ।

नोऽसाध्यां धमनीं वदन्ति मुनयो नाडीगतिज्ञानिनः ॥१७॥

If the pulse bears the characteristic features of *pitta* in the beginning, then that of *vāyu* and thereafter, that of *kapha,* if it shifts from its place very frequently, if it moves like a wheel, if it beats fiercefully, if it beats after pauses and if it is thready, then according to experts in pulse examination, such patients do not recover.

गम्भीरा या भवेन्नाडी सा भवेन्मांसवाहिनी ।

Gambhira (deep seated or thick) type of beating indicates that the pulse is carrying *māṁsa* (nutrients of muscle tissue).

14

ज्वरवेगेन धमनी सोष्णा वेगवती भवेत् ॥१८॥

In fever, the pulse is slightly hot to touch and it has a faster beat.

कामक्रोधाद्वेगवहा क्षीणा चिन्ताभयप्लुता ।

When a person is afflicted with passion and anger then the pulse beat is faster. If a person is afflicted with worry and fear, then his pulse becomes thready.

मन्दाग्नेः क्षीणधातोश्च नाडी मन्दतरा भवेत् ॥१९॥

If a person is suffering from *mandāgni* (suppression of the power of digestion) and *dhātu kṣaya* (diminution of tissue elements), then his pulse becomes very subtle to touch.

असृक्पूर्णा भवेत्कोष्णा गुर्वी सामा गरीयसी ।

लघ्वी वहति दीप्ताग्नेस्तथा वेगवती मता ॥२०॥

If the pulse is full of blood, then it is slightly warm in touch. If there is association of *āma*, then the pulse is heavy. If there is *dīptāgni* (strong power of digestion), the pulse is light in touch but it beats very fast.

चपला क्षुधितस्यापि तृप्तस्य वहति स्थिरा ।'

[योगरत्नाकर : नाडी परीक्षा : २२-२६]

If a person is hungry, then there is instability in the pulse beat. If, however, the person is satisfied with food, then there is stability in the pulse beat.

शीघ्रा नाडी [मलोपेता][15] दिनार्द्धेऽग्निसमो ज्वरः ॥२१॥

If the pulse beats very fast and if it appears to be covered with excreta, then within half day, the person will suffer from fever with high temperature.

[16] "मृतिकाले भवेन्नाडी शीर्णा डमरुवत् [?] ।"

दिनैकं जीवितं तस्य द्वितीये म्रियते ध्रुवम् ॥२२॥

At the time of death, the pulse beat resembles the beating of an old *ḍamaru* (a kind of pan). Such a person lives for only one day and he certainly dies on the second day.

मृत्युर्डमरुकस्यैव भवेदेकदिनेन च ।

[17] "मध्ये द्वादशयामानां मृत्युस्तस्य न संशयः ॥२३॥

If the pulse beat appears like the beating of a *ḍamaru* then the person succumbs to death in one day. He certainly dies within thirty six hours and there is no doubt about it.

शीतलं हृदयं नासा हस्तपादौ च शीतलं ।

नाडी वेगवती क्षीणा क्षणमेकं न जीवति ॥२४॥

If the heart, nose, hands and feet of a person become cold and if his pulse beat is very fast but subtle, then he does not live even for a moment.

दर्शनं स्पर्शनं [प्रश्नं][18] चतुर्थं नाडीलक्षणं ।

भिषग्रोगान् वदेत् पश्चान्मुनिरात्रेयभाषितम् ॥२५॥"

॥इति नाडीपरीक्षा॥

According to *Ātreya*, first of all the physician should examine the patient (disease) by *darśana* (direct observation), *sparśana* (touch), *praśna* (interrogation) and *nāḍī lakṣaṇa* (examination of characteristic features of pulse), and thereafter, he should determine the exact nature of the disease.

Thus, ends the description of the examination of pulse.

अथ मूत्रपरीक्षा

ब्राह्मे मुहूर्ते चोत्थाय आद्यधारां परित्यजेत् ।
19 शुभे पात्रे मध्यधारां कृत्वा मूर्ध्नांशुकावृताम् ॥२६॥

भास्करोदयवेलायां प्रकाशे स्थानके धृतम् ।
लोडयित्वा ततो मूत्रं परीक्षेत ततो धृतम् ॥२७॥

प्रमेहं मूत्रवर्णं च निरामं साममेव वा ।

Examination of Urine

The patient's urine should be collected when he gets up from bed in *brāhma muhūrta* (just before dawn). The first flow of the urine should be rejected, the middle *dhārā* (flow) of urine should be collected in a clean vessel. The mouth of this vessel should be covered with a clean cloth (to prevent the fall of dust, flies etc.). At the time of sun rise it should be brought to a lighted place. Holding the container, the urine should be stirred to see if there is *prameha* (obstinate urinary disorders including diabetes), the colour of the urine and its *nirāma* as well as *sāma* conditions.

तृणेनादाय तैलस्य विन्दुं मूत्रे कृते सति ॥२८॥

20 विकासि चेत्तैलमथाशु मूत्रे साध्यः स रोगी, न विकासितश्चेत् ।
स्यात्कष्टसाध्यस्तलगे त्वसाध्यो नागार्जुनेनैव कृता परीक्षा ॥२९॥

In a piece of straw oil should be collected and dropped on the surface of the urine. If the oil spreads instantaneously then the disease is curable. If it does not spread then the disease is difficult of cure. If the oil goes down the urine to settle at the bottom of the container then the disease is incurable. This method of examination of urine has been described by *Nāgārjuna*.

[21]"तृणेनादाय तैलस्य विन्दुं मूत्रयुगे सति ।

जायते बुद्बुदाः यत्र विकारः सोऽस्ति पित्तजः ॥३०॥

When the oil collected through a straw is dropped on the surface of the urine, if bubbles appear, then this indicates the disease caused by *pitta*.

स्निग्धं वसामलच्छायां वाते मूत्रं प्रजायते ।

तरीमुपरि बध्नाति तैलबिन्दुयुतं तथा ।

If the person is suffering from *vātika* disease, then the urine is unctuous and it looks like the waste product of *vasā* (muscle fat). The oil drop remains stagnant on the surface of the urine.

मूत्रे श्लेष्मणि जायन्ते समं पल्वलवारिणा ॥३१॥"

If there is aggravation of *kapha*, then the urine appears like the water of a *palvala* (muddy tank).

चर्पटितः

[22]नीलाच्छरूक्षहिमकृष्णनिभं (च वायौ) पीतारुणं तैलसमं च पित्ते ।

स्निग्धं कफाद्बहलं पल्वलवारितुल्यं स्निग्धोष्णरक्तबहलं रुधिरप्रकोपे ॥३२॥

According to Carpaṭi

Because of the aggravation of *vāyu*, the urine becomes blue, transparent, unctuous, cold and black. By the aggravation of *pitta*, the urine becomes reddish and it looks like oil. By the aggravation of *kapha*, the urine becomes unctuous, thick and like the water of *palvala* (muddy tank). If, there is vitiation of *rakta*, then the urine becomes unctuous, hot, red and thick.

मातुलुंगरसाभासं सौवीराभं जलोपमम् ।

प्रपाकरहितानां च मूत्रं चन्दनसन्निभम् ॥३३॥

If there is indigestion, the urine of the patient looks like the juice of *mātuluṅga*, *sauvira* (vinegar), simple water or sandalwood paste.

निरामवातादच्छं च श्वेतं चापि प्रजायते ।

Because of aggravated *vāta* in its *nirāma* condition, the urine of the person becomes transparent and white.

अजामूत्रविगन्धाढ्यं गन्धाढ्यं खरमूत्रवत् ॥३४॥

अजीर्णप्रभवे रोगे मूत्रं तण्डुलतोयवत् ।

In diseases caused by indigestion the urine of the patient looks like *tanḍula toya* (rice wash). It might have foul smell or excessive smell like the urine of a goat or a donkey.

यस्येक्षुरससंकाशं मूत्रं नेत्रे[23]ऽथ पिंजरे ॥३५॥

[24]"रसाधिकं विजानीयात् लंघनं तत्र कारयेत् ।

If the urine of a person appears like the sugar-cane juice and if his eyes are like *piñjara* (net-like or reddish) in appearance then it should be diagnosed that he is suffering from increase in *rasa dhātu*. To such patients *laṅghana* (fasting) therapy should be administered.

[25][नव]ज्वरे धूमवर्णं बहुमूत्र" प्रजायते ॥३६॥

During *nava jvara* (first stage of fever) the urine is smoky in colour and there is profuse urination.

पित्तानिले धूम्रजलाभकोष्णं श्वेतं मरुत् श्लेष्मणि बुद्बुदाढ्यं ।

तत् श्लेष्मपित्ते कलुषं सरक्तं जीर्णज्वरेऽसृक् सदृशं च पीतम् ।

If *pitta* and *vāyu* are aggravated, then the urine looks like smoke water and it is slightly warm to touch. If *vāyu* and *kapha* are aggravated, then the colour of the urine is white and there will be more of bubbles in the urine. If *kapha* and *pitta* are aggravated, then the urine is *kaluṣa* (cloudy) and red in colour. In chronic fever, the urine looks like blood and yellow in colour.

कृष्णमच्छं[26] विजानीयात्सन्निपातसमुद्भवम् ॥३७॥

If the urine is black and transparent, then it should be diagnosed that the patient is suffering from *sannipāta* (simultaneous vitiation of all the three *doṣas*).

ग्रन्थान्तरात्

कृष्णमूत्रमधःपीतमामवातकफोद्भवम् ।

According to another Text

If the urine is black in colour but there is yellow colour at the bottom, then the patient is suffering from *āmavāta* (rheumatism) and vitiation of *kapha*.

पीतं[27] रक्तं सफेनं च निरामज्वरसम्भवम् ॥३८॥

If the urine is yellow or red in colour and if it is foamy, then the patient is suffering from the *nirāma* stage of *jvara*.

छत्रिणी वारिसदृशं सहफेनं शिरोगदात् ।

If a patient is suffering from the disease of the head, then the urine appears like the water of an umbrella and it is associated with foam.

चिरात्प्रवर्तंते यस्य रूक्षं पीतं सितं तथा ॥३९॥

क्षमता लक्षणं तद्धि पथ्यादेवोपशाम्यति ।

If the urination takes place after a long time and if the urine is ununctuous, yellow and white, then this indicates the mild nature of the disease and it gets cured by *pathya* (wholesome diet) only.

वातरक्तोद्भवं कृष्णं बुद्बुदैः पिंजरप्रभैः ॥४०॥

If the patient is suffering from *vāta rakta* (gout) then his urine will be black in colour and there will be bubbles as well as *piñjara* (net like substance) in his urine.

अश्वमूत्रसमं मूत्रं भवेन्मण्डलकुष्ठतः ।

If a person is suffering from *maṇḍala kuṣṭha* (obstinate type of skin disease), then his urine will look like the urine of a horse.

ऊर्ध्ववाताबधः श्वेतं नीलं स्निग्धं तथोपरि ॥४१॥

If a patient is suffering from *ūrdhva vāta* (aggravation of *vāyu* in the upper part of the body) then the lower portion of the urine will be white in colour and the upper portion will be blue and unctuous.

गोपुरात्

अधस्तक्रप्रभं तैलवर्णं चोपरि लोहितम् ।

रक्तातिसारिणां मूत्रं छर्दितनृणां तथा ॥४२॥

According to Gopura

If a person is suffering from *raktātisāra* (blood diarrhoea) or *chardi* (vomiting) or facial paralysis, then the lower portion of his urine bears the appearance of either butter milk or oil and the upper portion appears red in colour.

अधो बहुलमारक्तमतीसारेषु जायते ।

In the case of simple *atisāra* (diarrhoea) the urine of the patient appears more red at the bottom.

सालस्यं श्वानमूत्राभं हरिद्राभं तथैव च ॥४३॥

कामला लक्षणं विद्धि पथ्यादेवोपशाम्यति ।

If the colour of the urine is yellow or like the urine of a dog and if there is laziness, then these are the signs and symptoms of *kāmalā* (jaundice) and the patient recovers by the intake of *pathya* (wholesome diet).

अल्पाल्पं कृष्णरक्तं च कृमिदोषसमुद्भवम् ॥४४॥

If the urination takes place in small quantities and if the colour of the urine is either black or red, then these indicate that the patient is suffering from *kṛmi doṣa* (infestation by intestinal worms).

मद्यवर्णं भवेन्मूत्रं रसं बहुतरं वदेत् ।

If the colour of the urine is like that of *madya* (alcoholic drink) then this indicates the increase in the quantity of *rasa*.

खरमूत्रसमं किञ्चित्पीतं बुद्बुदसन्निभम् ॥४५॥

हृच्छूलेन विजानीयात् नीलं स्यात्सन्निपाततः ।

Because of *hṛcchūla* (pain in the heart) the urine of the patient is like that of a donkey. It is yellowish in colour and there will be bubbles in it. The colour of the urine becomes blue in *sannipāta* (when there is simultaneous aggravation of all the three *doṣas*).

तैलबिन्दुर्यदा मूत्रे वृद्धिं याति नियोजितः ॥४६॥

मूत्रं च कृष्णतां याति क्षयरोगस्तदा भवेत् ।

If, the oil dropped over the surface of the urine spreads and if the colour of the urine is black, then these indicate that the patient is suffering from *kṣaya roga* (phthisis).

क्षयरोगे यदा श्वेतमसाध्यं च विनिर्दिशेत् ॥४७॥

If, a patient suffering from *kṣaya roga* (phthisis) passes urine of white colour, then this indicates the incurability of the disease.

मांसक्षालनपानीयतुल्यं भवति चोदरात् ।

If a patient is suffering from *udara* (obstinate abdominal diseases including ascites), then his urine looks like *māṁsa kṣālana toya* (meat-wash).

कृच्छ्रमूत्रमधः पीतमामवातकफोद्भवम् ॥४८॥

If the patient passes urine with difficulty and if the lower portion of the urine looks yellow, then he is suffering from *āmavāta* (rheumatism) and vitiation of *kapha*.

[In this connection, the first line of verse no. 38 may be seen—there appears to be some calligraphic errors].

ऊर्द्ध्वं श्वेतमधः पीतं मूत्रं स्यात्पादरोगतः ।

पानीयवर्णमुपरि पीतबुद्बुदसंयुतम् ।

28

हस्तपादसमुद्भूतदाहदोषोपशान्तये ॥४९॥

A patient suffering from the diseases of leg passes urine which is white above and yellow below. If the urine looks like water below and yellow above and if there are bubbles in it, then the patient is suffering from *dāha doṣa* (burning syndrome) of hands and feet. Such a disease generally gets cured.

हरिश्चन्द्रात्

खरमूत्रसमं मूत्रं पीतबुद्बुदसंयुतम् ।
नेत्रशूलेन जानीयान्नीलं चोदरपूर्वकं ॥५०॥

According to Hariścandra

If the urine is like that of a donkey, if it is yellow and if it is associated with bubbles then the person is to be diagnosed as suffering from *netra śūla* (pain in eyes). If there is association of *udara* (obstinate abdominal diseases including ascites), the colour of the urine is blue.

श्वेतवर्णं यदा मूत्रं रक्तबुद्बुदसयुतम्[29] ।
[30]"जायते तत्र जानीयाज्जिह्वादन्तगदो ध्रुवम् ॥५१॥

If the urine is white in colour and if there are red bubbles over it, then the patient should be diagnosed as suffering from diseases of tongue and teeth.

श्वेतरक्तान्वितं पीतमूद्र्ध्ववातेन जायते ।

The urine becomes white with reddish tinge in *ūrdhva vāta* (affliction of *vāyu* in the upper part of the body).

जलोदरसमुद्भूतं मूत्रं घृतकणोपमम् ॥५२॥

In *jalodara* (ascitis) the urine becomes like drops (*kana*=*small* pieces) of ghee.

पाषाणिकायां मूत्रं तु भवेत्कुंकुमपिञ्जरं ।

In *pāṣāṇikā* (stony inflammation of parotid gland) the urine of the patient looks netted and red like saffron.

श्वेतवर्णं यदा मूत्रं रक्तं बुद्बुदसंयुतम् ॥५३॥"

जायते नाऽत्र संदेहो ध्रुवं दंतविषस्य वै ।

If the colour of the urine is white and there are red bubbles, then the patient is undoubtedly suffering from *danta viṣa* (tooth-poisoning).

पीतं तथोपरिच्छायं कृष्णबुद्बुदसंयुतम् ॥५४॥

मूत्रं प्रसूति दोषेण ध्रुवं ज्ञेयं भिषक्तमैः ।

If the colour of the urine is yellowish and there are black bubbles in it then the patient is undoubtedly suffering from *prasūti doṣa* (post-partum infection).

मांसधावनपानीयतुल्यं[31] भवति चोदरात् ॥५५॥

Because of *udara roga* (obstinate abdominal diseases including ascitis), the urine looks like the water in which meat has been washed.

तोयवर्णं यदा मूत्रं पात्रे क्षिप्तं च तत्क्षणात् ।

[32]तैलवर्णं यदि भवेत्तदा याति यमालयम् ॥५६॥

If the original colour of the urine is like water but if it instantaneously changes to the colour of oil when kept in a pot, then the patient succumbs to death.

पीतवर्णं यदा मूत्रं तैलतुल्यं च बुद्बुदम् ।

मरणं प्राप्नुयात्तत्र ध्रुवं ज्ञेयं विशारदैः ॥५७॥

If the urine is yellow in colour and if there are bubbles like oil in it, then according to experts, the patient certainly succumbs to death.

शिवागमात्

पूर्वाशां वर्धते विन्दुरचिरात्सुखमेधते ।

दक्षिणाशां ज्वरो ज्ञेयस्तथारोग्यं क्रमाद्भवेत् ॥५८॥

According to Śivāgama

If the oil dropped over the surface of the urine immediately spreads towards the east, then the patient will recover from the disease. If the oil drop spreads to the South then the patient is suffering from *jvara* (fever) and he will gradually recover from the disease.

वारुण्यां प्रसरेद्विन्दुः सुखारोग्यं प्रचक्षते ।

If the oil drop spreads towards the direction of *Varuṇa* (West), then the patient recovers from the disease and gets happiness.

33 "उत्तरस्यां यदा तैलविन्दुः प्रसरते यदि ॥५६॥

आरोग्यं च तदा नूनं पुरुषस्य न संशयः ।"

When the oil drop spreads towards the North, then the patient undoubtedly recovers.

34 "ऐशान्यां वर्धते विन्दुर्ध्रुवं मासेन नश्यति ॥६०॥"

If the oil drop spreads towards the direction of *aiśāna* (North-East) then the patient succumbs to death within one month.

आग्नेयं च तथा ज्ञेयं नैर्ऋत्यां प्रसरेद्यदा ।

छिद्रितं च भवेत्पश्चात् ध्रुवं मरणहेतवे ॥६१॥

If the oil drop spreads towards the direction of *agni* (South-East) or *nairṛta* (South-West), and then, if holes appear in it, then the patient certainly succumbs to death.

वायव्यां प्रसरेद्बिन्दुः सुधापीतोऽपि नश्यति ।

If the oil drop spreads towards the direction of *vāyu* (North-West), then the person succumbs to death even if he has taken ambrosia.

तरते मज्जते विन्दुः भ्रमते च मुमूर्षुतां ॥६२॥

[35] "न जीवति ध्रुवं रोगी यथा सर्वाङ्गभाषिणे ।"

The oil drop sometimes floats, some times sinks and some times moves in the urine of a moribund patient. Such a patient never survives. [The implication of the term *sarvāṅga bhāṣiṇe* used in the text is not clear.]

विकासितं हलं कूर्मं [36]सौरिभाकारसंयुतम् ॥६३॥

कारम्भं मण्डलं चापि [37]शिरोहीनं नरं तथा ।

गात्रखण्डं च [38]शंखं च खड्गं मुशलपट्टिशम् ॥६४॥

शरं च [39]लकुटं चैव तथैव त्रिचतुःपथम् ।

बिन्दुरूपं भिषग्दृष्ट्वा न कुर्वीत क्रियां क्वचित् ॥६५॥

If the spreading oil drop takes the shape of *hala* (plough), *kūrma* (tortoise), *sauribha* (?), *kārambha*, *maṇḍala* (circle), man without a head, portion of human body, conch shell, sword, pastle and mortar, arrow, stick, crossing of three or four roads or *bindu* (drop), then the physician should not attempt treatment of such patients.

हंसकारण्डताडागं कमलं गजचामरम् ।

छत्रं च तोरणं [40]हर्म्यं सम्पूर्णं दृश्यते यदि ॥६६॥

आरोग्यता ध्रुवं ज्ञेया तदा कुर्यात्प्रतिक्रियाम् ।

If the spreading oil-drop takes the shape of swan, *kāraṇḍa*, pond, lotus, elephant, *cāmara* (tail of yak), umbrella, *toraṇa* (gate) and palacial building in complete form, then the patient will certainly get cured and such a patient should be treated.

तैलविन्दुर्यदा मूत्रे चल्लनी[41] सदृशो भवेत् ।।६७।।

कुक्षदोषं ध्रुवं ज्ञेयं प्रेतदोषसमुद्भवम् ।

If the spreading oil-drop takes the shape of a *callanī* (sieve), then it is because of *kukṣa doṣa* (?) and affliction by *pretas*.

"त्रिकोणे[42] शाकिणी दोषं गोत्रदोषसमुद्भवम् ।"

If the spreading oil-drop takes the shape of a triangle, then patient is afflicted by *śākiṇī* or *gotra doṣa* (fault of the clan).

नराकारं प्रजायेत किंवा स्यान्मस्तकद्वयम् ।।६८।।

भूतदोषं विजानीयाद्भूतविद्यां समारभेत्[43] ।

If the spreading oil drop takes the shape of a human being or two heads, then the patient is suffering from *bhūta doṣa* (affliction by evil spirits). The physician, in such cases, should take necessary steps to correct these evil spirits.

श्वेतधारा महाधारा पीतधारा महाज्वरः ।

रक्तधारा दीर्घरोगी कृष्णा च मरणान्तिका ।।६९।।

।।इति मूत्रपरीक्षा।।

If the stream of micturition is white, or big or yellowish then the physician should diagnose the patient as suffering from *mahā jvara* (acute fever). If the stream is red in colour then the patient is overcome by a chronic disease. If, however, the stream is black, then the patient succumbs to death.

Thus, ends the description of the examination of urine.

मलपरीक्षा

रुद्रतन्त्रात्

विकृताः मलभेदाश्च विज्ञेयाः धीमता खलु ।
वैद्यशास्त्रविधिज्ञेन पुरुषेण तु षोडशाः ॥७०॥
दुर्गन्धोऽपि विगन्धश्च श्यामो विट्त्रुटितः सितः ।
आरक्तः कपिलः शीतः शिथिलस्तु सफेनकः ॥७१॥
हरितो गुटिकाबन्धो धूम्रो विविधवर्णकः ।
कृष्णबद्धमबद्धं च एते भेदाः प्रकीर्तिताः ॥७२॥

Examination of Stool

According to Rudra tantra

An intelligent physician should know that there are 16 types of morbidities in the stool. These are as follows :

1. *Durgandha* (having foul smell in excess);
2. *Vigandha* (having no smell or having different type of smell);
3. *Śyāma* (bluish gray in colour);
4. *Viṭ-truṭita* (having broken pieces of stool);
5. *Sita* (having white colour);
6. *Ārakta* (having reddish colour);
7. *Kapila* (having brown or black colour);
8. *Śita* (cold to touch);

9. *Śithila* (having looseness);
10. *Saphena* (having foams);
11. *Harita* (having greenish colour);
12. *Guṭikā bandha* (scybalous stool);
13. *Dhūmra* (smoky);
14. *Vividha varṇaka* (having varieties of colour);
15. *Kṛṣṇa* (having black colour); and
16. *Baddha* and *abaddha* (stool which is both compact and loose).

वातपित्तकफदूषणेङ्गितैः ज्ञेयमेव सततं महात्मना ।
रोगपीडितशरीरिणो मलो[44] दृष्टिपातनिपुणेन[45] निश्चितः ॥७३॥

When a patient is suffering from diseases caused by the aggravation of *vāyu*, *pitta* and *kapha*, then the expert physician should directly observe the characteristic features of these *doṣas* in the stool.

वित्रुटितं फेनिलं च[46] मलं रोगी विमुञ्चति ।
तदाऽपि लक्षयेत्साक्षाद्वातादुदुष्टमनेकधा ॥७४॥

If the stool of the patient is broken and foamy then he is suffering from various types of *vāta roga*.

युक्तो हरितपीताभ्यां वर्णाभ्यां तु यदा मलः ।
पित्तव्याधिः स विज्ञेयो वैद्येन प्रतिजानता ॥७५॥

If the stool of the patient is either green or yellow in colour, then an expert physician should diagnose him as a case of aggravated *pitta*.

शीतं शुक्लं चातिसान्द्रं जले पक्वोऽपि[47] मज्जति ।

कफाद्रोमाञ्चयुक्तो ना मलं बहुनुदत्यपि ॥७६॥

As a result of the aggravation of *kapha*, the patient gets horripilation and he passes more of stool which is cold, white and exceedingly compact. If this stool is placed over a pot of water, it sinks.

[48]श्यामा श्वेता च [49]विष्ठा च जायते यदि रोगिणः ।

वातश्लेष्मविकारं तं लक्षयेद्भिषगुत्तमः ॥७७॥

If the stool is *śyāma* (bluish black) and white, then the physician should diagnose the patient as suffering from the disease caused by *vāyu* and *kapha*.

दुर्गन्धः शिथिलश्चैव विष्ठोत्सर्गः प्रदृश्यते ।

तदा जीर्णमलश्चात्र दोषज्ञैः परिकथ्यते ॥७८॥

If the stool has an exceedingly foul smell and if it comes out very loose, then a physician should diagnose this as a result of accumulation of stool in the colon since a long time.

पीतच्छायाभिसंसृष्टो बद्धो विट्त्रुटितो भवेत् ।

स दुष्टो वातपित्ताभ्यां सदैव स च लभ्यते ॥७९॥

If the stool has yellowish colouration and if it is compact but in pieces, then there is aggravation of *vāyu* and *pitta*.

आमवातपरिदूषितो मलः पीतकान्तिसहितः प्रजायते ।

दोषवर्धनपंथविचक्षते[50] दुष्टपित्तजनितो[51] गदो भवेत् ॥८०॥

If the stool is afflicted by *āma* and *vāyu* (?) and if there is yellowish colour in it, then the person is likely to suffer from a disease caused by *pitta*.

किंचित् श्यामः सफेनश्च दुर्धरो भुवि राजते ।

बाले शीतपरो भूत्वा शाकिनी[52] येन संश्रयः[53] ॥८१॥

If a child is afflicted by *śākinī*, then he passes stool after a feeling of cold in the body and the stool is bluish black, foamy and it spreads on the ground.

श्यामस्त्रुटितपीतश्च नीलश्वेतोऽथ दृश्यते ।

वातपित्तकफैरेवं वर्चो निर्णीयते दृढम् ॥८२॥

The stool becomes bluish black and broken by the aggravation of *vāyu*, yellow and blue by the aggravation of *pitta* and white by the aggravation of *kapha*. These characteristic features are beyond any doubt.

संग्राहप्रचुरो ह्रस्वश्चेतः प्रक्षीणबह्वतः ।

बस्तिं च दूषयेद्विष्ठा वद्धा संपद्यते ध्रुवम् ॥८३॥

If there is constipation, the patient becomes talkative (?), his mental power decreases; he becomes weak and his urinary bladder gets afflicted.

सिता महतिका पूतिर्विष्ठा यस्य प्रजायते ।

तस्माज्जलोदरारम्भो भिषग्भिः परिभाष्यते ॥८४॥

If a person passes stool which is white in colour and exceedingly foul in smell, then this according to physicians, is the beginning of his ascites.

श्यामा यस्य भवेद्विष्ठा क्षयस्तस्य भवेद्ध्रुवम् ।

कृष्णा श्यामा च दुर्गन्धा मृत्युस्तस्य न संशयः ॥८५॥

If a person passes stool which is bluish black in colour, then he certainly suffers from *kṣaya* (consumption). If his stool becomes black, bluish black and extremely foul in smell, then undoubtedly he succumbs to death.

भृशोष्णकुणपं कृष्णमरुणं वाथ पाण्डुरम् ।
मेचकं वा तत्क्षणेन मरणाय भवेच्छकृत् ॥
किमत्र बहुनोक्तेन भृशोष्णं मरणाय वै ॥८६॥

॥इति मलपरीक्षा॥

If the stool becomes exceedingly hot, *kuṇapa* (having smell of a dead body), black, reddish, *pāṇḍura* (yellowish white) and *mecaka* (greasy black) then the patient succumbs to death immediately. There is no use going into details. Exceedingly hot stool indicates the death of the patient.

Thus, ends the description of the examination of stool.

अथ नेत्रपरीक्षा

सरूक्षा धूम्रवर्णा च सरौद्रा च तथाचला ।
ज्वला चाभ्यन्तरे नेत्रे वातव्याधिंविनिर्दिशेत् ॥८७॥

Examination of eyes

If the eyes are dry, smoky in colour and fierceful, if the eye ball is mobile and if there is burning sensation inside the eyes, then the patient is suffering from diseases caused by *vāyu*.

हरिद्राखण्डसंकाशं रक्तं नीलं च वर्णकम् ।
54
दीपद्वेषि च संतप्तं पित्ते नेत्रं प्रकुप्यति ॥८८॥

If the eye is like a piece of turmeric, if its colour is red or blue, if the sight of a lamp (light) is not liked and if there is burning sensation, then there is aggravation of *pitta*.

जलार्द्रं विह्वलं श्वेतं ज्योतिर्हीनं चलान्वितम् ।

मन्ददृष्टिर्भवेद्यस्य स ज्ञेयः कफदोषतः ॥८९॥

If there is aggravation of *kapha*, there will be watering of eyes, there will be anxious look, the colour will be white, there will be no glaze in the eyes, the eye balls will be moving and the eye-sight will be weak.

55
"श्यामं निर्भुग्नसंजातं तंद्रामोहसमन्वितम् ।

सरौद्रं रक्तवर्णं च भवेच्चक्षुस्त्रिदोषतः ॥९०॥"

If all the three *doṣas* are aggravated, then the colour of the eyes will be bluish black, there will be fixed look, there will be drowsiness accompanied with unconsciousness, the eyes will look fierceful and they will be red in colour.

द्विलिंगभेदनिर्मुक्तं द्विलिंगपरिभावयेत् ।

If two *doṣas* are aggravated, then the characteristic features of both these *doṣas* will be manifested in the eyes.

एकदृष्टिः तथा रौद्रः द्वितीयं मिलितं यदा ॥९१॥

त्रिभिर्दिनैर्विजानीयात्स याति यमशासनम् ।

If one eye is fierceful and the other eye is closed then the person will succumb to death within three days.

कालं ज्योतिर्विहीने च जातेऽभ्यन्तरलोचने ॥९२॥

श्यामदृष्टिर्विशेषेण तस्य मृत्युरसंशयः ।

If the black portion of the eye (iris) loses its glaze, if the eye ball goes inside and if the vision is bluish-black, then the patient undoubtedly succumbs to death.

सरक्तं कृष्णवर्णं च रौद्रं च प्रेक्षते यदि ॥६३॥

इति लिङ्गं विजानीयान्मृत्युरेव न संशयः ।

If the eyes are red or black in colour and if the look is fierceful, then the patient undoubtedly succumbs to death.

एकदृष्टिरचैतन्यो विभ्रमः स्फुटतारकम् ।

एकाहे च विजानीयात्स याति यममन्दिरम् ॥६४॥

॥इति दृष्टिपरीक्षा॥

If there is fixed look, if the patient is unconscious and having delirium and if cracks have appeared in the pupil then he succumbs to death within one day.

Thus, ends the description of the examination of the eyes.

56

"जिह्वायां धावति प्राणः सूक्ष्मेन्द्रियप्रधानतः ।

जिह्वायां च विजानीयात् भोजने वचने यथा ॥६५॥

तस्मात्सर्वप्रयत्नेन जिह्वायाश्च परीक्षणम् ।

Examination of the Tongue

The *prāṇa* (elan vital) moves through the tongue. As it plays an important role in the intake of food and in speech, similarly, it is the most important among the subtle senses. Therefore, the tongue should be examined very carefully.

सज्वरं ज्वरमुक्तं वा सर्वं जिह्वा प्रकाशते ॥६६॥

वातपित्तकफाधिक्यं द्वंद्वजं सान्निपातिकम् ।

साध्यासाध्यविभागेन सर्वं जिह्वा प्रकाशते ॥६७॥

By the examination of tongue all the following conditions of the individual could be ascertained :

1. Whether the person is suffering from *jvara* (fever), or he has become free from it;

2. Aggravation of *vāyu*, *pitta* and *kapha* individually;

3. Aggravation of two *doṣas*, or all the three *doṣas* simultaneously; and

4 Curability and incurability of the disease.

जिह्वा वातात्प्रसुप्ता स्फुटितविकसिता शाकपत्रोपमा या ।

There will be numbness and cracks in the tongue and the tongue will be like a leaf of *śāka* if there is aggravation of *vāyu*.

पित्ताद्रक्ता सदाहा भवति विपचिता कंटकैर्व्याप्ता परीता ॥९८॥

By the aggravation of *pitta*, the tongue is red, there will be burning sensation in the tongue and it will be covered with thorn like growths.

गुरुस्थूलातिशीतासित बहलकफाशालै...............।

By the aggravation of *kapha*, the tongue is heavy, thick, excessively cold, white and thickly coated. [The verse is incomplete].

तु त्रिदोषजात..............................॥९९॥

रूक्षतिक्तोपमा जिह्वा कथिता मुनिपुंगवैः ।

परिदग्धा खरस्पर्शा जिह्वा स्रस्तांगजा[पुनः]॥१००॥

स्फुटिता संनिपातस्य कथ्यते ब्रह्मवेदिना ।

According to sages, in the *sannipāta* (when all the three *doṣas* are simultaneously aggravated), the tongue is ununctuous, bitter, *paridagdha* (as if burnt), rough to touch, *srastāṅga* (flaeid) and *sphuṭita* (having deep cracks).

एवं जिह्वापरीक्षा च ईश्वरब्रह्मणा कृता ।

लोकमध्ये प्रकाशाय हारीतमुनिनोदिता ॥१०१॥

॥इति जिह्वापरीक्षा॥

This method of examination of tongue was devised by Lord *Brahmā*. This was propagated among the worldly people by the sage *Hārita*.

Thus, ends the description of the examination of tongue.

परीक्षणं सुदन्तानां यदुक्तं परमेष्टिना ।

तथैव कथितं लोके हारीतमुनिनोत्तमम् ॥१०२॥

Examination of Teeth

The method of examination of teeth is described by the sage *Hārita* on the lines originally instructed by Lord *Brahmā*.

रदाः सप्तविधाः प्रोक्ताः श्यावाः रक्तासिताऽरुणाः ।

पीताः च रक्तसंस्रावाः दन्तमूलच्युताः तथा ॥१०३॥

The morbidity of teeth is of seven types viz., (1) *śyāva* (brown colour), (2) *rakta* (red colour), (3) *asita* (black colour), (4) *aruṇa* (reddish), (5) *pīta* (yellow), (6) *rakta saṁsrāva* (having bleeding) and (7) *dantamūla cyuta* (retraction of the gum from the roots of teeth).

नीलवर्णस्य दन्तस्य वातजातस्य लक्षणम् ।

नीलवर्णाः यदा दन्ता वातलाः विविधाः क्रियाः ॥१०४॥

The teeth become blue, as a result of the aggravation of *vāyu* and for correcting this condition, measures for the alleviation of *vāyu* should be adopted.

श्याववर्णाः यदा दन्ताः पित्तजाः विविधाः क्रियाः ।

Teeth become *śyāva* (brown) because of the aggravation of *pitta*. In such cases, measures for the alleviation of *pitta* should be adopted.

रक्तदंताः भविष्यन्ति श्लेष्मदन्ताः तथा गुणाः ॥१०५॥

If there is aggravation of *kapha*, then the teeth will become red (?) and they will have the other characteristic features of the *doṣas*.

वातपित्तासिताजाताः नीलश्यावाः सलक्षणाः ।

If there is simultaneous aggravation of both *vāyu* and *pitta*, then the teeth become black, *nīla-śyāva* (bluish brown) and there will be other characteristic features of these *doṣas*.

रक्तश्यावाः भवेत् दन्ताः मुखपाकं वदंति हि ॥१०६॥

The teeth become *rakta-śyāva* (reddish brown) in *mukha pāka* (stomatitis).

वातश्लेष्मविकारे तु दंताः जिह्वा विपच्यते ।

In the diseases caused by the simultaneous aggravation of *vāyu* and *kapha* there will be inflammation in teeth and glossitis.

पित्तश्लेष्मविकारेषु दंताः नासा स्रवन्ति च ।

In diseases caused by *pitta* and *kapha*, there will be exudation from the teeth and nose.

रदनं सदनं प्रोक्तं कल्पान्ते च विधीयते ॥१०७॥

Radana (tooth) is called *sadana* (a place of residence). [The meaning of the remaining *śloka* is not clear.]

दंतादीनां मलाढ्यत्वं प्रमेहात्[पूर्वलक्षणम्] ।

गुणागुणविभेदेन साध्यासाध्यं तथैव च ॥१०८॥

॥इति दन्तपरीक्षा॥

Adhesion of excreta in the root of the teeth is the premonitory sign of *prameha* (obstinate urinary diseases including diabetes). Depending upon the characteristic features of the teeth, the curability and incurability of a disease should be determined.

Thus, ends the description of the examination of teeth.

परीक्षणं नखानां हि वक्ष्येहं ब्रह्मणोदितम् ।

पादादौ विवरैर्युक्तं सर्वज्ञाय भिषग्वरैः ॥१०९॥

ततो परीक्षणं तेषां धातुदोषकृतस्तथा ।

सुवर्णस्य यथा रेखा तथा रेखा नखस्य चेत् ॥११०॥

Examination of Nails

Now the examination of nails of feet etc., as instructed by *Brahmā* will be described. They are examined with a view to ascertaining the morbidity in the *dhātus* and *doṣas*, and the presence of lines like those over a piece of gold.

वातपित्तकफं द्वंद्वं चतुर्थं सान्निपातिकम् ।

नखमध्ये तथा ज्ञात्वा सर्वशास्त्रेषु संमतम् ॥१११॥

One should ascertain the aggravation of *vāyu*, *pitta* and *kapha* and simultaneous vitiation of two *doṣas* or all the three *doṣas* by examination of nails according to the methods prescribed in all the medical texts.

नीलवर्णाः भवेद्वायुः रक्तवर्णाः सपैत्तिकः ।

पीतवर्णाः भवेत्छ्लेष्मः श्वेतवर्णाः समिश्रकः ॥११२॥

By the aggravation of *vāyu*, the nails become blue in colour. By the aggravation of *pitta*, the nails become either red or yellow in colour. The nails become white in colour by the aggravation of *kapha*. When two *doṣas* are aggravated simultaneously, then the characteristic features of both these *doṣas* are manifested in the nails.

नखाश्च नीलवर्णाभाः पीतरक्तास्तथैव च ।
वातपित्तपरीक्षा च कथिता मुनिपुंगवैः ॥११३॥
नीलाभं च यदा कृष्णं पीतवर्णं च दृश्यते ।
वातपित्तविकारेषु कथयंति यदा बुधाः ॥११४॥

If both *vāyu* and *pitta* are simultaneously aggravated, then the nails become bluish yellow or bluish red in colour. Bluish black and bluish yellow colours of nails are also caused by the aggravation of *vāyu* and *pitta*, according to great sages.

पीतं रक्तं यदा दृष्ट्वा नखानां च निरीक्षणम् ।
श्लेष्मपित्तं स्थितिस्तत्र कथयंति मुनीश्वराः ॥११५॥

The colour of the nails becomes either yellow or red by the aggravation of *kapha* and *pitta*.

रक्तं नीलं तथा पीतं हरितश्वेतनिर्मलः ।
सान्निपातः विजानीयान्मरणाय च देहिनाम् ॥११६॥

In *sannipāta*, (when all the three *doṣas* are simultaneously aggravated), if the colour of the nails becomes reddish blue, yellow, green, white and *nirmala* (free from any dirt), then the patient succumbs to death.

एवं नखपरीक्षां यो न जानाति चिकित्सकः ।
अपूज्यः सर्वलोकस्य [स भवेत् राजवर्जितः] ॥११७॥"

॥इति नखपरीक्षा॥

If a physician is not efficient in the above-mentioned method of examination of nails then he is despised by all people and the king should not entertain him.

Thus, ends the description of the examination of nails.

गुरोः सिद्धं कपालादिमन्त्रेशं द्वादशाक्षरम् ।

भूर्जे निजाऽसृजा लिख्य न्यसेदन्तः शरावयोः[57] ॥११८॥

संपूज्य जप्त्वा तन्मन्त्रं गुप्ते तत्स्थापयेन्निशि ।

प्रातरुत्थाय तत्पश्येद्विजानि द्वादशक्रमात् ।

यद्वर्णं नश्येत्तद्वर्षे तन्मासे तद्दिने मृतिः ॥११९॥

Prediction of the date of Death

Siddhi (perfection) should be attained in the *kapālādi mantra* with the help of the *guru* (perceptor). This *mantra* has twelve alphabets. This *mantra* should be written by the person in his own blood over a piece of *bhūrja patra*, which should be kept inside two *śurāvas* (earthen plates). Thereafter, oblation should be offered and the *mantra* should be recited repeatedly. The container having the *mantra* inside it should be kept in a secret place. In the morning after getting up from bed one should open the container and examine the twelve alphabets of the *mantra*. If any alphabet has become invisible then number should be counted. Death will occur in the same number of year or month or day.

कपालरुद्राय भगवते नमः ॥इति मंत्रः ॥१२०॥

Kapālarudrāya bhagavate namaḥ—this is the *mantra*.

सूर्यचन्द्रात्मकौ कृष्णशुक्लपक्षौ करौ स्मृतौ ।

क्षालयेत्तौ जलक्षीरघृतैस्तैलैस्त्रिवासरम् ॥१२१॥

कनिष्ठामूलपर्वादि चेष्ट्योर्ध्वं तेषु पर्वसु ।
तिथिर्नियोज्य ताः लाक्षारसेन परिरञ्जयेत् ।
58 यत्रेक्षते न तद्बिन्दुस्तिथौ तत्र मृतिर्भवेत् ॥१२२॥

॥इति नरपतिचर्यायां मृततिथिचक्रम्॥

Another method of Prediction

The hands of a person represent the *kṛṣṇa pakṣa* (black fortnight) and *śukla pakṣa* (bright fortnight) characterised by the energy of the sun and the moon respectively. These hands should be washed for three days with water, milk, ghee and oil. Beginning from the root of the little finger the *tithis* (names or numbers of the days of the fortnight) should be marked by spots. These fingers should then be smeared (coloured) with *lākṣā* (lac). If the spot in a particular phalange disappears then the patient will succumb to death on that particular day.

Thus, ends the *mṛta tithi cakra*, as described in *Narapati caryā*.

59 "आर्द्रादि मृगपर्यन्ते मध्ये मूलं प्रतिष्ठितम् ।
एवं क्रमेण विन्यस्य नाडीत्रयमतन्द्रितः ॥१२३॥
चन्द्रार्कजन्मनक्षत्रं एकनाड्यां यदा भवेत् ।
मृत्युं तदा विजानीयाद्रोगिणो नान्यथा भवेत् ॥१२४॥"

आ	पु	पु
पू	म	आ
उ	ह	वि
अ	वि	स्वा
ज्ये	मू	पू
ध	श्र	द्र
श	पू	उ
श	पू	उ
भ	अ	रे
कृ	रो	मृ

In three columns, twenty seven *nakṣatras* beginning from *Ārdrā* and ending with *mṛgaśirā* should be written carefully as given below having *Mūlā* in the centre. If the *candra* (moon), *arka* (sun) and *janma nakṣatra* (star of the time of birth) remain in one column then the patient succumbs to death, otherwise, he does not, die.

(6) *Ārdrā*	(7) *Punarvasu*	(8) *Puṣya*
(11) *Pūrva Phālgunī*	(10) *Maghā*	(9) *Aśleṣā*
(12) *Uttara Phālgunī*	(13) *Hastā*	(14) *Citrā*
(17) *Anurādhā*	(16) *Viśākhā*	(15) *Svāti*
(18) *Jyeṣṭhā*	(19) *Mūlā*	(20) *Pūrva Āṣāḍhā*
(23) *Dhanisthā*	(22) *Śravaṇā*	(21) *Uttarāṣāḍhā*
(24) *Śatabhisā*	(25) *Pūrva Bhādrapada*	(26) *Uttara Bhādrapada*
(2) *Bharaṇī*	(1) *Āśvinī*	(27) *Revatī*
(3) *Kṛttikā*	(4) *Rohiṇī*	(5) *Mṛgaśirā*

अथ रसार्णवात्

अथ प्रश्नावतारं च कृत्वा कुर्यात्क्रियां शुभाम् ।

भिषग्दीक्षासमायुक्तः,

According to Rasarṇava

The physician who has taken *dīkṣā* (initiation in a *mantra*) should initiate any auspicious act only after making *praśnāvatāra* (putting questions).

पूर्वोक्तं रसभैरवम् ॥१२५॥

समाहितमना[60] ध्यायेत् तदालीनं[61] समाचरेत् ।

अनाहते ब्रह्मरन्ध्रे मनः कृत्वा निरालये ॥१२६॥

करन्यासं पुरा कृत्वा अङ्गन्यासमनन्तरम् ।

यथाशक्तिः जपेन्मन्त्रं रसेन्द्रस्य समाहितः ॥१२७॥

He should meditate upon *Rasa bhairava* in the manner described before with concentration of mind and get submerged in it. During meditation, his mind should be in either *Anāhata, brahma randhra* or *nirālaya.* He should perform *karanyāsa,* and thereafter, *aṅganyāsa.* Having done so, he should recite the *mantra* of *rasendra* with concentration as much as he can.

चतुःकोणं पुरा[62] कृत्वा मध्ये षट्कोणमण्डलम् ।

हस्तमात्रं द्विहस्तं वा तण्डुलैर्विमलैर्लिखेत् ॥१२८॥

One should draw a square having four angles. Inside the square a hexagon should be drawn with the help of clean rice. The size of these drawings should be one or two *hasta* in length.

सुगन्धैर्लेपिते स्थाने [63]"पूजयेच्चन्दनादिभिः ॥१२९॥

कर्णिकायां न्यसेद्देवं[64] पूर्वोक्तं रसभैरवम् ।

षट्कोणे देवताषट्कं महाकालादि विन्यसेत्[65] ॥१३०॥

[रसार्णवः द्वितीयपटल : ९२-९६]

महाकालं महाबलमघोरं वज्रवीरकम् ।

[66] "प्रयत्नतः साधकेन्द्रो ह्यघोरं वह्निवीरकम् ।"

न्यसेत् क्रोधञ्च कङ्कालं मालामन्त्रैः समर्चयेत् ॥१३१॥

[रसार्णवः द्वितीयपटल : ९७]

A portion of it should be smeared with the fragrant pastes, and on this, one should inscribe the *mantra* (or *yantra*) with the help of pure rice. With the help of sandalwood paste, prayer should be offered to it. In the *karṇikā* (centre) the god *Rasa bhairava* should be located and in the six angles six gods viz., *Mahā kāla, Mahā bala, Aghora, Bajra viraka, Aghora* (?) and *Vahni viraka* should be located by the *sādhaka* (disciple or priest who is engaged in *sādhanā*). In addition, the *Krodha* (anger) *bhairava* and *Kaṅkāla* (skeleton or skull of a dead person) *bhairava* should also be placed there. The *mantra* should be recited with the help of a *mālā* (rosary).

67
ओं ह्रीं क्रें क्ष्णें क्ष्णुः ह्रीं ह्रीं ह्रीं ह्रूः हुं फट्-रसेश्वराय

महाकालभैरवाय रौद्ररूपाय कृष्णपिङ्गललोचनाय, अवतर

अवताराय जल्प जल्पाय शुभाशुभं कथय कथय कथय

कथापय २ महारक्षां कुरु २ कथापय कुरु २ कर्मणि

सिद्धिं देहि स्वाहा ॥१३२॥

The mantra

Oṁ, Hrīṁ, Kreṁ, Kṣṇeṁ, Kṣṇuḥ, Hrīṁ, Hrīṁ, Hrīṁ, Hrūḥ, Huṁ, Phaṭ—Raseśvarāya, Mahākāla bhairavāya, Raudra rūpāya, Kṛṣṇapiṅgala locanāya, Avtara, Avatārāya, Jalpa, Jalpāya, Śubhāśubhaṁ, Kathaya, Kathaya, Kathaya, Kathāpaya, Kathāpaya, Mahā rakṣāṁ, Kuru, Kuru, Kathāpaya, Kuru, Kuru, Karmaṇi, Siddhiṁ Dehi Svāhā.

68
महाकालभैरवाय हृदयाय नमः। महाबालभैरवाय शिरसे

स्वाहा। अघोरभैरवाय शिखायै वौषट्। वज्रवीरभैरवाय

कवचाय हुम्। क्रोधभैरवाय नेत्रत्रयाय वौषट्।

कंकालभैरवाय अस्त्राय फट्। सर्वत्र स्वाहान्तः।

एवमङ्गुलिन्यासः। एते मूलमंत्राः ॥१३३॥

Aṅga nyāsa

The *sādhaka* should touch the heart region by saying "*Mahākāla bhairavāya hṛdayāya namaḥ*", touch head by saying "*Mahābāla bhairavāya śirase svāhā*", touch the *śikhā* by saying, "*Aghora bhairavāya śikhāyai vauṣaṭ*", touch the arms by saying, "*Vajravīra bhairavāya kavacāya huṁ*" and touch the three eyes (one mystic eye in between the two eye brows in the forehead) by saying, "*Krodha bhairavāya netratrayāya vauṣaṭ*". He should then produce sound by clapping the back of the right hand over the palm of the left hand by reciting, "*Kaṁkāla bhairavāya astrāya phaṭ*". The term '*svāhā*' should be suffixed to all these *mantras*.

Aṅguli nyāsa should be performed in the same manner. These are the basic *mantras*.

एवं न्यासाक्षरैः कूटैर्गन्धपुष्पैश्च पूजयेत्[69] ।
पूर्णकुम्भं न्यसेन्मध्ये शरावं तंडुलैः सह ।।१३४।।
तस्योपरि न्यसेद्दीपं वर्ति मन्त्रैस्तु[70] मन्त्रयेत् ।
समानीय कुमारीं तु कुमारं[71] वा सुशोभनम् ।।१३५।।
एकद्वित्रिचतुःपञ्च यथालाभं समानयेत् ।
गन्धपुष्पैर्धूपदीपैर्नैवेद्येन च पूजयेत् ।।१३६।।
एकैकस्य न्यसेन्मन्त्रैर्हृदयाद्याश्च देवताः ।
ततो निरीक्ष्य तं[72] दीपं सर्वे[73] ते च कुमारकाः ।।१३७।।
पश्यन्ति देवतां दीपे ते कुमाराः शुभाशुभम् ।
सिद्धिं चाप्यथवासिद्धिं कथयन्ति कुमारकाः[74] ।।१३८।।
प्रश्नावतारं ज्ञात्वेति भिषक्कर्मसमाचरेत्[75] ।।१३९।।

[रसार्णव : द्वितीयपटल : ९८-१०३]

।।इति प्रश्नावतारः।।

In accordance with the above mentioned *akṣara nyāsa*, incense and flower, prayer should be offered. In the centre, an earthen jar full of water covered with a *śarāva* (earthen plate) full of rice should be kept. Over the *śarāva*, a *dipa* (lamp) should be placed. The wick of this lamp should be impregnated with the *mantra*. Thereafter, a beautiful girl or a handsome boy should be called. Their number may be one, two, three, four, five, or as many as available. They should be offered prayer with scents, flower, incense, lamp and *naivedya*. In each one of them, the gods should be placed by the help of *hṛdayādai nyāsa* etc. of the *mantra*. These boys and girls should then be asked to look at the flame of the lamp. They will be able to see the god inside it and will tell the auspicious and inauspicious events. They will also tell if the physician will succeed or fail in the treatment of the patient. Having ascertained this, the physician should initiate his treatment.

Thus, ends the description of *Praśnāvaṭāra*.

अथ योगरत्नावल्याम्

मार्गशीर्षस्य शुक्लायामेकादश्यां जितेन्द्रियः ।
आत्मनो वा परार्थे वा कालागमदिदृक्षया ॥१४०॥
उपवासेन वैकुण्ठीं द्वादशाक्षरदेवताम् ।
संलिख्य फलके सायं मलयोद्भववारिणा ॥१४१॥
हरिं तावत्समभ्यर्च्य शुचिस्तामवलोकयेत् ।
76
दृष्ट्वा सम्पूर्णविद्यस्तु कुशलं वत्सरावधि ॥१४२॥

According to Yoga ratnāvali

With a view to knowing the *kālāgama* (the nature of the time) for himself and for others, the physician should observe celibacy and keep fast on the eleventh day of the bright fortnight of the month of *mārgaśirṣa.* Then he should write over a *phalaka* (wooden plate) with the help of sandalwood water the god of *Vaikuṇṭhi dvādaśākṣara.* To that *Hari* (god)prayer should be offered, and with purity, the wise person should look at it for one year.

तस्याक्षराद्यभावेन मार्गशीर्षे गुरौ दिने ।

भूतायां च तिथौ यामे प्रथमे याति पञ्चताम् ॥१४३॥

If the first letter becomes invisible, then the patient succumbs to death in the first *yāma* (one *yāma*=3 hours) of *bhūta tithi* on a Thursday of the month of *Mārgaśirṣa.*

पौषस्य शुक्लपंचम्यां सायं भवदिने[77] ज्वरात् ।

विद्याद्द्वितीयं वर्णस्य लोपे स्यात्तु मरणं ध्रुवम् ॥१४४॥

If the second letter becomes invisible, then the patient being afflicted by fever, certainly succumbs to death in the evening of the *bhava dina* (Monday) on fifth day of *śukla pakṣa* (bright fortnight) of the month of *pauṣa.*

[78]पौर्णमास्याममायां वा [79]भानुवारेऽपराह्णके ।

ग्रहदोषात् ज्वरान्नाशं विद्याद्वह्न्यक्षरक्षयात् ॥१४५॥

If the third letter becomes invisible, then the patient being afflicted by evil planets and fever, succumbs to death during the afternoon of Sunday of *pūrṇimā* (full moon day) or *amāvasyā* (new moon day).

[80]"शुक्लायां फाल्गुनस्याथ नवम्यां दिवसार्धतः ।

शुक्रवारे ज्वरान्नश्येच्चतुर्थाक्षरसंक्षयात् ॥१४६॥

If the fourth letter becomes invisible then the patient being afflicted by fever, succumbs to death on Friday in the noon time of ninth day of the *śukla pakṣa* (bright fortnight) of the month of *Phālguna.*

चैत्रे भूतदिने भौमे सुप्रभाते विनश्यति ।

अतीसाराद्गते वर्णे[81] विद्यायाः पञ्चमे ध्रुवम् ॥१४७॥

If the fifth letter becomes invisible, then the patient being afflicted with diarrhoea, succumbs to death in the early morning of Tuesday having *bhūta tithi* in the month of *Caitra*.

वैशाखस्य त्रयोदश्यां सितायां गुरुवासरे ।

अवश्यं[82] म्रियते रात्रौ विद्यात्षष्ठाक्षरक्षये ॥१४८॥

If the sixth letter becomes invisible then the patient certainly succumbs to death at night of Thursday having *sitā tithi* during the thirteenth day of the fortnight in the month of *Vaiśākha*.

ज्येष्ठे भूतदिने मन्दे निशायाः प्रहरे गते ।

शोफक्षयात्क्षयं[83] याति सप्तमाक्षरलोपतः ॥१४९॥

If the seventh letter becomes invisible, then the patient being afflicted with oedema and consumption succumbs to death at, night after the passage of one *prahara* (3 hours) on a *bhūta* day and *manda* tithi in the month of *Jyeṣṭha*.

अष्टम्यामथ कृष्णायामाषाढे रविवासरे ।

मध्याह्ने यात्यतीसाराद्विद्यादष्टाक्षरक्षये ॥१५०॥

If the eighth letter becomes invisible then the patient being afflicted with diarrhoea, succumbs to death in the noon time of Sunday on the eighth day of *kṛṣṇa pakṣa* (black fortnight) in the month of *Āṣāḍha*.

आषाढे श्रावणे मासि सिते विष्णुदिने शनैः ।

निशायाः प्रथमे नश्येन्नवमाक्षरहानितः ॥१५१॥

If the ninth letter becomes invisible, the patient succumbs to death in the first part of the night on the day of *Viṣṇu* in the *śukla pakṣa* (bright fortnight) of the month of either *Āṣāḍhā* or *Śrāvaṇa*.

द्वादश्यामथ शुक्लायां रवौ भाद्रपदे निशि ।
सर्पतो याति पञ्चत्वं [84] दशमाक्षरलोपतः ॥१५२॥

If the tenth letter becomes invisible, then the patient being bitten by a snake, succumbs to death át night on Sunday on the twelfth day of the *śukla pakṣa* (bright fortnight) of the month of *Bhādrapada*.

आश्विनस्य तथाऽष्टम्यां कृष्णायामपराह्णतः ।
ज्वरोदरेण नाशः स्याद्यदा [85] रुद्राक्षरक्षये ॥१५३॥

If the eleventh letter becomes invisible then the patient being afflicted with *jvara* (fever) and *udara* (obstinate abdominal diseases including ascites) succumbs to death in the afternoon of the eighth day of *kṛṣṇa pakṣa* (black fortnight) of the month of *Āśvina*.

कार्तिके शुक्लपञ्चम्यामतीसाराद्विनश्यति ।
सत्यं [86] सूर्याक्षराभावादिति मे निश्चिता मतिः ॥१५४॥

If the twelfth letter becomes invisible, then the patient being afflicted with diarrhoea succumbs to death on the fifth day of the *śukla pakṣa* (bright fortnight) of the month of *Kārtika*.

श्रीनिवाससंहितायाम्

मुमूर्षुतद्बन्धुसुहृज्जनानां, पृष्टोऽपि मृत्युं कथयेत्तु न वै ।
दुखं महत्तत्कथनात्तु तेषां, चिकित्सितुं नापि मुमूर्षुं [87] मिच्छेत् ॥१५५॥

According to Śrīnivāsa saṁhitā

Even if requested by the moribund patient or his relatives or friends, the physician should not disclose about his death. If this is disclosed to them, then they will be extermely grieved. Such a a moribund patient should not be treated.

भूतप्रेतपिशाचाश्च रक्षांसि[88] विविधानि च ।
मरणाभिमुखं नित्यमुपसर्पन्ति मानवम् ॥१५६॥
तानि भेषजवीर्याणि प्रतिघ्नन्ति[89] जिघांसया ।
अमोघाः याः क्रियास्ता हि विफलाश्च भवन्ति हि ॥१५७॥

Towards a moribund patient, different types of evil spirits viz., *bhūtas*, *pretas*, *piśācas* etc., and *rākṣasas* are daily attracted. They counter-act the potency of drugs because of their desire to kill the patient. Therefore, even the most effective therapy fails to produce the desired result.

असाध्यं हि गदं दृष्ट्वा दृष्टारिष्टं भिषक्तमः ।
तीर्थे यत्नं प्रकुर्वीत दानं चैव विशेषतः ॥१५८॥
कुर्याद्वापि प्रतीकारं कथयित्वा निरालसः ।
गदोऽयं तीर्थसाध्यः स्याद्विष्णुः शान्तिःकरिष्यति ॥१५९॥

If a physician comes across a patient who is not curable or in whom bad prognostic signs and symptoms are manifested, then he should advise the patient to visit religious places and offer charity. He may also initiate treatment but before that, the patient should be informed without delay that the disease will be cured only by visits to religious places and Lord Viṣṇu will alleviate such a disease.

वैदिकोक्तं स्मरेन्मंत्रं सदा मृत्युंजयात्मकम् ।

विष्णोः सहस्रनामानि महाकालं स्मरेत्तथा ॥१६०॥

90

॥इति द्वादशाक्षरकालज्ञानविद्या॥

To overcome such situations one should recite the *Mṛtyuñjaya mantra* as described in the *Vedas*, the *Viṣṇu sahasra nāma* (one thousand names of Lord Viṣṇu) and *Mahākāla mantra.*

Thus, ends the description of *Kālajñāna* (determination of the time of death) on the basis of *Dvādaśākṣara mantra.*

॥इति श्री महाराजाधिराजटोडरमल्लविरचिते टोडरानन्दे आयुर्वेदसौख्ये नाडी-

91

परीक्षा-मूत्रपरीक्षा-नेत्रपरीक्षा-जिह्वापरीक्षादीपदेवतावैकुण्ठद्वादशाक्षरीकालज्ञान्

विद्याकथनं नाम षष्ठो हर्षः॥

Thus, ends the sixth Chapter of the *Āyurveda Saukhyaṁ* in *Ṭoḍarānanda,* composed by the great king Ṭoḍara malla which deals with the following important topics:

1. Pulse examination;
2. Urine examination;
3. Eye examination;
4. Examination of tongue;
5. Determination of the good and bad events by the help of the god in the form of a lamp; and
6. Determination of the time of death of a person on the basis of *Vaikuṇṭha dvādaśākṣara mantra.*

NOTES AND REFERENCES

1. "अचूचुरुद्यो————नेत्रचकोरचन्द्रः" पाठोऽयं द्वितीयषष्ठपुस्तकयोः नोपलभ्यते ।

2. "तच्चेष्ट्या———पंडितैः" पाठोऽयं षष्ठपुस्तके अधिकं भवति ।

3. "एकाङ्गुलं———वा शिराः" पाठोऽयं षष्ठपुस्तके अधिको भवति ।

4. 'कफस्यान्ते निजस्थाने' इति आदर्शपुस्तके पाठः ।

5. 'परीक्षा रत्नवच्चस्यात् अभ्यासादेव जायते' इति योगरत्नाकरे पाठः ।

6. 'काक-चालक-मण्डूकादिगतिं' इति द्वितीयपुस्तके पाठः ।

7. 'वह्निया' इति षष्ठपुस्तके पाठः ।

8. 'धमनी या' इति प्रथमपुस्तके पाठः ।

9. 'मन्दं मन्दं' इति योगरत्नाकरे पाठः ।

10. 'सूक्ष्मा' इति योगरत्नाकरे पाठः ।

11. 'नित्यं' इति षष्ठपुस्तके पाठः ।

12.

"शरीरं शीतलं यस्य नाडी सोष्णा च वेगधृक् ।
शंखनाडी जवोदर्कस्तस्यांतर्ज्वरमादिशेत् ॥१॥
ज्वरवेगेति
अर्धं विषाणायमाना सा कामान्क्रोधादुपप्लुता ।
क्षीणा चिताभयाभ्यां च सदा शोकेन जायते ॥२॥
गुर्विण्याः सुस्थिरा गुर्वी स्वगतिद्वयधारिणी ।
लघ्वी भवति दीप्ताग्नेस्तथा वेगवती सुखा ॥३॥
स्थिरा बलवती स्निग्धा सुखिन्नोबृंहितस्य च ।
नाडी दत्ताक्षियुगलं श्रमशोषेण जायते ॥४॥
भारधारणमूर्छां च भयशोकविसूचिकाम् ।
त्यक्त्वा वातामयानष्टशिरास्पन्दो न जीवति ॥५॥
यात्युत्सुका स्थिरात्यन्तं या च निर्मांसवाहिनी ।
याति सूक्ष्मवती वक्रा तामसाध्यां विनिर्दिशेत् ॥६॥
स्थित्वा नाडी क्षणे यस्य विद्युद्योतिरिवेक्षते ।
दिनैकं जीवति तदा नरो नैवात्र संशयः ॥७॥"

पाठोऽयं षष्ठपुस्तके अधिकमुपलभ्यते ।

13. 'पूर्वं पित्तगतिं प्रभञ्जनगतिं श्लेष्माणमाबिभ्रतीमत्यन्तं भ्रमणं मुहुर्विदधतीं चक्रादिरूढामिव । भीष्मत्वं दधतीं कलासु पतितां सूक्ष्मत्वमातन्वतीं नो साध्यां धमनीं वदन्ति मुनयो नाडीगतिज्ञानिनः ।" इति योगरत्नाकरे पाठः ।

14. 'स्थूला' इति प्रथमपञ्चमपुस्तकयोः पाठः ।

15. 'मलापाते' इति आदर्शपुस्तकेषु पाठः ।

16. "मृति———शीर्णडमरुवत्' पाठोऽयं षष्ठपुस्तके अधिकमुपलभ्यते ।

17. "मध्ये———पश्चान्मुनिरात्रेयभाषितम्" पाठोऽयं षष्ठपुस्तके अधिको भवति ।

18. 'स्पर्शे' इति आदर्शपुस्तके पाठः ।

19. 'शुभ्रे' इति प्रथमपुस्तके पाठः ।

20. क. 'विकाशि' इति द्वितीयपुस्तके पाठः।

ख. 'विकासितं तैलमथाऽशु मूत्रे साध्यः स रोगी न विकासितं चेत्' इति योगरत्नाकरे पाठः ।

21. "तृणेनादाय——पल्लवचारिणी" इति षष्ठपुस्तके अधिको पाठः ।

22. 'नीलं च रुक्षं कुपिते च वायौ पीतारुणं तैलसमं च पित्ते ।' इति योगरत्नाकरे पाठः ।

23. 'स्वच्छं च पित्ततः' इति षष्ठपुस्तके पाठः ।

24. "रसाधिकं———बहुमूत्रं" पाठोऽयं प्रथमपञ्चमपुस्तकयोः अधिकमुपलभ्यते ।

25. 'मलज्वरे' इति आदर्शपुस्तकयोः पाठः ।

26. 'कृष्णं पक्वं' इति प्रथमपुस्तके पाठः ।

27. 'पीताद्रक्तं" इति षष्ठपुस्तके पाठः ।

28. 'हस्तपादसमुद्भूतदाहदोषोपयाद्धितां' इति प्रथमपुस्तके पाठः ।

29. 'रक्तबुद्बुदपूर्वकं' इति प्रथमपुस्तके पाठः ।

30. "जायते——बुद्बुदसंयुतम्" पाठोऽयं षष्ठपुस्तके नोपलभ्यते ।

31. 'मांसधावनतोयाभं तुल्यं' इति द्वितीयषष्ठपुस्तकयोः पाठः।

32. 'नीलवर्णं' इति प्रथमपञ्चमपुस्तकयोः पाठः।

33. "उत्तस्यां———संशयः" पाठोऽयं षष्ठपुस्तके अधिकमुपलभ्यते।

34. "ईशान्यां———नश्यति" पाठोऽयं षष्ठपुस्तके नोपलभ्यते।

35. "व जीवतिध्रुवं———भाषिणे" पाठोऽयं षष्ठपुस्तके अधिकमुपलभ्यते।

36. 'सरमाकारसंयुतम्' इति पञ्चमपुस्तके पाठः।

37. 'नरं शिरविर्वर्जितं' इति प्रथमपुस्तके पाठः।

38. 'शस्त्रं' इति प्रथमपञ्चमपुस्तकयोः पाठः।

39. 'लगुडश्चैव' इति षष्ठपुस्तके पाठः।

40. 'रम्यं' इति षष्ठपुस्तके पाठः।

41. 'चालिनी' इति प्रथमपञ्चमपुस्तकयोः पाठः।

42. "त्रिकोणे———समुद्भवं" पाठोऽयं प्रथमपञ्चमपुस्तकयोः अधिकमुपलभ्यते।

43. 'समाचरेत्' इति पञ्चमपुस्तके पाठः।

44. 'ध्रुवं' इति प्रथमपञ्चमपुस्स्तकयोः पाठः।

45. 'विनिश्चितः' इति द्वितीयपुस्तके पाठः।

46. 'सफेनिलं विट् त्रुटितं' इति द्वितीयपुस्तके पाठः।

47. 'पक्वं निमज्जति' इति द्वितीयषष्ठपुस्तकयोः पाठः।

48. 'आमा' इति पञ्चमपुस्तके पाठः।

49. 'विप्रा' इति पञ्चमपुस्तके पाठः।

50. 'दोषवर्धनपंथविचक्षणो' इति प्रथमद्वितीयपञ्चमपुस्तकेषु पाठः।

51. 'दुष्टपित्तवशबुद्ध्यते गदः' इति प्रथमपञ्चमपुस्तकयोः पाठः।

52. 'सकिनी' इति षष्ठपुस्तके पाठः।

53. 'संशयः' इति द्वितीयपुस्तके पाठः।

54. 'पित्तद्वेषि' इति षष्ठपुस्तके पाठः।

55. "श्यामं———भवेच्चक्षुस्त्रिदोषतः" इति प्रथमषष्ठपुस्तकयोः पाठः।

56. "जिह्वायां ———इति नखपरीक्षा" पाठोऽयं षष्ठपुस्तके अधिकमुपलभ्यते।

57. 'निजाऽसृजालिख्यन्यसेदन्तशलाकया' इति षष्ठपुस्तके पाठः ।

58. 'यत्रैष्यते' इति द्वितीयपुस्तके पाठः ।

59. "आर्द्रादि———नान्यथा भवेत्" पाठोऽयं प्रथमपञ्चमषष्ठपुस्तकेषु उपलभ्यते ।

60. 'समाहितमाना' इति षष्ठपुस्तके पाठः ।

61. 'तदाहीनं' इति षष्ठपुस्तके पाठः ।

62. 'पुनः' इति आकरे पाठः ।

63. "पूजयेच्चन्दनादिभिः——— —सुगन्धलेपितस्थाने" पाठोऽयं षष्ठपुस्तके नोपलभ्यते ।

64. 'न्यसेद्देवि !' इति आकरे पाठः ।

65. पाठोऽयं रसार्णवे नोपलभ्यते ।

66. "प्रयत्नतः————वह्निवीरकम्" पाठोऽयं प्रथमपुस्तके रसार्णवे च नोपलभ्यते ।

67. ॐ ह्रीं क्रौं क्ष्लैं क्ष्लं ह्रीं ह्रीं ह्रीं ह्रीं ह्रूः हुं फट्— रसेश्वराय महाकालभैरवाय रौद्ररूपाय कृष्णपिङ्गललोचनाय, अवतार२ अवतारय२ जल्प२ जल्पय२ शुभाशुभं कथय२ कथापय२ महारक्षां कुरु२ रससिद्धि देहि । इति मालामन्त्राः । इति रसार्णवे पाठः ।

68. 'ॐ महाकालभैरवाय हृदयाय नमः । ॐ महाबलभैरवाय शिरसे स्वाहा । ॐ अघोरभैरवाय शिखायै वौषट् । ॐ वज्रवीरभैरवाय कवचाय हुम् । ॐ क्रोधभैरवाय नेत्राय वौषट् । ॐ कङ्कालभैरवाय अस्त्राय फट् । सर्व्वत्र स्वाहान्तम् । एवमङ्गन्यासाः एवमङ्गुलीन्यासान् कुर्य्यादादौ । एते षडङ्गे, पूजने च मूलमन्त्राः । इति रसार्णवे पाठः ।

69. 'समर्च्चयेत्' इति आकरे पाठः ।

70. 'मन्त्रैश्च' इति आकरे पाठः ।

71. 'चाशु शोभनम्' इति द्वितीयपुस्तके पाठः ।

72. 'तद्दीपं' इति आकरे पाठः ।

73. 'सर्व्वास्तत्र कुमारिकाः' इति आकरे पाठः ।

74. 'कुमारिकाः' इति आकरे पाठः ।

75. 'रसकर्म्मणि सञ्चरेत्' इति ग्राकरे पाठः।

76. 'वत्सरादपि' इति द्वितीयषष्ठपुस्तकयोः पाठः।

77. 'रुद्रदिने चिरात्' इति षष्ठपुस्तके पाठः।

78. 'पौषमास्याममायां' इति षष्ठपुस्तके पाठः।

79. 'नानुवारे' इति द्वितीयपुस्तके पाठः।

80. 'शुक्लायां———संक्षयात्' पाठोऽयं पञ्चमपुस्तके नोपलभ्यत।

81. 'वह्नो' इति षष्ठपुस्तके पाठः।

82. 'उत्पातक्षीयते' इति प्रथमपञ्चमषष्ठपुस्तकेषु पाठः।

83. 'शोहक्षयात्क्षयं' इति षष्ठपुस्तके पाठः।

84. 'हानितः' इति प्रथमपञ्चमपुस्तकयोः पाठः।

85. 'रुद्राक्षरक्षयः' इति द्वितीयषष्ठपुस्तकयोः पाठः।

86. 'सूक्ष्मतरा' इति षष्ठपुस्तके पाठः।

87. 'चिकीर्षितुं' इति द्वितीयपुस्तके पाठः।

88. 'यक्षांसि' इति प्रथमपञ्चमपुस्तकयोः पाठः।

89. 'प्रजिघ्नन्ति' इति द्वितीयपुस्तके पाठः।

90. 'द्वादशाक्षरविद्याकालज्ञानम्' इति द्वितीयपुस्तके पाठः।

91. 'वरणद्वादशाक्षरी' इति प्रथमपुस्तके पाठः।

INDEX

GLOSSARY

Abaddha

The stool which is not hard in consistency i.e. loose. This is one of the sixteen morbid conditions of stool to be examined by the physician.

Abādhā

Also written as *ābādha*. This term is used here as a synonym of 'disease'. This is used to imply 'pain' (*Suśruta* : *Cikitsā* 24 : 1) and diseases of the body and mind in general (*Suśruta* : *Sūtra* 24 : 12).

Abandhyā

Also written as *avandhyā*. Some plants produce seeds and others do not. The former category is called *abandhyā* i.e. fertile.

Abhayā

This is one of the synonyms (types) of *harītakī* (*Terminalia chebula* Retz.). This causes fearlessness because it promotes positive health and prevents as well as cures diseases.

Abhimāna

One of the psychic attributes implying 'ego'. Saints are free from this. But a common household person do possess it. It is controlled by *sādhaka* type of *pitta* located in the heart.

Abhiśaptaka

A group of diseases caused by the *abhiśāpa* or curse of great saints and preceptors when they are angry because of the wrong behaviour of a person. Normally, saints and preceptors are free from anger. But they become angry when a person's behaviour far exceeds the socially approved norms and affects the well-being of the people. Such diseases are normally not amenable to ordinary therapies. These can be cured only if the person changes his behaviour and obtains the blessings of those saints.

Abhiṣyandin (dravya)

The drug, diet or drink which causes heaviness by obstructing the channels of circulation because of sliminess and heaviness is called *abhiṣyandin*. Curd is an example of this category.

Abhyaṅga

Massage over the body with the help of oil etc. Often medicated oil is used for this purpose. Massage of the body is indicated both for healthy persons and patients—in the former it prevents deseases and produces sturdiness of the body, and in the latter, it cures deseases. It is specifically useful for deseases caused by *vāyu*. It is contra-indicated in the *sama* condition of the desease, among others.

Ācāra

This term generally implies different types of regimens that should be followed during day and night and in different seasons. Improper regimens cause aggravation of the *doṣas*. This term is used in this text to indicate common household activities which a lady should avoid during her period of menstruation.

Acintya

A thing which is unthinkable. It is used here as an epithet of the Universal Soul or *ātman*. The exact nature of the *ātman* is not perceivable with the help of the ordinary mind. It is realised only by the saints of very high order.

Ādāna

This is the period of the year in which the energy of the living beings and other non-living material on the earth gets absorbed. This is also called *uttarāyaṇa* which includes three seasons namely *śiśira* or late winter, *vasanta* or spring and *grīṣma* or summer. The *śiśira* season starts from the month of *māgha* (approximately middle of January) and the *grīṣma* season ends in *āṣāḍha* (approximately middle of July). The period of *ādāna* is dominated by the qualities of *agni* (fire). The following table provides the comparative view of the classification of the year :

Ayana	Seasons	Months according to Hindu Calender	Months according to English Calender
Uttarāyaṇa (*ādāna kāla* or the period of absorption)	1. *Śiśira* (late winter)	I *Māgha* II *Phālguna*	January-February February-March
	2. *Vasanta* (spring)	I *Caitra* II *Vaiśākha*	March-April April-May
	3. *Griṣma* (summer)	I *Jyeṣṭha* II *Āṣāḍha*	May-June June-July
Dakṣiṇāyana (*visarga kāla* or the period of elimination)	1. *Varṣā* (rainy season)	I *Śrāvaṇa* II *Bhādrava*	July-August August-September
	2. *Śarat* (autumn)	I *Āśvina* II *Kārttika*	September-October October-November
	3. *Hemanta* (early winter)	I *Mārgaśirṣa* II *Pauṣa*	November-December December-January

Āḍhaki

The botanical name of this plant is *Cajanus cajan* (Linn.) Millsp. It is cultivated through out India as a pulse crop. It aggravates *vāyu* when taken in excess.

Ādhibhautika
Ādhidaivika
Ādhyātmika

Duḥkha or miseries, including diseases are classified into three categories. Those arising out of external objects are called *ādhibhautika*. Miseries or diseases arising out of providencial causes are called *ādhidaivika*. Such of the diseases and miseries as are caused by the vitiation of *doṣas* in one's own body are called *ādhyātmika*, in the present context. In general Sanskrit literature, the term *ādhyātmika* means "spiritual or things concerning the soul". This classification of diseases has been accepted and described in detail in *Suśruta : Sūtra* 24 : 4. According to *Caraka* (*Vimāna* 6 : 3), diseases are classified into two categories or groups on the basis of five different criteria, as follows :

Criteria of classification	*Groupings of diseases*
1. Prognosis	I Curable II Incurable
2. Intensity	I mild II severe
3. Location	I mental II physical
4. Nature of the causative factors	I endogenous II exogenous
5. Site of origin	I having origin from *āmāśaya* (stomach) II having origin from *pakvāśaya* (colon).

Causes of diseases are of three types, namely, excessive utilisation, non-utilisation and wrong utilisation of objects (of senses), acts and time. For example, excessive gazing at the highly illuminous substance would constitute excessive utilisation of the visual objects. Not looking at anything at all would amount to its non-utilization. Similarly, its wrong utilisation would be to see things too close or too far away or things that are awful or terrifying or are surprising, contemptuous, frightful, deformed and alarming.

Excessive utilisation of auditory objects would be to hear uprorious noise coming out of thunder and kettle drum, loud cries etc., its non-utilisation would be not to hear anything at all; hearing of harsh words, news about the death of friends, assaulting, insulting and terrifying sounds constitute the wrong utilisation.

Smell of exceedingly sharp, acute and intoxicating odours constitute an excessive utilisation of olfactory sense faculty; not to smell at all is its non-utilisation; its wrong utilisation is the smell of exceedingly putrid, unpleasant, dirty, putrified and cadaverous odour and poisonous gas.

Similarly, excessive intake of various substances having various tastes would amount to over-utilisation of gustatory sense faculty; not to use it at all amounts to its non-utilisation. Factors which are described in the *Caraka : Vimāna* 1 : 21 except *rāśi* will constitute its wrong utilisation.

Excessive use of exceedingly cold and hot bath, massage and unction etc., amounts to over utilisation of the tactile sense faculty, not to use it at all is its non-utilisation; the use of bath, massage and unction and other hot and cold substances without observing the prescribed order, touch of uneven place, dirty objects, bacteria and injurious touch constitute its wrong utilisation.

Ādibala pravṛtta

Diseases caused by the vitiation of the sperm and ovum of the parents and inherited by the offspring belong to this category.

Adṛṣṭa

Literally, this word means an unseen factor. In the present context, it is used to imply the factor which is responsible for the combination of the sperm and the ovum which helps in conception and procreation of a child. It is the "Individual soul" which transmigrates from one body to the other along with *sūkṣma śarīra* or the astral body which enters into the uterus of the mother and helps in the combination of the ovum and the sperm for the procreation of a child.

Agada

The term "*gada*" means a disease. Agents which make the body free from diseases are called *agada* in general. It has however, a specific meaning in the present context, according to which it implies "the treatment of different types of poisons". *Agada tantra* or *Agada kriyā* means the science or the specialised branch of Ayurveda which provides description of different types of poisons and the knowledge for their cure.

Agastya

He is one of the great saints, who along with others, originally propounded Ayurveda for the benefit of living beings. Discovery of many rejuvenating recipes is attributed to him. This is also the name of a medicinal plant which is botanically known as *Sesbania grandiflora* Pers. In the present context it is used to indicate the star Canopos. This star arises in the sky on the seventh day of the second half of the *Bhādrapada*. Its rays have a strong detoxicating effect on the water. Therefore, the water exposed to the rays of this star is considered to be free from any defects and it is healthy for the individual.

Aghora

Literally, this term means "not terrific". It is an euphemistic title of lord Śiva, who is the god of medicine. According to tradition, *Aghora mantra* should be recited before the beginning of the purification of mercury. In the present context, a ritual has been prescribed for the prediction of good and bad events in which *Aghora mantra* is to be recited.

Agni

This term is generally used in Ayurveda to indicate the power of digestion. It is also used as a synonym of *pitta*. In a broad sense, it implies all the digestive and metabolic functions of the body. Enzymes which are responsible for the digestion of the food, its metabolism and assimilation in each and every cell of the body are called *agni*. The similarities and distinctive features between *pitta* and *agni* are described in *Suśruta saṁhitā* and quoted in this text. The south-east direction is known as the abode of *agni* in *ādhidaivika* parlance. For the treatment of some of the diseases, fire or heated objects are used. This is called "*agni kriyā*". As one of the five basic elements which constitute this universe, it is called *agni mahābhūta*. The entire universe is also classified into two categories, namely, *agni guṇa* or heating attribute and *saumya guṇa* or cooling attribute. The sun is considered to be the controller of the heating attributes of the universe and the moon is the controller of the cooling attributes. Taken together, the universe is called *agni ṣomiya*.

Agnyāśaya

This is described as one of the abdominal viscera in which *agni* is located. It is located above the *āmāśaya* (stomach including small intestine) and towards the left side of the umbilicus. It is supposed to excercise control over all the enzymatic activities in the body. There is a great deal of controversy regarding the exact indentification of this important organ. However, many ayurvedic scholars hold the view that this term *agnyāśaya* stands for pancreas.

Aguru

Ref : Materia Medica of Ayurveda—the first volume of this series.

Ahiphena

Ref. *Aphuka* in Materia Medica of Ayurveda—the first volume of this series.

Ajaptari

This is a very uncommon Sanskrit word. In the present text it is used to mean "more effective" or "more in quantity".

Akasmikā

Lit. this term means "accidental". In this text it is used to imply a group of diseases which occur accidentally as a result of the displeasure of the gods (*daiva bala saṁbhūta*). It has been explained that such accidental diseases are manifested because of the maturity of the results of the past evil deeds (*karma*). These evil deeds might have been performed in the previous years of the present life or during the *pūrva janma* or past-life.

Akṣa

This term is used as a synonym of several drugs like *bibhitaka* (*Terminalia belerica* Roxb.), *rudrākṣa* (*Elaeocarpus ganitrus* Roxb.) and a type of *sarṣapa* (*Brassica campestries* Linn. var. rapa). According to the explanatory note given in this text, it is used here to mean *sauvarcala* or sonchal salt which is prepared by boiling soda with emblic myrobalan.

Akṣara nyāsa

The term '*akṣara*' lit. means 'imperishable'. It generally implies a syllable or a letter. A *mantra* is composed of many such letters. Before this *mantra* is recited, it is necessary to impregnate the body including its various limbs and organs by the alphabets or letters of the *mantra* and this is called *akṣara nyāsa*.

Ālocaka pitta

This is one of the five varieties of *pitta*. It is located in the eyes and helps in the perception of vision. Bhela has described two varieties of it viz., (1) *cakṣu vaiśeṣika* which helps in the perception of vision; and (2) *buddhi vaiśeṣika* which while located between the two eye brows helps in the perception, memory, intellect and instinctive activities.

Āma

Lit. this term means "uncooked material". In the context of medicine it means the product of improper digestion and metabolism. The mucus that is passed along with stool in dysentery is generally called *āma*.

All diseases are caused by the suppression of *agni* or the activities of the enzymes responsible for digestion and metabolism. This *agni māndya* causes *āma* formation in different levels. It circulates in the body and gets mixed up with the *doṣas* and *dhātus*. Such *doṣas* are called *sāmā doṣa*. While circulating in the body to perform their physiological activities, such *sāma doṣas*, because of the changes in their composition, get obstructed in the channels (*srotas*). This results in the vitiation and obstruction of these channels which produces the diseases. In the beginning of each internal disease, the *doṣas* are invariably in the *sāma* stage. Therefore, the patient is advised to keep fast which prevents further accumulation of *āma*. Once this first stage is over, the patient is given drugs for the *pācana* (cooking or metabolic transformation) of this *āma*. This *āma* can also be removed from the body by elimination therapies like *vamana* (emesis) and *virecana* (purgation). Depending upon the nature of this *āma* and channel of circulation involved, different types of diseases are manifested in the body. *Śuṇṭhī* (*Zingiber officinale* Rosc.), *pippalī* (*Piper longum* Linn.) and *marica* (*Piper nigrum* Linn.) are collectively called *trikaṭu* or three pungent drugs. They are considered to be the best drugs for the *pācana* of *āma*. Therefore, in most of the recipes used in ayurveda, these three drugs are invariably added.

Drugs dominated by *agni*, *vāyu* and *ākāśa mahābhūtas* are endowed with attributes for the *pāka* of *āma*. Generally pungent and bitter drugs are dominated by these *mahābhūtas*. Astringent, saline and sour drugs are partially dominated by these *mahābhūtas*. Sweet taste, on the other hand is dominated by *pṛthvī* and *jala mahābhūtas*. Therefore, drugs and diet having sweet taste produce more of *āma*. Such drugs are generally prohibited in the beginning stage of a disease.

Āmalaka(*ī*)

Botanically this drug is called *Emblica officinalis* Gaertn. It grows wild in the mixed deciduous forests of India. It is often cultivated in gardens and home yards. It's fruit is rich natural source of vitamin-C. It is popularly used as a rejuvenating agent in different forms. *Cyavana prāsa* is the most popular preparation (in linctus form) of this fruit. There is a mythological story behind this preparation according to which the great sage Cyavana took this preparation during his old age and become young again.

Harītakī (*Terminalia chebula* Retz.), *bibhītakī* (*Terminalia belerica* Roxb.) and *āmalakī* (*Emblica officinalis* Gaertn.) are collectively called *triphalā* (three important fruits). Apart from their rejuvenating effect, they promote the power of resistance of the body against diseases. Therefore, these fruits are added to many ayurvedic recipes. These drugs have special attributes to promote eye sight. Therefore, in different forms, these fruits are used to correct refraction errors of eyes and to prevent as well as cure cataract.

Āmāśaya

Lit. the receptacle of *āma* or undigested food. This is one of the fifteen *koṣṭhāṅgas* or viscera of the abdomen and thorax. It is the *mūla* or controlling organ of the channels carrying food.

According to Caraka, this is located between the two nipples and the umbilicus. Suśruta has described its location as above the *pittāśaya*. Both *kapha* (*kledaka*) and *pitta* (*pācaka*) are located in it. Cakrapāṇi has clarified that the upper part of the *āmāśaya* is the abode of *kapha* and the lower portion is the abode of *pitta*.

According to modern anatomy *āmāśaya* is both stomach and the upper portion of the small intestine. This term is also used in some places to imply the stomach alone.

Diseases are of two categories viz., *āmāśayottha* or those arising out of *āmāśaya* and *pakvāśayottha* or those arising out of *pakvāśaya*. Diseases of the former category are dominated by *kapha* and *pitta* and for their treatment emesis and purgation therapies are generally administered.

Āmavāta

Description of this disease generally simulates rheumatism even though both these conditions are not exactly the same. This disease is described in the *Caraka saṁhitā* only in brief. Its detailed description is available only in later ayurvedic works like *Mādhava nidāna*.

Vitiated *vāta* afflicted by *āma* is responsible for the causation of this disease and drugs which counteract both of them like castor oil and *guggulu* are used in its treatment.

Amṛtā

This is one of the synonyms of *guḍūci* (*Tinospora cordifolia* Miers). It is also used as a synonym of many other drugs like *harītaki* (*Terminalia chebula* Retz.), *āmalaka* (*Emblica officinalis* Gaertn.), *indra vāruni* (*Citrullus colocynthis* Schrad.) and *dūrvā* (*Cynodon dactylon* Pers.).

Amṛta

Lit. this term means immortal or imperishable. In the text it is used to imply the mythical ambrosia which was produced at the time of the churning of the ocean by the gods and the demons and this is supposed to confer immortality, everlasting youth and beauty.

Aṁśūdaka

The water which is exposed to the rays of the sun and the moon. According to the description provided in this work, the water which is exposed to the rays of the Star Canopus along with the sun and the moon is called *aṁśūdaka*. It is very healthy and free from all blemishes.

Anāhata

This is one of the six *cakras* of *Yoga*. It is located in the region of the heart. It has twelve petals over which letters from *Ka* to *Ṭha* are located with a bindu above them which is of vermilion colour. This *cakra* has the colour of the flower of *bandhūka*. In its pericarp is the hexagonal *vāyu maṇḍala*, of a smoky colour, and above it *sūrya maṇḍala*, with the *trikoṇa* lustrous as ten million flashes of lightning within it. Above is the *vāyubīja*, of a smoky hue, seated on a black antelope, four-armed and carrying the goad (*aṅkuśa*). In his (*vāyu bīja's*) lap is three-eyed *īśa* like *haṁsa* (*haṁsābha*). His two arms extended in the gestures of granting boons and dispelling fear. In the pericarp of this lotus, seated on a red lotus, is the *śakti kākinī*. She is four armed, and carries the noose (*pāśa*), the skull (*kapālā*), and makes the boon (*vara*) and fear-dispelling (*abhaya*) signs. She is of a golden hue, is dressed in yellow raiment, and wears every variety of jewel and a garland of bones. Her heart is softened by nectar. In the middle of the *trikoṇa* is *śiva* in the form of a *bāṇa liṅga*, with the crescent moon and *bindu* on his head. He is of a golden colour.

He looks joyous with a rush of desire. Below him is the *jīvātmā* like *haṁsa*. It is like the steady tapering flame of a lamp. Below the pericarp of this lotus is the red lotus of eight petals, with its head uplurned. It is in this (red) lotus that there are the *kalpa* tree, the jewelled altar surmounted by an awning and decorated by flags and the like, which is the place of mental worship.

Concentration in this *cakra* during the process of meditation endows the *yogi* with the special power of speech, among others.

Aṅga nyāsa
Aṅguli nyāsā

Impregnation of different organs of the body and fingers with the letters of the *bija mantra*, This is generally done along with *akṣara nyāsa* before the actual recitation of the *mantra*.

Antaḥ parīmārjana

Therapies are broadly classified into two categories, namely *antaḥ parimārjana* and *bahiḥ parimārjana*. The former involves the cleaning of the body internally by the help of emesis, purgation etc. and the latter involves cleaning the exterior of the body by the application of ointment, massage, bath etc. By the process of *antaḥ parimārjana* the *malas* or waste products of the body are taken out through the stomach or colon.

Antra

It is of two types namely *kṣudrāntra* or small intestine and *bṛhadantra* or large intestine.

Anupāna

It generally means the drink that is used after the food. This also means the drinks which are taken after the intake of medicines. Vehicles like honey and ghee are also used *along with* the medicines. For different types of *doṣas* different types of *anupānas* are prescribed. These *anupanas* supplement and accentuate the effects of original medicines.

Anuvāsana

The medicated enema which is prepared by adding oil is called *anuvāsana*. Sometimes ghee, muscle fat and bone-marrow are added to it. This type of medicated enema is generally given for a longer period and it does not produced any adverse effect even if retained inside the body beyond one day. This alleviates *vāyu* and produces nourishing effect in the body.

Āpta
Āptopadeśa

The enlightement and refined persons who are absolutely free from the effects of *rajas* and *tamas* by virtue of the power of penance and knowledge and who are always in possession of an uninterrupted knowledge pertaining to the past, present and future are called *āptas* (authorities). They are also called *śiṣṭa* (gentlemen) and *vibuddha* (enlightened persons). Their testimony is beyond any doubt. Their statements are based on the *vedas* and other scriptural material in agreement with the *vedas*. It is the most authentic source of knowledge.

In the context of medicine the statement of the patient has the similar status.

Āpyāyanī

The umbilical chord which provides nourishment to the foetus is called *apayāyanī nāḍi*.

Ariṣṭa

The signs and symptoms which are indicative of the imminent death are called *ariṣṭa*. The term *riṣṭa* is also used for similar purposes. Appearance of such signs certainly leads to death in some cases. In some others, death can be avoided by the performance of rituals and use of potent medicines.

Ārtava

Lit. this term means seasonal or periodical phenomena. In ladies it implies the menstrual flow. This term is often used to mean the ovum (*strī bīja*) which is responsible for conception. It is considered to be the *upadhātu* of *rasa*. *Śoṇita*, *rajaḥ*, *strī bīja* and *strīś ukra*—these terms are also used as synonyms of *ārtava*.

Artha

This is one of the four-fold internal desires of human beings —the other three are *dharma* (performance of religious rites), *kāma* (satisfaction of sex desire) and *mokṣa* (salvation). Lit. the term *artha* means wealth and the objects of senses.

Āsava

The medicine or drink prepared by fermentation is called *āsava* or *ariṣṭa*. In the former medicines and liquids including water are used as such, and in the latter these are boiled and then processed. This is a general rule but there are many exceptions.

In *āsavas* and *ariṣṭas* sweet things like honey, jaggery and sugar are added for alcoholic fermentation. The flowers of *dhātaki* (*Woodfordia fruticosa* Kurz) are added to *āsavas* and *ariṣṭas* for fermentation. To initiate this process *kiṇva* (yeast) is added. In ideal conditions 14% alcohol is generated in this process. But in ordinary *āsavas* and *ariṣṭas*, the alcoholic content is generally—7% to 10%. This alcohol works as a preservative. It also keeps dissolved some of the therapeutically effective components of the drugs added to the recipe.

Aśmarī

This is commonly used to indicate the "stone in the urinary bladder" and other parts of the urinary system. Stone in gall bladder etc., is also called *aśmarī*. It is of four types viz., *vātika*, *paittika*, *ślaiṣmika* and *śukraja*.

Aśoka

Bot. *Saraca indica* Linn. This plant grows in the forests of Central and Eastern Himalayas, Bengal and Western Peninsula. This plant is specifically indicated in female diseases like menorrhagia. It is also useful for healthy women because it produces resistance against the occurence of such diseases. This is also cultivated as a garden plant because of its beautiful flowers.

According to Rāmāyaṇa, Sītā was kept in captivity by Rāvaṇa in a garden of *aśoka*.

Āsthapana

This is one of the two types of medicated enema. It is also known as *nirūha basti*. It restores youth and keeps the *doṣas* (specially *vāyu*) in their respective places for which it is called *āsthāpana basti*. Normally decoctions etc. are used for the preparation of this enema.

Aśvagandhā

Ref. Materia Medica of Ayurveda—the first volume in this series.

Aśvamedha yajña

A celebrated ritual, the antiquity of which reaches back to the Vedic period in which horse is sacrified. Sometimes the horse is not actually immolated but kept bound during the period of ceremony. It is stated that performance of one hundred such rituals entitles the performer to displace Indra from the dominion of *svarga.*

Aśvins

The twin celestial physicians who propounded ayurveda in this mortal world through Indra. They learnt ayurveda from Prajāpati. The Aśvins are described in the Vedas as the gods of medicine. The term is invariably used in dual number (Aśvinau) in Sanskrit.

Atasi

Ref. Materia Medica of Ayurveda—the first volume in this series.

Atmā(an)

The Soul which transmigrates from one body (after death) to another through *sūkṣma śarira* or astral body. It is the union of this soul with the sperm and the ovum in the mother's womb which results in conception. The union of physique, senses, mind and the soul is called *āyus* or the life.

It is of two categories viz., the *Paramātman* or the Universal Soul and the *Jivātman* or the Individual Soul. The former is *nirguṇa* or free from attributes. Various qualities are attributed to it only when it comes in contact with the senses and the mind. The *Paramātman* is *yoga pratyakṣa* i.e. it can be realised or perceived during *samādhi* only.

Avanti

This is the name of a state in the ancient and medieval India. Many important historical events are associated with this state. This is the modern Ujjain in Madhya Pradesh. It is considered to be one of the seven sacred cities of the Hindus. Death in this city gives salvation and eternal happiness.

Ayana

Ref. *Ādāna.*

Āyuḥ

Union of the physique, senses, mind and soul is called *āyus* or life. Its synonyms are *dhāri*, *jivita*, *nityaga* and *anubandha* Ref. *Ātman.*

Badarodaka

A sour drink prepared of *badara* (*Zizyphus jujuba* Lam.).

Bala

It is the synonym of *ojas* which is the essence of all the seven *dhātus*. Its nature can be ascertained from the individual's ability to perform exercise. *Bala* or strength of the individual naturally increases during *visarga kāla* or the time of elimination and decreases during *ādāna kāla* or the time of absorption.

Bāṇa

Bot. *Avicennia officinalis* Linn.

Bandhūka

Bot. *Pentapetes phoenicea* Linn.

Basti

Basti cikitsā

Basti means the urinary bladder. Medicated enema which was being administered in old days with the help of the bladder of animals is also called *basti*. Even though some modern devices are being adopted for administering this medicated enema now a days, in some parts of India, traditional *vaidyas* are still using the urinary bladder of cattle for administering *basti*.

It is classified into several categories as follows :

(*a*) Two types viz., *nairūhika* and *snaihika*
(*b*) Three tyes viz., *āsthāpana*, *anuvāsana* and *uttara basti*
(*c*) Three types viz., *karma basti*, *kāla basti* and *yoga basti*
(*d*) Three types viz., *doṣotkleśaka*, *doṣa śodhaka* and *doṣa śāmana*.

Basti is the best among the therapies for the alleviation of diseases caused by *vāyu*. In view of its therapeutic efficacy some physicians describe *basti* as *cikitsārdha* (half of entire therapeutics). *Basti* is specially useful for rejuvenation. Along with appropriate drugs, *basti* has aphrodisiac and nourishing effects also.

Bhallātaka

Ref. Materia Medica of Ayurveda—the first volume of this series.

Bhalli

A kind of arrow.

Bharata

Name of a celebrated hero and monarch of India who was the son of Duśyanta and Śankuntalā. He was first among the twelve *cakravarties* or universal emperors.

Many other historical persons are also known by this name. The son of Daśaratha and brother of Rāmacandra was also Bharata.

Bhasma

Metals and minerals including some plant and animal products are used in the form of *bhasma* which is prepared by adding other drugs and burning. This pharmaceutical process makes these metals non-toxic, assimilable and therapeutically more effective. *Rasa śāstra* in which details of these processes are described became very popular among the physicians after the advent of Buddhism, specially after Nāgārjuna.

This term is also used to mean common ash which the outcome of the burning of plants etc.

Bhasmaka

In this text it is used to imply the name of a city. In ayurveda, this term is generally used to mean the gluttonous appetite which is caused by over-digestion inasmuch as the patient suffering from this ailment always remains hungry inspite of his taking frequent heavy meals.

Bhīma

In this text *bhima* is described as the name of a medicinal plant. In the note that is given under the text, it is explained as *yukā* which is equally vague.

In *nighaṇṭu* texts, *bhīma* is described as the synonym of *amla vetasa*.

Bhūrja patra

Bark of *Betula utilis* D. Don. The term *patra* generally means leaf. Here it means the leaf like bark. In ancient India bark of this plant was in use for the purpose of writing. Even now this is used for writing sacred *mantras* etc.

Bhūta

A good or evil spirit or the ghost of a deceased person.

Bilva

Ref. Materia Medica of Ayurveda—the first volume of this series.

Brahmā

The impersonal universal spirit manifested as a personal creator and the first of the triad of personal gods—the other two being Viṣṇu and Maheśvara. He is the original propounder of ayurveda. He brought to his memory this science of medicine and then taught to Prajāpati (to Bhāskara according to *Brahma Vaivarta Purāṇa*).

Brahmā composed ayurveda as one of the upavedas of the Atharva veda. It consisted of one hundred thousand *ślokas* divided into one thousand chapters. But considering the short span of life and inadequate intelligence of man he recast the book into eight divisions.

Several recipes are attributed to him.

Brahma dundubhi

A type of kettle drum.

Brahma randhra

A suture or aperture in the crown of the head through which the Soul escapes on death.

Brahman

The divine essence or source from which all created things emanate, or with which they are identified and to which they return at the time of dissolution.

Bṛhaspati

Name of the god in whom piety and religion are personified. He is the chief offerer of prayers and sacrifices. He is the priest or *purohita* of the gods. In later times he was known as the god of wisdom and eloquence to whom various works are ascribed.

Bṛhati

Ref. Materia Medica of Ayurveda—the first volume in this series.

Brihi

Also written as *vrihi*. It is a variety of paddy (*Oryza sativa* Linn.). The size (breadth) of this paddy is used as the unit of linear measurement. The size of different layers of skin is described in this and other ayurvedic texts according to this unit.

Cakora

N. of the bird—Greek pheasant (*Perdix rufa*).

Çakra vāka

N. of the bird—Ruddy sheldrake (*Anas cascara*).

Campaka

Candana

Ref. Materia Medica of Ayurveda—the first volume in this series.

Carma dala

This is a type of skin disease characterised by itching eruptions.

Cātaka

N. of the bird—Tree sparrow (*Passer montanus*).

Cavya

Bot. *Piper chaba* Hunter.

Citraka

Dāḍima

Ref. Materia Medica of Ayurveda—the first volume of this series.

Dadhi

Milk coagulated by acid—curd.

Dadru

A type of skin disease—ring worm which is manifested by the vitiation of *pitta* and *kapha*.

Dahana

This term generally means *agni* or fire. In this text it is used to indicate a part of the moon's course or the constellation called *kṛttikā* (?)

This term is also used for drugs like *citraka* (*Plumbago zeylanica* Linn.) and *bhallātaka* (*Semecarpus anacardium* Linn.)

Ḍākini

A female imp attending the goddess *Kāli*. She feeds on human flesh. At times she afflicts human beings and the treatment of such conditions is called *Bhūta cikitsā*.

Dāmana

N. of a flowering tree. Ref. Materia Medica of Ayurveda—the first volume of this series.

Darbha

Bot. *Desmostachya bipinnata* Stapf. This is a variety of *kuśa*.

Dauhṛda

During the fourth month of pregnancy, foetal heart starts functioning. Heart is the seat of the mind. During this period the mental activities of the mother affects the child's mind. This is called *dauhṛda* or the bicardiac stage. Certain dos and don'ts are prescribed for the mother during this period. The likings and desires of the mother during this period should not be ignored. Even if she desires to take unwholesome food etc., these should be given to her but these food and drinks should be mixed with such drugs as would make them harmless. Ignoring the desires of the mother during this period is exceedingly harmful for the child.

The physical and psychic nature of the offspring can be predicted from the desires of the mother during this period.

Dhanvantari

Dhanvantari is the name of the physician of the gods and the god of medicine. He appeared on the earth as Divodāsa, the King of Kāsī surnamed Dhanvantari. Lit. this term means the person who has excelled in the science of *dhanu* or surgery. He imparted the knowledge of surgery to the sages like Suśruta Aupadhenava, Vaitaraṇa, Aurabhra, Puṣkalāvata, Karavīrya and Gopura rakṣita. *Purāṇas* are replete with reference to the god Dhanvantari, specially to his original birth and achievements. Many recipes are attributed to him. Several other physicians of the later period had also the name Dhanvantari.

Dhātri

It is one of the synonyms of *āmalaki* (*Emblica officinalis*

Gaertn.). It is generally used to mean a midwife or caretaker of the child. In ancient India *dhātris* were being employed for the breast feeding of the child. This practice is current in some parts of the country even now. Method of examination of a suitable *dhātrī* is elaborated in ayurvedic classics.

Dhātu

Dhātvagni

Tissue elements which sustain the body. Even *doṣas* and *malas* in certain contexts are described as *dhātu* because they also help in the sustenance of the body.

Classification of tissues in ayurveda is different from the modern medical classification. These are seven in number viz., *rasa* (chyle and plasma), *rakta* (hemoglobin fraction of the red cells of the blood), *māṁsa* (muscle tissue), *medas* (fat tissue), *asthi* (bone tissue), *majjā* (bone marrow—both white and red) and *śukra* (semen in general and sperm in males and ovum in females in particular). Each of these *dhātus* has *upadhātus* and *malas*.

These *dhātus* are of two categories viz., *poṣaka* or *asthāyi dhātus* (nutrient material of tissues) and *poṣya* or *sthāyi dhātus* (tissues themselves). There are *agnis* or enzymes specific to each of these *dhātus*. They are called *dhātvagnis*. They help in the synthesis of *poṣaka dhātus* from the *anna rasa* which after absorption from the intestines has become homogeneous by the action of the five *mahābhūtagnis*.

Moities of the *pācakāgni* are present in each of these *dhātus*. They convert the *poṣaka dhātu* into the *poṣya* or *sthāyi dhātu*. Increase or decrease of these *pācakāṁśas* cause decrease and increase of the *dhātus* respectively.

Each *dhātu* has its channels of circulation, and through these channels the *poṣaka dhātus* are carried to the *poṣya dhātus*.

Dipyaka

Bot. *Apium graveolens* Linn.

Divya

It is one of the synonyms of *lavaṅga* (*Syzygium aromaticum* Merr.).

Doṣa

This term is derived from the root *duṣ*, which means 'to vitiate' others. *Vāyu, pitta* and *kapha*—these are the three *doṣas* in the body. They regulate all the physiological and physico-chemical activities of the body. They remain in a definite proportion in a healthy body. Any change in this equilibrium results in disease and decay. This equilibrium is disturbed by the intake of improper food and drinks and regimens including physical as well as mental activities. When a disease is manifested as a result of the disturbance in this equilibrium, drugs are administered either to alleviate the aggravated *doṣas* or to eliminate them from the body. Even if a person is adopting proper diet and regimens, the equilibrium tends to get disturbed because of certain natural effects like the seasons. To prevent occurence of diseases certain precautions are to be taken during different seasons which is called *ṛtu caryā*. Drugs and elimination therapies are, therefore, prescribed to be used during different seasons even by a healthy person. *Doṣas* pervade the entire body including the nails and tips of hair.

Rakta is also considered to be one of the *doṣas* in the texts of surgery.

Human body is the abode of several categories of germs. Some of them are helpful and most of them are harmful. But they produce their harmful effects, they grow and multiply only when the equilibrium of *doṣas* is disturbed. Similarly to cure an infective condition the ayurvedic physician does not attempt to kill the germs. Ayurvedic medicines bring about the equilibrium of *doṣas* and create an environment in the tissues in which germs find it difficult to thrive and they die their natural death.

Sometimes *vāyu, pitta* and *kapha* are translated as wind, bile and phlegm which is wrong and misleading. *Tridoṣa* theory of ayurveda is different and distinct from the humoral theory of the ancient Greek medicine.

Drākṣā

Bot. *Vitis vinifera* Linn. The dried fruits of this plant are called *kismis* or *munakkā* and they are extensively used in ayurvedic recipes for their cooling and nourishing effects.

Dravya

Dravya or matter is of nine categories viz., *pṛthvi, ap, tejas, vāyu, ākāśa*, soul, mind, time and space. The entire universe is composed of these nine categories of matter. The first five *dravyas* are called *mahābhūtas*. These *bhūtas* are of two types viz., *sthūla bhūtas* or gross elements and *sūkṣma bhūtas* or subtle elements. The latter is also called *tanmātrās* which are the quantas of energy and each one of the former is composed of all the five *tanmātrās*. For example *pṛthvi mahābhūta* (gross) is composed of 50% of the *pṛthvi tanmātrā* and 12½% of each of *ap tanmātrā, agni tanmātrā, vāyu tanmātrā* and *ākāśa tanmātrā*. Combination of five *tanmātrās* to form the *sthūla bhūta* or *mahābhūta* is called *pañcī karaṇa*.

In medical parlence, the term *dravya* is generally used for a drug or ingredient of diet as well as drinks.

Duḥkha

Pratikūla vedanā or unfavourable stimulus is called *duḥkha* or misery including disease.

Eṇa

Eraṇḍa

Ervāruka

Ref. Materia Medica of Ayurveda—the first volume of this series.

Galagaṇḍa

Tumour on the side of the neck or goitre.

Gaṇḍamālā

Swelling of the glands of the neck.

Gandharva

Gandharvas are the celestial musicians or heavenly singers who form the orchestra at the banquets of the gods. They constitute one class into which the higher form of creation is divided—the other three are *Sarpas, Apsarās* and *Pitṛs*. These Gandharvas along with *Piśācas* are considered to exercise evil effects on human beings and the specialised branch dealing with the treatment of such afflictions is called *Bhūta vidyā*.

Gaṇeśa

N. of the god of wisdom who removes obstacles. Hence, he is invoked at the commencement of all undertakings and at the opening of all compositions with the words *namaḥ*. He is represented as a short fat man with a protuberant belly, frequently riding on a rat. He has the head of an elephant having only one tusk.

Garbhādhāna

Cohabitation with a view to procreating a child.

Gaullāla(ka)

N. of a flower.

Gāyatrī mantra

N. of a hymn composed in *Gāyatrī* meter having 24 syllables arranged generally in a triplet of eight syllables each.

Ghoṇā

This term generally means nose. In this text, this is used to indicate the foamy secretion from the mouth.

Ghuṇākṣara nyāya

Holes done by an insect (*ghuṇa*) in a piece of wood may accidentally take the shape of an alphabet (*akṣara*) or an object. Similarly, a thing which is not designed but which is achieved accidentally is called the attainment by *ghuṇākṣara nyāya*.

Go

Cattle in general and cow in particular. A cow is considered to be an auspicious animal by the Hindus.

Gokarṇa

An animal having ears like those of a cow. A cow-eared deer (*Antilope picta*).

Gotra doṣa

People belonging to a particular clan are prone to get afflicted by certain diseases. This is called *gotra doṣa* (defect in the clan).

Grāhi

Drugs which cause obstruction to physiological motions of organs in the body. Generally this means a drug which causes constipation.

Guḍūci
Guggulu
Haṁsa
Hareṇu
Haridrā
Hariṇa
Haritaki

Ref. Materia Medica of Ayurveda—the first volume of this series.

Hata

This term means 'killed'.

Hāyanaka

It is a variety of *śāli* (*Oriza sativa* Linn.).

Hita

This term means 'beneficial'. In this text this term is used as a synonym of 'therapy'.

Hṛdaya

Lit. this term means "the centre". In the medical texts it is used to mean the heart. Unlike modern science, in ayurveda heart is considered to be the seat of the mind and all mental functions of the person are controlled by this organ.

Hṛdayādi nyāsa

Impregnation of the vital organs of the body like heart etc., with the *bija mantra*, alongwith *aṅguli nyāsa*, *akṣara nyāsa* etc., this (*hṛdayādi nyāsa*) is invariably performed before the actual recitation of a *mantra*.

Hriṁ (ह्रीं)

This is one of the *bijas* (seeds) of a *mantra*. 'Ha' (ह) is Śiva, 'ra' is Prakṛti, 'ī' is Mahāmāyā, '*nāda*' is the mother of the universe and *bindu* (˙) means the dispeller of sorrow. This *bija* is generally used to worship the goddess Bhuvaneśvarī.

Hrūḥ (ह्रूः)

This is one of the *bījas* of a *mantra.*

Hūṁ (हूं)

This is one of the *bījas* of a *mantra.* 'Ha' is Śiva, ū is Bhairava, *nāda* is *para* or supreme and *bindu*(ं) means dispeller of sorrow.

Ikṣu

Ref. Materia Medica of Ayurveda—the first volume of this series.

Itkaṭa

This drug is not properly identified. Perhaps it is Bot. *Sesbania bispinosa* Faucet and Rendle.

Jaṁbu

Ref. Materia Medica of Ayurveda—the first volume of this series.

Japa

Repeated recitation of a *mantra* with the concentration of mind on the object (god or goddess) of contemplation is called *japa. Mantras* are composed of *bījas* and their repeated recitation creates a vibration inside the body which endows the person with supernatural powers and attainments.

Jāti phala
Jāti puṣpa
Jimūta
Jīraka
Kadalī
Kadamba
Kākamācī
Kakubha
Kalāya
Kalhāra
Kaliṅga

N. of drugs.

Ref. Materia Medica of Ayurveda—the first volume of this series.

Kapālādi mantra

This *mantra* is used to predict the time of death of a person. Oṁ *Kapālarudrāya bhagavate namaḥ* – this is the *mantra*.

Kapha

Kena jalena phāyate vardhate iti kaphaḥ. The *doṣa* which expands by watsy elements is called *kapha*. This is one of the three *doṣas*. It helps in the adhesion of different organs of the body (*Śliṣ āliṅgane*). The phlegm that comes out from the throat in bronchitis, pharyngitis, laryngitis etc., is also called *kapha*. These two *kaphas* are different from each other. The latter is only an excreta and it does not help in the physiological activities of the body like the former. It pervades all over the body. It is classified into five categories and locations as well as specific functions of these varieties are described in detail.

Kara nyāsa

Impregnation of the hands with the *bijas* of a *mantra*. This, alongwith *akṣara nyāsa* and *hṛdayādi nyāsa* is invariably performed before the recitation of a *mantra*.

Karaka

Small variety of *dāḍima* (pomegranate).

Kārambha

The meaning of this term is not clear. If the actual reading is *kārabha* then the meaning is the "shape of a camel".

Karira
Karkandhu
Karṇikā
Karpūra
Kāśa
Kāsamarda (*ka*)
Kaseruka
Kastūrī

Ref. Materia Medica of Ayurveda—the first volume of this series.

Kāya

This term means 'body'. It is derived from the root *ciñ*

which mean "to get nourished" or "to grow". Growth of the body continues right from child-hood to the ripe old age. Because of excessive catabolic process in old age for which the tissues are destroyed more in comparison to the growth that in old age, the growth is not perceptible.

The term *kāya* also means *jāṭharāgni*. This implies that the enzymes responsible for digestion and metabolism work constantly during the whole life and stoppage of the functioning of the activities of these enzymes results in death.

Keśava

N. of Viṣṇu or Kṛṣṇa. Lit. one having long and beautiful hair.

Ketaki

Ref. Materia Medica of Ayurveda—the first volume of this series.

Khaḍga

Sword.

Khañjariṭa
Kharjūra
Kiṁśuka
Kodrava
Kola

N. of drugs.
Ref. Materia Medica of Ayurveda—the first volume of this series.

Koṅkaṇa

N. of a region, in the Western part of the Southern peninsula of India.

Koradūṣa
Kovidāra
Kramuka

N. of drugs.
Ref. Materia Medica of Ayurveda—the first volume of this series.

***Krīṁ* (क्रीं)**

This is one of the *bijas* of a *mantra*. '*Ka*' means *kāli*, '*ra*' is

Brahmā, '*i*' means Mahāmāyā, *nāda* is the mother of the universe and bindu(˙) is the dispeller of sorrow. This *bīja* is generally used for worshipping the goddess Kālikā.

Kṛṣṇa

Lit. this term means 'black'. But it is used to mean the name of the celebrated incarnation of Viṣṇu. Sometimes He is identified with Viṣṇu Himself. He is often represented as a young and amorous shepherd with flowing hair and a flute in his hand. He preached Śrīmad Bhagavad-gītā.

Kṛṣṇātreya

In ayurvedic literature, there is the description of four Ātreyas viz., Punarvasu Ātreya, Bhikṣu Ātreya, Dattātreya and Kṛṣṇātreya. Kṛṣṇātreya was perhaps different from Punarvasu Ātreya. The former belonged to the school of Surgeon's where as the latter was dealing with Internal medicine.

Kṛtamāla

Ref. Materia Medica of Ayurveda—the first volume of this series.

Kṣṇeṁ

Kṣṇuḥ

The *bījas* of a *mantra*.

Kṣudrā

Ref. Materia Medica of Ayurveda—the first volume of this series.

Kubera

The celestial treasurer of the wealth in the heaven.

Kukṣa doṣa

The actual implication of this term is not clear. It is perhaps the same as *kukṣi doṣa* which means defects in the lower abdomen.

Kulaka

N. of a flower.

Kulattha

Kuṁkuma

Kumuda

Kunda

N. of drugs and flowers. Ref. Materia Medica of Ayurveda—the first volume of this series.

Kuṅnala

N. of a flower.

Kunta

A spear or a lance.

Kuṣṭha

Obstinate skin diseases including leprosy.

Kuṭaja

Ref. Materia Medica of Ayurveda—the first volume of this series.

Kuthaka

A veriegated cloth used for bed sheet etc.

Lasuna
Lavali
Lavaṅga
Lodhra

Ref. Materia Medica of Ayurveda—the first volume of this series.

Loha

The term *loha* or *lauha* commonly means iron. But it is also used to mean all metals and minerals in general.

Madana (phala)
Mādhavi

Ref. Materia Medica of Ayurveda—the first volume of this series.

Madhura phala

Fruits having sweet taste.

Mahākāla mantra

Mahākāla is the name of one of the forms of Śiva in his character as destroyer. The *mantra* recited to propitiate this form is called *mahākāla mantra.*

Mahā māṣa

The wild variety of *māṣa* (*Phaseolus mungo* Linn.) which is bigger in size.

Mahābhūta

Pṛthvī, *jala*, *tejas*, *vāyu* and *ākāśa* are the five *mahābhūtas* or basic elements composing the universe. The animal body as well as the drugs and diet are composed of these *mahābhūtas*. But in different objects they remain in different proportions. In the human body these *mahābhūtas* are present in the form of *doṣas*, *dhātus* and *malas*. *Doṣas* control the physiological and physico-chemical functions in the body. *Dhātus* or tissue elements form the body matrix. *Malas* are the waste products (digestive and metabolic) which get eliminated from the body after subserving certain useful purposes. From the derangements in the functions of *doṣas*, *dhātus* and *malas*, the physician can determine the state of the *pañca mahābhūtas* in the body.

To correct these disturbances or diseases, such of the drugs, diet and drinks including regimens are administered as are capable of maintaining the equilibrium of *pañca mahābhūtas* in the body—they should replenish the decreased *bhūtas* and decrease the excessive only.

The *mahābhautik* composition of a drug can be ascertained from its taste, *guṇas* (attributes), *vīrya* (potency) and *vipāka* (taste that emerges after digestion). Thus, the exact *mahābhautika* requirement of the living being is supplied through these drugs, diet and drinks. Diet and drinks are regularly used by a healthy person to replenish the loss of *mahābhūtas* caused by the actions of the enzymes which are going on continuously in the body.

The *pañca mahābhūtas* in drugs, diet and drinks are made homologous, absorbed and assimilated by the help of *agnis* (enzymes).

These *mahābhūtas* viz., *pṛthvi*, *ap*, *tejas*, *vāyu* and *ākāśa* are often mistranslated as earth, water, fire, air and ether. May be in the earth, *pṛthvi mahābhūta* is predominantly present. But the concept of *pṛthvi mahābhūta* is different from earth.

The atoms of different basic elements of modern physics can be classified into five categories of *mahābhūtas*. Each atom has also these five *mahābhūtas* (in the form of *tanmātrā*) in it.

Mahendra

Synonym of Indra.

Mahiṣa

Buffalo.

Makaranda

Mālatī

Ns. of flowers.

Mālava

N. of a kingdom in ancient India.

Mallikā

Mandāra

Ref. Materia Medica of Ayurveda—the first volume of this series.

Māndhātā (ṛ)

Name of a king in ancient India.

Mantha

Drink prepared of the roasted corn-flour.

Mantra

That is called a *mantra* by the meditation (*manana*) on which the *Jiva* acquires freedom from sin, enjoyment of heaven and liberation and by the aid of which a person attains in full the fruits of *dharma*, *artha*, *kāma* and *mokṣa*. It is called *mantra* because it is performed by mental process (*mananāt*). *Mananāt trāyate* is *māntraḥ* i.e., *mantra* gives liberation if meditated upon.

A *mantra* is composed of letters. Letters and their combinations as syllables and words are all forms of manifested *śabda* i.e. Brahman. They are each and all forms of creative stress as uttered by the mouth, heard by the ear and conceived by the mind. But what are ordinarily called *mantras* are those particular sounds which are used in worship and practice (*sādhanā*) which consist of certain letters arranged in a definite sequence of sounds of which the letters are the representative signs.

The relations of *varṇa, nāda, bindu*, vowel and consonant in a *mantra* constitute the *devatā* in various forms. Certain *vibhūti* or aspects of the *devatā* are inherent in certain *varṇas*. The *mantra* of a god is that letter or combination of letters which reveals the god or goddess in the consciousness of the *sādhaka* who has evoked it by *sādhanā-śakti*. The form of a particular god or goddess, therefore, appears out of the particular *mantra* of which that god or goddess is the *adhiṣṭhātā* or *adhiṣṭhātrī*. The *mantra* is intoned in a particular way according to the requirements of the *varṇa* (letter) and the *svara* (rhythm). Therefore, the *mantra* becomes effective only when it is recited in its original form and its translation into any language does not produce any such effect. For this reason a *mantra* when translated ceases to be a *mantra*, that is the sounds heard and uttered in translation are not the body of, and do not evoke the god or the goddess. Thus, the *mantra* is not merely an individual's thinking but a particular sound-body of consciousness. *Mantra* is a mass of radiant energy representing the body of the god or the goddess.

Manuṣya

This term means 'human being' or 'man'. The implication of this term as is used in this text is not clear.

Mārdvika

The alcoholic drink prepared of *mṛdvikā* or grape.

Marica

Ref. Materia Medica of Ayurveda—the first volume of this series.

Marma

The vital organ which when injured causes death or excruciating pain.

Maruva (ka)
Māṣa
Mastu
Masūra
Matsya
Mātuluṅga

Ref. Materia Medica of Ayurveda—the first volume of this series.

Mayūra

Peacock.

Mitrā-varuṇau

N. of two gods who together uphold and rule the earth as well as the sky, promote religious rites and avenge sins. They are considered to be the protectors of truth and light.

Mṛdvīkā

Mṛṇāla

Ref. Materia Medica of Ayurveda—the first volume of this series.

Mṛtyuñjaya mantra

The *mantra* recited to propitiate Lord Śiva specially during serious illness to prevent death and for the recovery of the patient.

Mudga

Ref. Materia Medica of Ayurveda—the first volume of this series.

Muhūrta

An astrological term for the measurement of time which is 30th part of a day and equivalent to 48 minutes.

Mūlaka

Muśalī

Nāga keśara

Ref. Materia Medica of Ayurveda—the first volume of this series.

Naiṣadha

An inferior variety of *śāli* (*Oriza sativa* Linn.)

Naivāla

N. of a plant.

Nala

Ref. Materia Medica of Ayurveda—the first volume of this series.

Nārāca

An arrow made of iron.

Navami

Ninth day of a lunar fortnight.

Nīlotpala

Nimba

Ref. Materia Medica of Ayurveda—the first volume of this series.

Nimeṣa

Unit of time which is equivalent to the time taken for twinkling or shutting of the eyes.

Nipa

Also written as *nīpa*. It is a variety of *kadamba* (*Anthocepalus cadamba* Miq.).

Nirālaya

It's meaning is not clear. Perhaps it is used in this text as an epithet of *brahma randhra.*

Nirūha (ka)

This is a type of medicated enema consisting of decoctions of drugs etc.

Niṣpāva

Nīvāra

Ref. Materia Medica of Ayurveda—the first volume of this series.

Ojas

The essence of all the seven categories of *dhātus* or tissue elements is called *ojas*. It is responsible for the strength and vitality in the body.

Oṁ (ॐ)

The *mantra* '*oṁ*' is composed of three letters viz., अ (*a*), उ (*u*) and म् (*m*). Of these, the first two vowels coalesce to form ओ (*o*). Over the ओ(*o*) is written the sign *candra* (moon like shape) which is the *nāda* and *bindu* (dot). *Nāda* and *bindu* are the two aspects of the Mother or Great Power (*Mahā śakti*). She is both the efficient and the material cause of the universe. अ (*a*), उ (*u*) and म् (*m*) represent the trinity of will (*icchā*), knowledge (*jñāna*) and action (*karma*) in the form of Brahmā, Viṣṇu and Rudra.

Padma kaṇṭaka

N. of a skin disease. It is like the thorns of a lotus stalk.

Pañca kola

Pippali (*Piper longum* Linn.), *pippali mūla* (root of *Piper longum* Linn.), *cavya* (*Piper chaba* Hunter), *citraka* (*Plumbago zeylanica* Linn.) and *nāgara* (*Zingiber officinale* Roscoe.)—all these five drugs taken together in equal quantity are called *pañca kola*.

Pañca sāraka

N. of a drink prepared of *drākṣā*, *madhūka*, *kharjūra*, *kāśmarya* and *paruṣaka* all the equal quality. This drink is cooled and added with camphor before use.

Pañca svara

The implication of this term used in this work is not clear.

Pañci karaṇa

Causing *mahābhūtas* to contain all the five basic elements. During the process of creation *pañcabhūtas* are created from the *pañca tanmātrās*. Each *mahābhūta* is again a conglomeration of all the five *bhūtas*. For example, *pṛthvi mahābhūta* is composed of 50% of *pṛthvi* and 12½% of each of *jala*, *agni*, *vāyu* and *ākāśa*. This process of formation of *mahābhūtas* is described in the *Vedānta* as *pañci karaṇa*.

Pāpmā

Lit. this means 'sin'. In this work, and in other ayurvedic classics this is described as one of the synonyms of disease.

Pāribhadra

Pāṭalā

Ref. Materia Medica of Ayurveda—the first volume of this series.

Pathya

Lit. this term means 'wholesomeness'. In this work, this term is also used as a synonym of 'therapy'.

Patita

A fall or a thing that has fallen.

Paṭola

Paṭolī

Ref. Materia Medica of Ayurveda—the first volume of this series.

Phaṭ

A mystical syllable used in an incantation.

Pīlu

Piṇḍālu

Ref. Materia Medica of Ayurveda—the first volume of this series.

Pitta

The term '*pitta*' is derived from the root '*tap*' which means '*santāpa*' (to produce heat), *dāha* (to burn, digest and metabolise) and *aiśvarya* (to endow with higher mental activities). Thus, *pitta* does all these functions inside the body through the help of enzymes. It is often mistranslated as 'bile' which forms only a small fraction of the total concept.

It is of five types and locations as well as functions of all these five types are described in detail in ayurvedic literature.

Prabhāva

Action of a drug can be generally explained on the basis of their *rasa* (taste), *guṇa* (attributes), *vīrya* (potency) and *vipāka* (taste that emerges after digestion). Actions of some drugs cannot be explained on the basis of these concepts. Such actions of drugs are attributed to *prabhāva* which lit. means "specific action". This is the result of *vicitra pratyayārabdha.* Specific actions of *mantras* and gems also belong to this category.

Prāṇa

It is the "process of living" of all creatures including plants. It is described as an unpenitrable phenomena free from sound, touch, vision, taste and smell. One of the categories of *vāyu* is also called *prāṇa* which controls the activities of vital organs of the body. In yoga, control of *prāṇa vāyu* is given a lot of importance because it is responsible for all the mental activities. Control of the mind is essential for *samādhi* and other higher forms of super-natural achievements. Control of *prāṇa* through different breathing exercises is called *prāṇāyāma* which also cures many psychic and psycho-somatic diseases. *Prāṇāyāma* is essential for arousing the hidden energy in the man called *kuṇḍalinī śakti.*

Praśamana

Lit. this term means 'alleviator'. In ayurvedic literature this is used as one of the synonyms of 'therapy'.

Praśnāvatāra

This is a tantric practice in which after certain rituals are performed to propitiate the god or the goddess, the priest or the *sādhaka* is put questions about the future well-being of a person and they predict the future events with the help of the god or the goddess.

Prasṛti

It is a unit of measurement—approximately 96 gms.

Prastha

It is a unit of measurement—approximately 768 gms.

Pravāla

Tender leaves or coral.

Praveṇī

A piece of coloured woolen cloth.

Prāyaścitta

Lit. 'atonement' for the previous misdeeds. In ayurvedic literature this term is used as one of the synonyms of 'therapy'.

Priyaṅgu

Pṛṣata

Ref. Materia Medica of Ayurveda—the first volume of this series.

Pṛthukā

Rice scalded with hot water, dried and then ground in a mortar for flattening and dehusking is called *pṛthukā.*

Pṛthula

Thick.

Pūjā

Offering prayer to the gods.

Punnāga

Ref. Materia Medica of Ayurveda—the first volume of this series.

Purāṇa

N. of a group of classics depicting the events of the past compiled by Veda vyāsa. These are 18 in number.

Rajas

(a) One of the three attributes of mind—the other two being *sattva* and *tamas. Rajas* represent the quality of passion.

(b) The menstrual blood and ovum in woman. It is often used as a synonym to *ārtava.*

Rākṣasa

Rākṣasas are divided into three classes viz., one being of a semi-divine benevolent nature, the second, corresponding to titans or relentless enemies of the gods and the third answering to nocturnal demons, imps, fiends and goblins going about at night, haunting cemeteries, disturbing sacrifices and even devouring human beings.

Raktotpala

Ref. Materia Medica of Ayurveda—the first volume of this series.

Rasendra

The master of *rasa* (mercury) i.e. Lord Śiva.

Rāśi

A sign in zodiac, one-twelfth part of ecliptic, an astrological house.

Rasona

Ref. Materia Medica of Ayurveda—the first volume of this series.

Ratha

Car or cart.

Recana

Purgative.

Roga

The term *roga* is derived from the root '*ruj*' which means "to give pain". Generally this term indicates 'a disease'.

Rohi (ta)

N. of a type of fish (Red carp fish).

Ṛṣi

One who has super human power to visualise phenomena is called a *ṛṣi* (*Ṛṣi darśanāt*).

Rudra

The fierceful form of Lord Śiva.

Ruru

Swamp deer (*Rucervus durancelli*).

Ṣāḍava (ka)

A preparation of green fruits of *āmra* fermented after boiling with *guḍa* etc., and added with oil, *elā* and *nāgara* is called *ṣāḍava* or *rāga ṣāḍava*.

Sahadevī

Saindhava

Śāka

Ref. Materia Medica of Ayurveda—the first volume of this series.

Śākhā mṛga

Animals who live on the branches of trees like monkeys.

Śākiṇī (nī)

A female imp attending Kālī who feeds on human flesh.

Śakti

A spear or a lance.

Śakunta

N. of a bird of prey called "blue jay".

Śāla

Śāli

Ref. Materia Medica of Ayurveda—the first volume of this series.

Śāli grāma

Also written as *Śāla grāma*. It is the name of a sacred stone worshipped by *Vaiṣṇavas*. This stone is pervaded by the presence of Lord Viṣṇu. These stones are black in colour and are generally found in the river *gaṇḍaki*.

Śālmali

Śālūka

Ref. Materia Medica of Ayurveda—the first volume of this series.

Sāma doṣa

A *doṣa* (*vāyu, pitta or kapha*) associated with *āma*.

Śamana

A drug which alleviates *doṣas*.

Śamī

Saṁ (ṅ) kha

Ref. Materia Medica of Ayurveda—the first volume of this series.

Saṁśamana

Same as *śamana*.

Saptāhva

It is a synonym of *saptaparṇa* Bot. *Alstonia scholaris* R. Br.

Sārāmbu

A drink prepared of the extract of the white variety of *khadira* (*Acacia catetu* Willd.)

Sārasa

N. of a bird—the Indian or Siberian crane.

Sarasvatī

N. of the goddess of learning and speech.

Sarja

N. of a medicinal tree—Bot. *Vateria indica* Linn.

Sarṣapa

Ref. Materia Medica of Ayurveda—the first volume of this series.

Śaṣkulī

A large round cake prepared of rice, sugar and sesamum and cooked in oil or ghee.

Ṣaṣṭhī

Sixth day of the lunar fortnight.

Śatāvarī

Ref. Materia Medica of Ayurveda—the first volume of this series.

Sattva

(a) mind.

(b) One of the three attributes of the mind—the other two being *rajas* and *tamas*. *Sattva* stands for purity, wisdom etc.

Sauvarcala

Sonchal salt.

Sauvīra

A sour drink—vinegar.

Siddha

Great saints who have accomplished supernatural faculties viz., *aṇimā*, *mahimā*, *laghimā*, *garimā*, *prāpti*, *prākāmya*, *īśitva* and *vāśitva*.

Sidhma

A type of skin disease—leucoderma.

Sidhu

A type of alcoholic drink. It is prepared in two different ways viz., by boiling (*pakva rasa*) and without boiling (*śīta rasa*).

Siṁha

Lion.

Simīvāli

Also written as Sinīvālī. N. of a goddess. She is described as broad-hipped, fair-armed and fair-fingered. She is the presiding deity for fecundity and easy birth.

Sindhu

(a) N. of a state in ancient India—the modern Sindh.

(b) N. of an edible plant.

Sitā tithi

A day in the light half of the lunar month.

Śivā

This is the synonym of many medicinal plants like *āmalaki*, *harītakī*, blue variety of *dūrvā* and *haridrā*.

Śleṣmā (an)

See *Kapha*.

Ślīpada

N. of a disease-elephantiasis.

Smṛti śāstra

Texts on the Hindu law and social as well as moral practices.

Snāyu

(a) This is described in this text as the name of a plant alongwith *taskara*. It is perhaps a calligraphic error and *taskara snāyu* is the name of one medicinal plant which is also called *kāka nāsā*. (See the Foreword to this book).

(b) Ligament.

Śoṇita

This term is generally used for ordinary blood. But, at times it is used to mean the menstrual blood. It is also used to mean the ovum.

Śrīdāma

Sudāma who is the friend of Kṛṣṇa.

Śrīvaka

N. of a flower.

Śrīkhaṇḍa

N. of a flower—sandal-wood.

Śrīparṇa

N. of a flower.

Śṛṅgāṭaka

Ref. Materia Medica of Ayurveda—the first volume of this series.

Śūdra

One of the four castes among the Hindus—the other three being *brāhmaṇa*, *kṣatriya* and *vaiśya*.

Sugandhāmalaka

Ref. Materia Medica of Ayurveda - the first volume of this series.

Śukra

The seventh category of *dhātus* (tissues). Generally it is used for semen in general. But it is also used for sperm in particular.

The ovum of the woman is also called *śukra*. Some scholars also hold another secretion from the genital tract of the woman as *śukra*. But this *śukra* does not help in conception. If two women indulge in sexual intercourse, ejaculation of this *śukra* may also result in conception. But in that case the foetus will be devoid of any bone.

Preservation of this vital fluid by celibacy etc., is regarded as an essential factor for both physical and mental health. Excessive indulgence in sex and resultant wastage of this vital fluid is considered to cause many serious diseases like tuberculosis and even death.

Śukra (sperm) which is also described as *bija* is described to have its parts and sub-parts (*bija-bhāga* and *bīja bhāgāvayava*). Any morbidity is these parts or sub-parts of sperm results in the death of or disease in the offspring.

Śukta

A sour drink or a type of vinegar.

Śuṇṭhī
Surā
Sūraṇa

Ref. Materia Medica of Ayurveda—the first volume of this series.

Svāhā

A mystic syllable denoting an exclamation used in making oblations to the gods.

Śvitra

Leucoderma.

Śyāmāka

Bot. *Echinochloa frumentacea* Linn.

Tālamūlī

Bot. *Curculigo orchiaides* Gaertn.

Tanmātrā

These are the subtle elements. They are five in number namely, *pṛthvī tanmātrā, ap tanmātrā, tejas tanmātrā, vāyu tanmātrā* and *ākāśa tanmātrā*. These five *tanmātrās* are formed by the permutation and combination of the three attributes of *prakṛti* namely *sattva, rajas* and *tamas*. These five *tanmātrās* are in the form of quantas of different types of energy. They conglomerate in different proportions to constitute *mahābhūtas* or basic elements of the matter.

Tapasvī(n)

Saints who are dedicated to different forms of *tapas* or penance.

Taskara

In this text *taskara* is used as the name of the plant alongwith *snāyu*. There appears to be a calligraphic error. *Taskara snāyu* should be one word which is a synonym of *kāka nāsā*. (see the discussion in the Foreword of this book).

Tila

Ref. Materia Medica of Ayurveda—the first volume of this series.

Tithi

A lunar day. The first fifteen *tithis* during the moon's increase constitute the light half (*śukla pakṣa*) and the remaining fifteen *tithis* constitute the dark half (*kṛṣṇa pakṣa*).

Tittira
Tittiri
Trapuṣa
Trivṛtā
Tryūṣaṇa

Uddālaka

Ref. Materia Medica of Ayurveda—The first volume of this series.

Upadhātu

Subsidiary tissue element or metals of lesser importance.

Uparasa

Gandhaka, tālaka, kāśīsa, śilā, kaṁkuṣṭha, rājāvarta and *gairika*—these seven minor mineral products are called *uparasa* or subsidiary *rasa.*

Utpala

Ref. Materia Medica of Ayurveda—the first volume of this series.

Vāṇa

An arrow.

Varāha

Pig (*Sus scrofa*).

Varaka

N. of a plant. Bot. *Panicum miliaceum* Linn.

Vāta

This term is derived from the root '*vā*' which means motion (*gati*) and sensation of stimulation (*gandhana*). Therefore, lit. *vāta* means the factor in the human body which is responsible for all the movements and perception of sensation. This term is mistranslated as wind or air. Some people get mislead by such translations and believe that the flatus or the gas which accumulates in the abdomen and passes out through the anus is the *vāyu* or *vāta* described in ayurveda. In fact the flatus is entirely different from the concept of *vāyu* of ayurveda.

Among the three *doṣas*, it is the *vāyu* which is the most powerful and it controls the functioning of both *pitta* and *kapha*. *Basti* or medicated enema is the best therapy for the cure of diseases caused by *vāyu.* Oil (til oil) is the best drug for the alleviation of *vāyu.*

Vāyu represents the sensation that passes through the nervous system to different parts of the body. *Vāyu* has five divisions. Locations and functions of these five varieties of *vāyu* are described in detail in ayurvedic literature. The six *cakras* (centres of energy) also represent different aspects of *vāyu*. In *yoga śāstra prāṇāyāma* or breath control is described to regulate the functioning of this *vāyu*. *Vāyu* also controls the mind and its functions. Thus, by the practice of *prāṇāyāma* a person can effectively control his mental activities.

Vaṭaka

Vatsaka

Vakula

Ref. Materia Medica of Ayurveda—the first volume of this series.

Vallī phala

Name of a group of creepers whose fruits are used in medicine namely *ikṣvāku, jīmūta* etc.

Vāyu

See *vāta*.

Veṇu

Bamboo.

Visa

The stalk and the root of the lotus.

Viṣa

Poison.

Viṣṇu

N. of one of the three principal Hindu deities—the other two being Brahmā and Maheśvara. Brahmā is considered to be the creator, Viṣṇu the preserver and Maheśvara, the destroyer. Although Viṣṇu comes second in the rank of the triad, he is identified as the supreme deity by his worshippers.

Viṣṇu sahasra nāma

One thousand names of Lord Viṣṇu which are recited to endow auspiciousness on a person and to make him free from diseases and untimely death.

Vyādhi

A synonym of disease (*roga*).

Yakṣa

N. of a class of semi-divine beings who are the attendants of Kuvera. They at times cause demoniacal possession of human beings and the treatment of such possessions is called *Bhūta vidyā.*

Yakṣmā

Synonym of the disease (*roga*).

Yama

N. of the god who presides over the *pitṛs* and rules the spirits of the dead.

Yāma

Unit of time equivalent to three hours.

Yantra

A mystical diagram possessing occult power.

Yava

Grain of barley.

Yavaka

A variety of barley.

Yagavāhi(n)

A drug or vehicle which carries and accentuates the effects of the original drug to which it is added.

Yoginī

A female demon or any being endowed with magical power. She is the attendant of the goddess Durgā.

Yūthikā

Ref. Materia Medica of Ayurveda—the first volume of this series.